CW00621622

HEALTH VISITI

HEALTH VISITING

Edited by
GRACE M. OWEN
MPhil, BSc(Soc), SRN, SCM, HVTutor, RNT
Head of the Department of Nursing
and Community Health Studies,
Polytechnic of the South Bank, London

Foreword by
ELAINE E. WILKIE
OBE, BA, FRCN, SRN, HVTutor
Formerly Director of the Council for
the Education and Training
of Health Visitors, London

SECOND EDITION

BAILLIÈRE TINDALL · LONDON

Published by Baillière Tindall,
a division of Cassell Ltd,
1 St Anne's Road, Eastbourne BN21 3UN

© 1983 Baillière Tindall
a division of Cassell Ltd

First published 1977
Second edition 1983

ISBN 0 7020 0981 4

Typeset by Inforum Ltd, Portsmouth
Printed and bound in Great Britain
by Woolnough Bookbinding,
Wellingborough, Northants

British Library Cataloguing in Publication Data

Health visiting—2nd ed.
   1. Public health nursing—Great Britain
   2. Home care services—Great Britain
   I. Owen, Grace M.
   362.1'0941   RT97
   ISBN 0–7020–0981–4

Contents

Contributors

Ann Burkitt, MSc, SRN, SRMN, Dip.Health Ed, Dip.Further Ed, Senior Lecturer in Health Education, Polytechnic of the South Bank

June Clark, BA(Hons), MPhil, SRN, HVCert, Health Visitor, West Berkshire Health District. Part-time lecturer, Department of Nursing and Community Health Studies, Polytechnic of the South Bank

Paula Crouch, BA(Ed), SRN, DipHV, HVTutor, RNT, Health Visitor, Harrow. Member of the Health and Welfare Committee, British Dyslexia Association

Susan Freeman, SRN, DipHV, CHNT, NDNCert

Jean Gaffin, JP, BSc(Econ), MSc, Organizing Secretary, Child Accident Prevention Committee

Sheila Jack, BA(Hons), SRN, SCM, QIDNS, HVTutor, RNT, Principal Lecturer in Community Health Studies, Polytechnic of the South Bank

Margaret Kerr, SRN, DipHV, HVTutor, Lecturer in Community Health Studies, Polytechnic of the South Bank

Maureen Lahiff, SRN, SCM, BTA, Cert, HV, CHNT, RNT, Senior Lecturer in Nursing Studies, North East Surrey College of Technology; Lecturer in Nursing Studies, University of Surrey

Grace M. Owen, MPhil, BSc(Soc)(Hons), SRN, SCM, HVTutor Cert, RNT, FRCN, Head of the Department of Nursing and Community Health Studies, Polytechnic of the South Bank

Elizabeth Raymond, SRN, SCM, QN, HVTutor Cert, T Cert Ed, RNT, Senior Lecturer in Nursing Studies; Course Director: Modified Postgraduate Health Visitor Course at Polytechnic of the South Bank

Foreword

It is five years since the original publication of this book, based closely on the training and examination introduced by the Council for the Education and Training of Health Visitors in 1964. It was then my privilege to write a foreword, a particular pleasure for one who had been closely involved in the design of the new and somewhat revolutionary training pattern. In 1977, direct involvement in training had only just finished with my retirement. Now, in 1983, it is possible to survey from a greater distance, and perhaps more objectively, the way in which these early plans have matured.

The aim of the Council in the Sixties in designing a system of training was the identification of the knowledge base of health visiting skills and the setting of these in broad areas of study. Educational principles, however, are developed in a context and it is that context which is important when we look at the present state of the development of health visitor education. Both 1977 and 1983 have been periods of considerable uncertainty, in each, health visitors experienced major change. Following the reorganization of the National Health Service, the employment structure altered from one of incorporation within local health authority staffs to becoming part of the national health service. This was accompanied by the virtual disappearance of the supporting structure of the Medical Officer's departments. In the Eighties the change has been even greater, along with colleagues in nursing and midwifery, health visitors are seeing the end of the various statutory bodies previously concerned with the establishment and maintenance of standards of training and practice.

New thinking on the preparation for health visitors working in an integrated service, as for their colleagues in the curative areas of that service, will follow. In the meantime a restatement of the principles upon which training has been based, along with appropriate updating as in this edition, provides the reassurance necessary for the continuing consolidation of the health visitors' skills by students and practitioners alike. In the light of the changing context it is particularly important that the new editions should incorporate more discussion of the implications of integration for the future of health visiting, and such discussion emphasizes the need for research which is considered under that heading. Research can be seen as the natural outcome of the original effort of twenty years ago to establish the knowledge base of health visiting. Now, that statement must be expanded and subjected to effective examination and analysis so that further progress can be made.

Looking back over the upheavals and interprofessional problems of the health visitors function, the development of new education, begun so optimistically in 1962, is seen to have maintained a steady progress and can look forward equally optimistically to the next decade. This book can make a major contribution to that progress.

Elaine E. Wilkie
1983

Preface

Health Visiting was first written by a group of lecturers who worked together as a team on the health visitor's course in the Department of Nursing and Community Health Studies at the Polytechnic of the South Bank. The authors included several health visitor tutors with specific areas of expertise, and others who made a contribution to teaching on the course.

The book was produced primarily as a reference book for health visitor students, in an attempt to give an introduction to health visiting as a profession, and as an aid to gaining an understanding of the course as a whole, and insights into specific aspects of the syllabus. However, in a broader perspective, a wide range of professionals in the integrated health and welfare services find this book of interest. Within the caring services there is a need to understand and appreciate the role and function of other professionals. Social workers, doctors, teachers and those in all fields of nursing find this need for understanding met by reading this book.

This revised edition remains basically the same as the first edition, but has been brought up-to-date in the light of current developments, and the questions, booklists and references have been adjusted accordingly. It was thought wise to retain the original approach in the text until such time as the new Statutory Bodies had formulated policy and plans for new developments, and until the Council for the Education and Training of Health Visitors had made changes in the curriculum.

The philosophy of approach is one of seeking to see the developing role and function of the health visitor, and the educational process of the course within the wider context of the social and administrative structure, showing how theoretical studies can be applied to the practice of health visiting. The use of too much factual material that could become out of date very quickly has been avoided, while greater emphasis has been placed on general principles that are likely to be applicable within the changing social structure, anticipating that there will be advancement in knowledge in relation to health care, or even changes of emphasis within the objectives of the health visitors couse itself, in the not too distant future.

References to material quoted within the text are given at the end of each chapter, with other additional titles suggested for further reading, and in some instances where applicable a few questions have been added as possible topics for discussion, essays, or examples of examination questions. Where new expressions, terminology or concepts are introduced they are printed in italics on the first occasion. This provides the student with an opportunity to ensure that they are fully understood and interpreted before proceeding further with the subject.

The book is divided into four parts. Part I centres upon the growth and development of health visiting as a profession, with special reference to relationships with other caring professions, and particularly within the context of the development of nursing education, and, then, picks up the theme of the role, function and image of the health visitor in the present day and develops the discussion on the day-to-day work of the health visitor. Part II concentrates particularly on the health visitors course, outlining the philosophy, aims and objectives of the course, and offering a general approach to study for potential students. There is an introduction to theoretical studies relating to the five main sections of the health visitors syllabus, showing the relevance of the subject material to health visiting practice. Part III deals in more detail with the actual work the health visitor does. The sphere of work is discussed first of all, including the various places in which health visiting is carried out and some of the appropriate methods of doing the work in these locations. Another chapter looks at the people served and some of the groups which occupy much of the health visitor's time. Some of the places and groups in need may change, as the administrative and social structures change, but the family, parents and children, the home and the community are likely to remain at the heart of health visiting. The same can be said of health education which remains fundamental to all health visiting and merits a full discussion in the final chapter of Part III. Finally Part IV looks at the future of health visiting.

The major areas of the syllabus are covered fairly comprehensively. Aspects requireing a relatively small input from lecturers in a specialist area that is constantly changing have not been included, but some indication has been given in references to journals where students may find factual material that should be up to date. It is hoped that students may find that the examples and suggested approach to study together with the references and questions provide a framework for study and are helpful in applying theory to practice.

The book is intended to be used not as a substitute for tutorial work or teaching in a specific subject area but rather as a complement to any health visitors' course curriculum and also to provide a stimulus for students who wish to study the subjects in greater depth. It has also been found to be a useful reference book for fieldwork teachers who are seeking to keep in touch with the content and philosophy of the course; and also for those preparing to be community health tutors and looking for a comprehensive approach to course preparation and planning. Obviously some areas have been left unexplored but we hope the ground covered here will give a sense of direction for students and provide stimulation for further studies in health visiting. The authors hope that this revised edition will continue to meet the needs of the wide range of interested readers.

Acknowledgements

Grateful acknowledgement for permission to reproduce material is made as follows: to The Council for the Education and Training of Health Visitors for Fig. 2 and Table 1; to The Treasury for Fig. 3 taken from Economic Progress Report no. 135 (July 1981); to Cambridge University Press for Fig. 4 taken from 'Thoughts on poverty and its elimination' from the *Journal of Social Policy* (1972), 1, 2; to the Office of Health Economics for Figs. 5, 7, 8, 9 and 10; to HMSO for Fig. 6; to Croom Helm Publishers for Fig. 11; to HMSO for Figs. 12, 13, 14 and 15; to DHSS for Table 4 taken from *Health and Personal Social Services Statistics for England and Wales, 1972*, London: HMSO; to OPCS for Table 5 taken from Occupational Mortality Decennial Supplement 1970–1972, England and Wales; and to the Health Visitors Association for extracts from Health Visitor, **48**, 9. HMSO material is Crown copyright and is reproduced by permission of the Controller of Her Majesty's Stationery Office.

The authors would also like to acknowledge their appreciation for all the encouragement they have received from their colleagues and friends during the production of this book.

Grace M. Owen
1983

I. Health Visiting

1. The Development of Health Visiting as a Profession

Grace M. Owen

The origins of health visiting can be traced back for just over 100 years, years which have seen a period of rapid social and educational evolution. Despite considerable changes in environmental conditions, patterns of health and disease and the development of the welfare services, the fundamental reasons for the health visitor remain essentially the same as they were in the early years.

In 1893 Florence Nightingale contemplated the training of lady Health Missioners to give instruction, among other things, in 'the management of health of adults, women before childbirth, infants and children' (Nightingale 1954). In 1971, The Royal College of Nursing Working Party noted an essential part of the health visitor's work was home visiting, 'concerned with the principles of healthy living, building up families and individuals' personal resources so that they can better cope with the normal crises of life. She (the health visitor) is in a position to detect the earliest signs of ill health, abnormal development or social distress . . . undertake the developmental assessment of children . . . and give long-term guidance and support' (Royal College of Nursing 1971). This, it would seem, is an extended version of Florence Nightingale's original vision in 1893.

Although the basic objectives of health visiting may have changed little, because of the complexities of modern society and the advancement of health care, the skills and knowledge required to meet the needs are of a very different nature. It is, however, because the basic objectives are so similar to those of the founders that it is useful for the student to know something of the origins of the service and to be able to trace the forces that have shaped its historical development, and that have made it the kind of profession, with all its paradoxes, challenges and potential, that it is today.

Readers will most likely be aware of some of the uncertainties that have beset health visitors on many occasions in recent years. Such phrases as the 'uncertain health visitor' (Jefferys 1965), or the 'dilemma of identity in health visiting' (Hunt 1972), have been heard only too frequently, and with perhaps more emphasis than necessary, and the dilemma was by no means solved by the publication of the Report of the Committee on Nursing (HMSO 1972). But in spite of all this, the health visitor still exists, with the same title; there is still a need to be met, and a very firm place for the health visitor in the present structure and future developments of the health services in the United Kingdom.

It is quite possible that some of the origins of the uncertainties of recent years had their roots in the early course of events and students will find that a perspective on the background helps them to understand and appreciate some of the present situations and gives a sense of direction for the future. Therefore, it is important to consider some of the historical events that were significant in development and to see the emergence of today's health visitor in the context of the growth of other caring professions.

As the student gets involved in the health visitor's course and is introduced to the nature of the work, and also in the process of reading this and other books on health visiting, it is quite likely that a sense of identity in health visiting will be acquired. This is often a very personal acquisition, as most health visitors would agree on what they *do*, and on their aims and objectives in their work, but one of the attractions of health visiting is that there are many different ways of interpreting these in meeting human need.

THE EARLY YEARS

Although the early evidence seems conflicting, most sources suggest that the origins of health visiting were to be found in the local efforts of some voluntary workers in trying to meet a need among the underprivileged and neglected members of society in the Manchester and Salford area. In 1852 the formation of the Manchester and Salford Sanitary Reform Association was established 'to give information to the poor and aid the aged and feeble' (McCleary 1935*a*). It had a female branch, the Ladies Sanitary Reform Association, which was particularly concerned with the dissemination of health knowledge among women and children, from 1862.

Dowling (1973a) suggests, however, that there were already 134 'Bible women' type of sanitary missionaries at work in London and Aberdeen, and he explores the influences of Mrs Renyard and Mrs Fison on the employment of Bible women, in an attempt to 'bridge the gulf that separated the upper and lower strata of society'. These women were selected from the 'better informed and Christian women of the lower middle class' (News Item 1962).

These events took place in the wake of the 1848 Public Health Act which had established the first medical officers of health and stimulated or reflected a public awareness of the plight of the poor, and particularly the need to improve the standards of cleanliness and hygiene.

One thing that does emerge clearly from all the early records is that it was thought at first that standards could be improved by didactic teaching and charitable works, talking and distributing tracts, soup, blankets and whitewash and that this could be most effectively carried out by a respectable and kind, motherly woman rather than by educated ladies. The inadequacy of this approach soon became apparent and gave way to a less didactic and more educative method. It was, of course, not surprising that the first approach failed, since it was likely that many of the recipients of the pamphlets distributed could have been illiterate at that time.

The establishment of the Ladies Sanitary Reform Association in 1861 led to the first official appointment of a 'respectable working woman' to go from door to door among the poorer classes of the population to teach and help them as opportunity offered. She was to carry carbolic powder, explain its use and leave it where accepted, direct attention to the evils of want of fresh air and impurities of all kinds and give hints on infant-feeding and the clothing of children; also where sickness was found, to assist in promoting comfort, urging the importance of cleanliness, thrift and temperance on all occasions (Hale et al. 1968).

MacQueen points out that the Manchester/Salford development could be justified as different from the other voluntary efforts and therefore as the *real* origin of health visiting on two accounts. First of all it succeeded when, between 1862 and 1890, six of the staff of the Manchester and Salford Sanitary Association were transferred to the Manchester Public Health Department and the lady missioners of the Association became known as the 'sanitary visitors'. The following year the Association changed its own branch title to the 'Ladies Health Society' and the sanitary visitors became 'health

visitors'. The second justification was that in this particular development the health visitor was envisaged as a 'health teacher and
counsellor rather than a nurse' (MacQueen 1962).

The employment of the sanitary visitors had spread after 1862
to many areas, records showing a similar growth in Yorkshire,
Brighton and Glasgow among other places. In the Glasgow area
four women were appointed as assistant sanitary inspectors and
their duties were to include the instruction of the poorer classes in
cleanliness in person and home and to give lessons in sewing and
bedmaking and domestic duties (Dowling 1963). In 1863 Arthur
Ransome had been urging the training of nurses, some of whom
could be used as sick visitors to the poor in their homes. In 1871
the President of the Association of Medical Officers in London
suggested every town and village should have a Sanitary Aid Agency
and every medical officer should have a competent 'woman teacher'
at his disposal to instruct women in the details of disinfection.

The Social Forces Shaping Health Visiting
Health visiting could thus have 'taken off' in any one of several
different directions: nursing, health teaching, counselling, teaching
or sanitary inspection, and indeed health visiting today is a combination of some of the skills from all of these occupations. As the Royal
College of Nursing Working Party Report on the Role of the Health
Visitor so aptly puts it, 'The individual skills of the health visitor are
not peculiar to health visiting, it is the combination (of skills) which is
unique' (Royal College of Nursing 1971), and the kind of combination that emerged could well have had its roots in these origins in
the early years and in the fact that (as MacQueen suggests) they were
'successful' by the criteria of that day. That there was a specific need
to be met is obvious from the health reports of that period. In 1871
the infant mortality rate was 158 per 1000 live births (see Chapter 7);
213 in fact in Manchester and 246 in Liverpool, where one child in
every four died before reaching the age of one year. In 1900 the
infant mortality rate was still 150. By 1880 the Manchester sanitary
missioners were receiving simple lectures on clothing, diet, and
ambulance work and in 1882 all the women attending a course had
passed an examination set by Dr Emrys Jones, and thus the first
stirrings towards 'training' visitors began (Dowling 1963).

It is interesting to see the progress over these 30 years set against
other aspects of social change during the same period. The 1848
Public Health Act and the creation of medical officers of health had

already been noted and subsequently the 1871 Act created the local sanitary authorities setting the scene for environmental reform. The 1858 Medical Act had brought together the physicians', surgeons' and apothecaries diploma under the umbrella of one medical qualification and the 1860s saw the establishment of the general practitioner and the British Medical Association and thus the pattern of modern medical practice was set. The same period saw the foundation of a School of Nursing at St Thomas' Hospital by Florence Nightingale with 15 probationers in 1860, to set the pattern of nursing schools for future years, and in the early 1860s Rathbone's District Nursing Services were started in Liverpool.

These were also the years during which the early stirrings of the struggle for the emancipation of women were beginning and it is likely that they gave an impetus to the growth of 'respectable' occupations for women, particularly for those in the middle classes. In 1861, 72.5 per cent of teachers were women and with the 1870 Education Act, teaching became an even more popular choice for women. The year 1874 saw the foundation of the London School of Medicine for Women to provide for the education of women doctors. A number of schemes for training midwives had already been in existence and although the battle for statutory recognition was a tough one (11 Bills were put before the House in the last decade of the century) success came in 1902 with the first Midwives Act setting up the Central Midwives Board.

Florence Nightingale's vision for training nurses extended also to health visitors and she persuaded the North Buckinghamshire Technical Education Committee to start on training courses for health missioners. Sixteen women were selected for a course of 16 lectures, 12 took the examination at the end and 6 passed (McEwan 1951). Three of them became the first qualified health visitors to be appointed by Buckinghamshire County Council as full-time health visitors. Florence Nightingale had already a clear-cut distinction in her approach when in 1891 she wrote:

> It seems hardly necessary to contrast sick nursing with this (health visiting). The needs of home health bringing require different but not lower qualifications and are more varied. She (the health visitor) must create a new work and a new profession for women (Nightingale 1892).

Thus by the turn of the century the pattern of the health visitor's work and employment was beginning to be established with a tendency to include some of the skills of teaching, medicine, counselling, environmental health practice and nursing. Increasingly it seemed that the bias was moving towards those with a nursing background and yet it was recognized that the skills required were distinct from those of nursing. By 1908, Manchester was recruiting health visitors from trained nurses only and many authorities were asking for the certificate of the Central Midwives' Board in addition.

THE MATERNITY AND CHILD WELFARE ERA

The social legislation and consequent changes of the first decade of the twentieth century could have been an additional influence on the way health visiting developed. There was a growing sense of public concern about the high infant mortality rate and experience in Huddersfield in 1905 (Hale et al. 1968) had shown the value of notification of new births which enabled the health visitor to call and give guidance on infant management. A Notification of Births Act in 1907, although permissive, encouraged many more areas to adopt the system which became universal and compulsory in 1915. This was an important factor in providing the health visitor with inform-ation about new births and creating access to the homes at a time of need. It must be realized, however, that from the very start the health visitor had no legal right of entry and her home visiting has always been based on establishing a successful relationship as a friend and counsellor.

Another influence at that time was the growing interest in the development of the infant welfare movement along the lines already established in France. Although as McCleary (1935b) pointed out, it was natural for health visitors to become linked with infant welfare, they had existed independently before it became popular. This interest in infant welfare grew even more as the concern with reducing the infant mortality rate became paramount, and a re-duction in the rate from 108.7 in 1911 to 90.9 in 1915 reinforced the belief in health visitors and encouraged the local government boards to open more maternity and child welfare centres. By 1918 (Dowling 1973b), there were 700 local authority centres and 578 voluntary ones and there were 751 full-time and 760 part-time health visitors employed in connection with these centres. The Maternity and Child Welfare Act of 1918 clarified the situation by making it the responsibility of every council to establish maternity and child welfare committees, and gave them powers to provide services. By the end of World War I over 3000 health visitors were employed.

This emphasis on maternity and child welfare grew alongside the work of the school nurses. The 1870 Education Act had, for the first time, brought together all children of school age compulsorily for a few years of life. The discovery of the fact that over 50 per cent of the Boer War recruits were unfit for service had alerted public conscience to the need for some attention to be paid to preventive measures while children were still at school as a 'captive' group. Rowntree's work in York (1922) had also drawn attention to the prevalence of poverty and these factors gave impetus to the 1906 Education (Provision of Meals) Act and also the 1907 Administrative Provisions Act which made it a duty of local authorities to provide for the medical examination of all children attending elementary schools and to make the necessary arrangements for treatment. Naturally this necessitated the appointment of school nurses. Much of the school nurses' work at that time consisted of instruction on cleanliness, treatment of minor ailments and medical inspections. It is interesting to see how this service was to change and develop because the extent to which the care of the school child has been part of the health visitor's work has fluctuated from time to time over the years and varied with different local authorities, and remains a controversial area even to this day.

Early Training for Health Visitors

London was the first authority to demand a professional qualification for health visitors following the London County Council (General Powers) Act of 1908 which gave the metropolitan boroughs power to appoint health visitors. This was followed by the Health Visitors (London) Order of 1909 which laid down that their required qualifications should be: either (1) a medical degree; (2) the Central Midwives' Board Certificate; (3) General Nursing Training and the Health Visitors' Certificate of an Organization approved by the Board; or (4) previous duties in local authority service (Hale et al. 1968). Once again this shows a trend towards preference for a person with a nursing background.

By 1907 there were several alternative schemes for training prospective health visitors. Bedford College for Women and Battersea College (now the University of Surrey) offered two-year courses for those without previous qualifications and a six-month course for nurses. The Royal Sanitary Institute (now the Royal Society of Health) introduced a course in biology, hygiene, nursing, infant care, disease prevention, first aid and statistics together with some practical training. It was not until 1919, however, that these standards set for London were to become general throughout the country, when a Ministry of Health circular to local authorities established these general requirements throughout the country. The health visitor had come to stay (Clark 1973).

The war years had seemed to intensify the concern with maternity and child welfare and more efforts were concentrated on the establishment of antenatal clinics and home visiting as the care of expectant and nursing mothers and young children became the responsibility of the major local authorities. Likewise, concern for the care of the school child grew with the establishment of clinics and medical and cleanliness inspections.

It is interesting to trace this emergence of the health visitor as a 'well baby' nurse, or the 'lady from the welfare' as she came to be called. Clark (1973) points out that the present-day stereotype of the health visitor could well have been established in this post-war era, but this was the public image held and it was not necessarily the same as the formal definition of her role (as will be seen later). Perhaps it differed less radically from the health visitor's perception of her own role and function at that time.

QUALIFICATION AND PROFESSIONAL CONSOLIDATION

The formation of the Ministry of Health in 1919 helped to formalize the existing patterns of practice and training. The Ministry of Health and the Board of Education were jointly responsible for a scheme for a two-year course of training and a one-year course for trained nurses, graduates or women with three years' experience of health visiting. The way in which these training patterns evolved must also be seen in context of the struggle for State Registration in the nursing profession. The midwife's position had been formally recognized in 1902, by statutory provision, which firmly established her as a practitioner in her own right, while legislation had continued to improve the social and financial provision for health care and domiciliary services.

Many historians have described the evolution of the professional nurse, and health visitor students may be interested to refresh their knowledge by reference to Hector's account (1973) in the context of the changing role of women and their occupations and the ensuing controversy over the value of state registration. It seems that the medical profession was largely in favour, apart from a few dissenting individuals, but it is interesting to note Florence Nightingale's comment to Sir Henry Verney, on the preponderance of doctors involved in the decision-making process about nursing education (Hector 1973). As with midwifery, a succession of Bills was introduced between 1904 and 1914 only to be rejected and it was not until the Ministry of Health was set up in 1919 that the final impetus came for the passing of the Nurses Act and the setting up of the General Nursing Council, with the ultimate result of State Registration in 1925. The Ministry of Health was then requiring that health visitors should also be midwives and, by 1928, that they should hold the Certificate of the Royal Sanitary Institute which was designated the official examining body. The health visitors course was to be six months for all trained nurses and midwives, and a two-year course for others. This was to remain the pattern until 1938 when midwifery training was divided into two parts and possession of Part I only became acceptable for health visitors.

The period between the two World Wars, then, was one of consolidation and establishment of health visiting practice. There were no dramatic changes in legislation or administration, but there was a general concentration of health visiting work on maternity and child welfare aspects in the home, clinic and school setting. This doubtless reinforced the 'stereotype' already noted, and some writers have seen this as an undesirable development in terms of the health visitor's public image (MacQueen 1962; Clark 1973). There is no doubt, however, that the need for this kind of visitor still existed and was justified by some of the dramatic improvements in the health of young children. The infant mortality rate fell from 163 in 1899 to 51 in 1939 (MacQueen 1962) while diseases such as rickets, rheumatic fever, scarlet fever and diphtheria, shown to be killers in the early 1900s, were by the 1950s reduced in severity to minimal proportions, there being no deaths from diphtheria or scarlet fever in 1957. It is important not to imply causal relationships where factual evidence is hard to establish. Much of this improvement could have been due to improved social welfare provision, school meals, social insurance, immunization and medical care. At the same time, however, the health visitor must have made a considerable contribution, particularly in terms of facilitating the use of provisions and services and communication of knowledge on infant-feeding and health care. It should be remembered that at that time the mass media was less influential than at the present time and the health visitor was in a position to communicate with those who needed her knowledge and skill.

A Joint Consultative Committee (HMSO 1943) set up during World War II outlined the duties of the health visitor to include maternity and child welfare duties, the school medical services, tuberculosis visiting, the control of infectious diseases and social work—caring for the family as a unit. This gave a new sense of direction to post-war developments, as an almost imperceptible change had come about during the war years, moving from the 'well baby nurse' to the 'family visitor'.

THE ALL-PURPOSE FAMILY VISITOR

In the wake of World War II there came the inevitable burst of legislation for reform, including the Education Act, the Children Act, the National Insurance Acts, the National Health Service Acts, the latter giving the statutory responsibility for the provision of health visiting to the county councils and county boroughs. The National Health Services (Qualifications of Health Visitors and Tuberculosis Visitors) Regulation of 1948 (Statutory Instrument no. 1415) required the appointment of qualified health visitors to all health visiting posts, full or part time.

The School Health Service (Handicapped Pupils') Regulations (1945), had the effect of clarifying the health visitor's responsibilities within the new School Health Service structure and the other legislation had further implications for her work in the field of child care, aftercare and care of the elderly and those suffering from mental disorder. Departmental circulars re-emphasized that her work was now concerned with the entire household, including the preservation of health and health education in cooperation with the general practitioner, district nurse and sanitary inspector. Once again a broad field of interest was indicated but still no clearly defined functions, apart from a general hint that they were mainly educative.

One other development of the early post-war years of considerable professional significance was the beginning of the preparation of health visitor tutors. A one-year full-time course was set up at the Royal College of Nursing in 1945 including among other subjects educational psychology, teaching methods, training school management and professional development. MacQueen (1962) suggests this initiated the improvements in health visitor training in subsequent years, as the tutors gradually took over responsibility for course administration and tutorial preparation of students. The Roll of Tutors set up by the Royal College of Nursing eventually became the responsibility of the Council for the Training of Health Visitors and later other methods of preparation for tutors were approved.

By 1950 there were 32 health visitor courses training about 700 students annually. The training centres were either organized by local authorities or were set up in educational establishments. Course lengths varied from just over six to nine months. The majority of students were state registered nurses with at least Part I midwifery training and thus would have followed at least four years' preparation for health visiting; in fact many would have taken up to five years (Ministry of Health, Department of Health for Scotland and Ministry of Education 1956).

By 1953 it was apparent that there was a general shortage of health visitors and also that some clarification of the work and changing role within the National Health Service was needed. This led to the setting up of a Working Party under the chairmanship of Sir Wilson Jameson, with the terms of reference:

> To advise on the proper field of work, recruitment and training of health visitors in the National Health Service and School Health Service (Ministry of Health 1956).

The Jameson Report was published in 1956 and every student should be familiar with its main recommendations as it laid the foundations of present-day health visiting and training. The Report outlined and defined the main function of the health visitor as 'health education and social advice' (para. 293, Ministry of Health 1956) having 'full regard to the needs of the family and the part played by other workers'. The health visitor should 'act as a common point of reference and a source of family information—a common advisor in health teaching and a common factor in family welfare . . . She could be in a real sense a general purpose family visitor' (page viii, Ministry of Health 1956).

The Report brought together for the first time a wealth of information of a statistical and descriptive kind about health visiting and led to the setting up of the Council for the Training of Health Visitors in 1962. It was, however, difficult even in retrospect to

disentangle from the recommendations a very clearly defined outline of the role and function of the health visitor, and 'health
education and social advice' was open to so many different interpretations by local authorities and individual health visitors. The
'all-purpose family visitor', attractive as it sounded, became a somewhat diffuse concept which could possibly have led to some of the
uncertainties of the next decade. It was left to the newly formed
Council after 1962 to set about the task of clarifying the role and
creating the 'new breed of health visitor' (Hill 1971; see Chapter 3).

One of the recommendations of the Jameson Report which was to
influence the shape of things to come was the idea of the 'group
advisor', an experienced health visitor who was to act in a general
advisory capacity, with responsibility to organize the practical training of student health visitors and arrange experience for nurses and
other students in the community. This was the first positive attempt
to create a 'career' grade for health visitors and was the forerunner
of the fieldwork instruction and the promotion ladder set up by the
Mayston structure of the sixties (Department of Health and Social
Security, Scottish Home and Health Department and the Welsh
Office 1969).

One point often overlooked is the fact that the Report queried the
value of the institutional hospital nurse training (which provided
little opportunity for treating patients as whole persons) as a
basis for health visitor training. The long period spent in curative
nursing, it was observed, could make it difficult for students to
adjust to a preventive outlook.

There were, however, some nursing skills which were recognized
as being usefully carried over into health visiting. Part I midwifery
training spent mainly in hospital gave little introduction to 'normal'
childbirth and was even less useful to the student. This comment was
the basis for the preparation of the subsequent obstetric course.

Attention was drawn to the early proposals for integrated courses
which could be set up as experiments under the 1949 Nurses Act.
These could enable students to follow a specially designed course,
integrating experience in nursing, midwifery and health visiting
and preparing them for qualification in each field. More will be said
of these experiments later. The important point here, however, is
that the Report came down firmly in favour of the fact that in spite of
the disadvantages, nursing training was an essential prerequisite for
health visiting.

Nurse Training as a Basis for Health Visiting

This issue was to be raised as a controversial topic many times in subsequent years and correspondence columns of professional journals show evidence of heated arguments. However, the Council, when established, reinforced the findings of the Report in all its early literature and the same line was to become apparent in the Report of the Committee on Nursing in 1972, once again generating a great deal of discussion. This is not the place to enter into the various aspects of the argument, but it is important for the student to be able to see that it has its roots in history and to see the forces that have shaped the present situation. This does not suggest that change should not be considered in response to changing need, but shows that these two major Reports in 1956 and again in 1972 have seriously considered the issues involved.

Other Influential Factors

MacQueen points out that one factor emerges with great clarity from the accounts of the post-war era and the years following the publication of the Enquiry into Health Visiting (Ministry of Health 1956). It would have been so easy for the health visitor to disappear from the scene in the post-war reorganization. There were many 'straws in the wind' that could have changed the course of events. A number of experimental schemes were set up by enterprising local authorities to employ 'specialist' health visitors (Ministry of Health 1956). These would carry very small general caseloads and be responsible also for a specific field of work demanding some special expertise, such as care of diabetics or the elderly, health education or psychiatric care, within a wider geographical area. This idea was generally deprecated by the Jameson Report, but it has fluctuated in popularity and in various forms over the years, and is tending to reappear in the present day rather on a parallel with the concept of the clinical nurse consultant in the hospital setting.

Another controversial point has been the question of 'combined duties'. In some rural areas it is a very practical proposition for one professional worker to combine the midwifery, district nursing and health visiting in a geographical area and this can be done quite successfully, given good consideration of services and team work. Arguments have been put forward from time to time for a combination of the role of health visitor and community nurse on the grounds that this could provide better continuity of care and communications and would be a more rational use of manpower

(Buckoke & Irvine 1971). This point of view, however, disregards the fact that there are relatively few professionally trained people who choose to combine these roles or feel able to adapt to the situations and acquire the different sets of skills required to meet different needs.

The evolution of the social worker, particularly in the post-war years, was to pose another possible threat to health visiting. With the apparent lack of a clearly defined role for the health visitors and a definition of 'health education and social advice' it was not surprising that where the work of the social worker appeared to run parallel with that of health visitors, confusion should arise. The Health Visiting and Social Work Act (Training) 1962, acknowledged in statute that the two kinds of worker were necessary. It created twin councils with a joint secretary and chairman and some mutual members, which was in essence a recognition of a separate identity for both professions. Health visiting was by then a well-established profession, with its own standards, code of practice, training schools, courses and examinations. Social work was just setting out in 1962 to establish itself. Much of the ensuing uncertainty and threatening situations were understandable, but quite unjustified and unnecessary when seen in the context of statutory provision for social need and the professional identity of the two groups.

Health visiting has survived these conflicts and emerged with a more clearly defined role and status and a unique set of skills, having weathered the storms of doubt and found a firm place within the integrated health service.

HEALTH VISITING AS A PROFESSION

It will have become apparent by this time that as the picture of the growth of health visiting takes shape and unfolds, the words 'profession' and 'professional' have been used with increasing frequency. It is therefore relevant to break away from the historical perspective at this point to look at the sociological perspective and clarify the use of the concept of 'professional development'. Some students, however, may prefer to leave reading this section of the discussion until later in the course when they have encountered some of the issues and begun to establish a sense of professional identity for themselves.

Readers will be aware that a variety of definitions exists and whether nursing and health visiting can strictly be called 'professions' is a frequently debated question. Most writers are generally agreed that the criteria for recognition of a profession include a code of conduct which is transmitted within a formal educational preparation, leading to a recognized qualification, and specific skills which are linked with, and based on, a body of theoretical knowledge. Students wishing to pursue the sociological aspects of professionalization may be interested to study some of the more theoretical approaches. Prandy (1965) suggests that professionalization includes aspirations for prestige and status, and Jupp (1972) rather supports this approach in his discussion on status inconsistency, suggesting as he does that the recent establishment of nursing studies in universities is an attempt to resolve the inconsistency between the 'status quo' and full professional status.

McFarlane (1970), however, sees professional education as something more than just a striving towards status and points out that nursing education for professional practice equips the individual with skills and knowledge, enabling the fullest development of potential and contributing towards the care of the patient, service and the community.

Hunt (1972) looked extensively at this question specifically in relation to health visiting on the basis of the following characteristics common to all professions.

1. A core of specialist abstract theory as a basis for practice.
2. Acquisition of knowledge acquired through a long period of education.
3. Motivation to service rather than for gain.
4. The exercise of control over recruitment, training, qualification and standards of practice.
5. An ethical code of behaviour.

Each profession, however, develops its own unique set of skills.

On the basis of her study, Hunt suggests that health visiting is an occupation involved in the process of professionalization and that it falls more strictly into the category of the 'semi-professions'. She discusses the 'dilemma of identity in health visiting', as being possibly due to the fact that health visitors share a tenuous sense of identity with those engaged in curative nursing. She demonstrated clearly that 93 per cent of her sample appreciated the nurse training in their background—an interesting point in relation to some of the foregoing discussion on the historical perspective and recent arguments. It should be recognized, however, that her study was done in Scotland and similar research in other parts of the United Kingdom could show regional variations.

Greenwood's definition of a profession is a useful one to include here, giving as it does an accompanying framework for analysis. He includes five attributes and characteristics of a profession (Greenwood 1967).

1. A systematic body of knowledge.
2. Professional authority, including professional competence which highlights the layman's ignorance and protects the public from unauthorized practice.
3. Community sanction or approval, which confers on it certain rights and privileges including the right to set its standards of training and qualification.
4. A code of ethics partly formal and partly informal governing the behaviour of its members.
5. Professional culture which relates to values, norms, symbols and images handed down within the profession.

Greenwood suggests that most established occupational groups show all of these attributes and others show none at all, and that occupational groups can be arranged along a continuum, the well-recognized professions being at one end and the least skilled jobs at the other. Doctors, for example, appear to be consistently high on every dimension. It is usually held that points 2 to 5 are true for nursing (and health visiting could be added here) but that it fails to meet the first one entirely as yet. Greenwood points out the need for intellectual as well as practical experience in gaining professional competence.

On the basis of this definition it could possibly be argued that health visiting is now moving more fully into professionalization. Health visiting courses are now based mainly in further or higher educational establishments in this country and there is a rapidly growing interest in research and research appreciation among health visitors themselves. Stimulus is being added to this as young graduates complete the more recently established degree courses and other health visitors gain degrees later in their careers. The Council for the Education and Training of Health Visitors has a research function as one of its responsibilities and the first research monograph was published in 1974 (Gilmore et al. 1974). The

Council also has records of a number of research projects completed or in progress, and relating to health visiting.

There is quite a considerable amount of research based on disciplines related to health visiting and of value to the profession, but it is only comparatively recently that health visitors themselves have begun to attempt to identify their own skills or evaluate their own work and training or to produce a theoretical approach to any of these problems. Examples of some of the early attempts to identify aspects of health visiting can be seen in Clark's study, *A Family Visitor* (1973) and Marris's report on the Work of Health Visitors in London (1969; see Chapter 12).

At the present time we lack basic tools for the job, such as the criteria for assessment and evaluation of health visiting skills or even a profile of health visiting. Such studies as do exist demonstrate clearly the interesting and challenging field that lies ahead for those interested in research in health visiting.

Health Visiting as a Stimulus to the Growth of Nursing in Higher Education

One point of interest emerges here, which is often overlooked, and that is the recognition of an association between the present growth of intellectual activity within the nursing profession as a whole and the training of health visitors. The foregoing account has referred to the setting up of some of the earlier courses for health visitor training, in educational establishments, for example Battersea College and Bedford College. This link has in fact increased over the years and since the Council was set up in 1962 all health visitors courses have gradually moved into the education sector.

It was in the colleges and universities where health visiting-linked courses were initiated that the first movements in the United Kingdom came to combine with nursing education. Rienkemeyer (1968) points out that the British nursing profession was reluctant to allow nursing to be taken over by universities and equally the universities were wary of accepting the status of nursing as an academic discipline. It often goes unnoticed that the first few links came where there were qualified health visitor tutors in post, or connections with health visiting courses.

The first Director of the Nursing Studies Unit set up at Edinburgh University in 1956 was Elsie Stephenson, State Registered Nurse, midwife and health visitor. In 1960, for the first time in the United

Kingdom, student nurses could study for a BSc. or MA degree with their basic nursing course and this included an introduction to health visiting (Scott Wright 1973). The next three developments came in the form of the integrated courses already referred to earlier in this chapter. In 1957 a course pioneered by Pat O'Connell, Health Visitor Tutor at Southampton University and linked with St Thomas' Hospital (the Nightingale School), combined nursing and midwifery with health visiting (O'Connell 1978). A joint planning committee between Hammersmith Hospital, the Queen's Institute of District Nursing and Battersea College of Advanced Technology (later Surrey University), and including Rosemary Hale, Health Visitor Tutor at the College, launched an integrated course at the same time as the previous one, to include nursing, midwifery, district nursing and health visiting qualifications. In 1959, Manchester University followed with a similar kind of course leading to a Diploma in Community Nursing, and Elaine Wilkie, a health visitor tutor was appointed to establish the course. These three experimental courses, all including health visiting, were, together with the Edinburgh Nursing Studies Unit, to form the spearhead for subsequent growth in the wider field of higher education for nurses. The courses at Manchester and Southampton now have degree status and the BSc. (Human Biology) with a nursing option at Surrey University was initiated by the team of tutors working on the integrated course.

Thus the placing of health visitors in the higher education sector was to prove quite a significant factor in the course of events for British nursing in its move towards professional status in terms of Greenwood's definition, and movement towards the more intellectual aspects of nursing education. There are now a number of universities and polytechnics offering degree-linked courses or degrees in nursing or nursing studies, some including a health visitor component.

The growth of nursing and health visiting in higher education is sometimes viewed with caution by those who fear that practical skills will be obscured and neglected as students are introduced to the different stimulation of the educational world. It is, however, essential that there should be an intellectual basis for the practice of professional skills and also in order to evaluate their effectiveness.

The Influence of the 'Public Image of the Nurse'
Before leaving this topic it is worth returning briefly to Hunt's

suggestion that the health visitors' 'dilemma' is in some way linked with the tenuous sense of identity with nursing—using nursing in its clinical sense (Hunt 1972). It is often implied that health visitors themselves are responsible for their own uncertainties, but there is another side to the coin.

Anderson (1973) draws attention to the powerful influence of the 'views of the public in relation to the image of the nurse', and that these views can promote or impede progress.

The Report of the Committee on Nursing comments that the image of the nurse 'retains an inhibited image which belongs to the late nineteenth century'—that of the 'Lady with the Lamp' (paras. 81–83). We have already noted Florence Nightingale's famous phrase used when describing early health visiting, 'I use the word nursing for want of a better', and yet the Report implies she had much to do with the created public image, which has been handed down, 'the familiar association of the nurse with pain, suffering and death, and the tendency to place her (almost always her rather than him) within the setting of a hospital, impede an understanding of the great variety of jobs nurses actually do' (HMSO 1972). Such was the strength of the nineteenth century attitudes that some of the most basic of them have survived vast changes in medical and social history.

American and Canadian writers have recorded similar phenomena across the Atlantic. One comment was that 'the popular image of the nurse was that of a floor nurse, to the exclusion of any concept of the public health nurse' (Davis et al. 1966). It was observed that most recruits to nursing came with the image of the hospital nurse in mind, although by the time they graduated public health nursing had gained in popularity. Much the same pattern of development, incidentally, can be seen in both Canada and the United States as in the United Kingdom, in that the public health nurses there are trained in educational establishments, and this entry into the universities ultimately led to the setting up of the first degree programmes in nursing.

It is recognized in all these countries that other factors have also affected the public image of the nurse, including the doctor/nurse relationship, the role of women in society, the class element and the authoritarian hierarchy.

An interesting aside in this context is seen in the difficulties some health visitors have experienced in the battle over wearing uniform and the kind of clothing worn that was acceptable for the working image. In some areas the navy blue, brown or grey suit has been the accompanying mark of office for the health visitor even in very recent years. All this could well be connected with the fact that the popular image of the nurse remains for many people that of a relatively young girl in uniform. The many male nurses, nurse teachers and managers, health visitors and occupational health nurses are far less often included in the general picture. It is, therefore, difficult to establish any concept of nursing apart from one in the context of hospitals.

In contrast to this the International Council of Nurses' definition of a nurse in 1973 was revised as follows:

> A nurse is a person who has completed a programme of basic nursing education and is qualified and authorized in his/her country to provide responsible and competent professional service for: the promotion of health, the prevention of illness, the care of the sick and rehabilitation . . . (International Council of Nurses 1973).

As Chapman (1974) points out, the activity of nursing became tied to a medical model and has developed along those lines. The Report of the Committee on Nursing indicates that new relationships are being created which are changing images and they will change even further with integration. The vast majority of health visitors now see themselves as nurses with an extension of some of their basic skills, which together make up a new, specific and unique set of skills for health visiting and which in turn now fits quite happily into the new international definition of a nurse.

Clark (p. 98) describes a parallel situation in relation to the stereotype of health visiting, showing a lack of congruence between the health visitors' perception of their role and the stereotype of health visiting held by other groups, such as patients, clients, general practitioners and social workers. She describes the differences between these images (which have been reinforced by the method of statistical record keeping) and the actual situation in reality and goes on to discuss the origins of the public image in some of the past situations already referred to here (Clark 1973).

THE PRIMARY CARE TEAM IN THE INTEGRATED HEALTH SERVICE

It can thus be seen that many social pressures exist, which tend to preserve the 'status quo', and retain vestiges of past images and stereotypes, but also the forces of social change have to be reckoned with at the same time. The moves towards an integrated health service in 1974 created further opportunities for recognition of the role of the primary care team and reinforced the value of the already firmly established links with general practice units. Over the last 10 or 15 years there has been a gradually increasing movement towards health visitors working in liaison with, or attached to, general practice teams. This has opened up opportunities for better understanding of respective roles and functions of doctors, nurses, midwives, health visitors and social workers, and has also made a contribution towards improved working relationships and communications.

Clark (1973) in her discussion of the growth of health visitor attachment to general practice units, observes some of the changes which have occurred in the general practitioners' perception of the health visitor's role, and points out that organizational changes have in fact led to greater mutual understanding, more frequent consultation and better use of resources. However, Gilmore and her colleagues in 1974 still found a high proportion of health visitors who thought their functions were misunderstood, or not fully appreciated by general practitioners, particularly in relation to primary prevention, and also noted the *laissez-faire* approach to communications that still existed.

There are also other significant changes which have taken place in recent years in the working relationships between the medical profession and health' visitors. In the early years of health visiting, their value in preventive medicine was recognized and fully appreciated by the most progressive medical officers of health who became and remained for many years their employers. The changes in administrative structure, culminating in the health service reorganization of 1974 made subtle alterations in the working relationships between doctors and nurses at managerial level, who now have distinctive and specific roles and responsibilities at all levels, in regional, and district teams; and nurses and health visitors have acquired responsibility for management of their own professional staff.

The Report of the Committee on Nursing comments on the effects of both general practitioners attachment and the reorganized health service and these are partly instrumental in introducing the public to a new conception and image of the nurse.

Other existing misconceptions of roles and stereotypes between health visitors and social workers are also described by Clark, particularly as they are related to some of the confusion that has been described. The Report stresses the need for a multidisciplinary approach to avoid overlap of functions, and improved understanding of roles, and it is already apparent that structural changes are having some effects in this direction as uncertainties which have dominated the scene for so long begin to be resolved. At the same time, however, there is much to be done by all members of the team, both at field and administrative levels in terms of improving communications between professionals.

THE NEW BREED OF HEALTH VISITOR

The new breed of health visitor became a popular description of the health visitor of the sixties and seventies. The influence of the Council set up in 1962 gradually began to make itself apparent in shaping a course of preparation for the job, particularly as the newly planned syllabus came into being after 1966. This, and the Council's role, will be discussed more fully in Chapter 3, but it is relevant here to point out that its members included experienced health visitors from teaching and management posts, also medical practitioners with community experience and educationalists, and to note the significance of their contribution to future developments. Evidence of the new image of the health visitor emerging and of the changing philosophy can be seen in some of the Council's literature produced during the last decade. An interesting glimpse of health visiting as it was at the beginning of the 1960s can be found in Akester and MacPhail's account of health visiting in Leeds (1963). All nine illustrations included show health visitors in uniform: seven of these showing her at work illustrate her working with mothers and babies or young children. By contrast the literature and publicity leaflets produced by the Council began to show the wide range of work with all age groups and in different situations and to present the image of an attractive and often younger health visitor, with a distinct individuality of her own as the uniform disappeared.

The Report of the Royal College of Nursing Public Health Committee published in 1969 (Royal College of Nursing 1969), outlining the future trends, unfortunately aroused some misgivings about the lack of clarification between the roles of community nurse and health visitor. It was, however, followed quickly in 1971 by a working party report on the role of the health visitor (Royal College of Nursing 1971) which gave a positive and clearly defined picture of the unique and specific skills of health visiting, and saw the health visitor as being firmly placed in a key position in the community health team. The Council's own leaflet on the role and function of the health visitor (Council for the Education and Training of Health Visitors 1967), combined with other informative literature, gradually helped to build up the newly emerging image of the family visitor, and made a substantial contribution to clarifying her role in the team. One aspect which should not be ignored at this point is the increasing role of the mass media, particularly television, in presenting the new image to the general public.

Controversy has raged around the question concerning the suitability of the new syllabus in preparing the student for the job she has to do. This was obviously an important issue and one difficult to evaluate. Loveland, in 1971, described the work of health visitors in one urban and one rural area and concluded that the bulk of health visitors' work in these two areas was still with mothers and young children and the family, although where general practitioners attachment existed, work with the elderly and chronic sick was substantially increasing. She concluded that the one health visitor course under consideration in her study was, in fact, preparing the students adequately for the job they were expected to perform, but new skills may need to be more fully developed to meet changing patterns of need.

Clark (1973) recorded in Berkshire that the health visitor most commonly visited families with young children, although 29 per cent of visits were in fact made to households without children, 18 per cent being to the elderly and 11 per cent where there were neither young children nor elderly people.

Marris, reporting on the work of health visitors in London, looked at a random sample of London health visitors in 1969, and showed that a large proportion of time was still allocated to work with mothers and young children. Mothers with first babies accounted for 17.3 per cent of this, 17.5 per cent was spent with mothers with second babies and 15.6 per cent with children not at school. These were by far the three highest proportions recorded, showing that approximately 50 per cent of time was spent primarily on these groups (Marris 1969). This report obviously made no attempt to assess the quality of service given, but, like Clark's study in Berkshire, makes a valuable contribution to indicating what the health visitor actually does. Both studies looked at the topics most frequently covered and found that although different classifications were used, it is evident that child management, including infant-feeding, health problems, child care and development were by far the most frequent.

Some of the most interesting human situations obviously never fit the statistical records but the Appendix of Marris's report makes interesting reading, listing under 'unusual visits':

Collection and delivery of unwanted furniture
Directing van driver
Children's home open-day
Harvest festival attended

and various other items which demonstrate the health visitor's involvement in the life of the local community.

A comprehensive view of the health visitor of the seventies as seen by the Health Visitors Association described her work in the context of current changes and was followed by an account of her position as it then stood in relation to the School Health Service (Health Visitors Association 1975). It also showed some aspects of the potential career development for health visitors at the time. Other avenues for health visitors with different interests and skills are available for work in different kinds of specialization (such as the geriatric field), attachment to general practice units, or with emphasis on health education, while for those interested in teaching there are opportunities to become fieldwork teachers or qualify as tutors, with subsequent openings in the field of further or higher education.

HEALTH VISITING IN THE SOCIAL CONTEXT

In this chapter an attempt has been made to set the growth of health visiting as a profession within the wider context of social change and the growth of other caring professions, particularly considering it in terms of the relationship with developments in nursing as a whole. It is clear that although the fundamental objectives of health visiting are very similar to those of early years, the application of skills to the task in hand has been modified and adapted in response to the needs of the people and community to be served.

The *model* shown in Fig. 1 gives a *sociological perspective* for viewing health visiting practice and education in the wider context of society as a whole. More will be said of the use of sociological models in

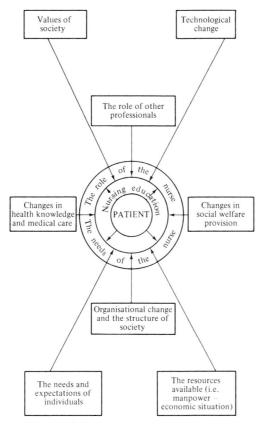

Fig. 1. A model for studying nursing and health visiting education and training.

Chapter 4, but students may find this a meaningful and relevant one to begin with. It illustrates some of the possible relationships between pressures and constraints on professional practice, and the kind of educational process preparing the potential student for qualification. At the centre, or hub of the situation, there is obviously the patient or client, with specific or differentiated needs and expectations, which in turn are influenced by social, psychological and environmental pressures. It could be assumed that the kind of professional practice and skills that emerge do so in response to those needs and expectations, and that the education process prepares the student for that role.

The model shows, however, that in the context of the wider social structure and system there are other influences and pressures at work, such as the counter role of other professionals in the team, existing social, health and welfare provisions, legislative structure and the current state of knowledge in health care. These in turn meet the pressures of current technological change, the pressures of the economic situation and resources available, the current values of society and again the needs and expectations of the people concerned. Values, in particular, will influence the way in which resources are allocated in terms of provision of health care in relation to need. For example, decisions have to be made between spending money on developing expensive new units for sophisticated surgery or diverting money into preventive aspects of health care, or educating individuals to accept more personal responsibility for health care within the family and community (see Chapter 6).

As the course progresses students will find themselves faced with a bewildering number of alternatives and apparently unanswerable questions. A study of the different disciplines within the course will contribute different points of view in appreciating the kind of dilemma facing society. The universalism/selectivity argument in social policy, or criteria for evaluation of need and assessment of priorities in medical care, or the concept of *relative deprivation* in sociology, are examples of various approaches which may help the student to gain insights into the nature of social problems, and indeed to the possible constraints and influences affecting health visiting as a profession.

Human need and human nature, however, are constant factors in the situation, and these always help to shape the kind of work required of health visitors. Future trends will be discussed more fully in Chapter 12. For the present, a fitting note on which to conclude this chapter may be found in the Report of the Committee on Nursing. At the time of writing the full implementation of the Report is still to be developed by the new Statutory Bodies set up under the Nurses, Midwives and Health Visitors Act of 1979. The passage through Parliament of the Bill leading up to this act was a stormy one. The proposals threw into stark relief the many different professional interests within the nursing profession, and health visitors found themselves actively involved in political lobbying to establish their identity and to ensure it was safeguarded within the new legislation. Under the provision of the Act, a United Kingdom Central Council was set up and four National Boards for Nursing, Midwifery and Health Visiting with the intention of forming an integrated structure to replace the existing separate statutory bodies concerned with education.

The Boards and the Central Council started work in the autumn of 1980 and with an enormous task ahead of them, to set up a single professional register, and for the time being they are working in parallel with the existing education and training bodies, until such time as they are sufficiently established to enable the new machinery to take over existing functions and to formulate new schemes for Nursing Education.

The health visitor is firmly recognized, however, in the shape of things to come and although the Report originally used the terminology of 'family health sister', later departmental circulars recognized the more appropriate and more popular title of health visitor as being more generally accepted and it is likely to be retained.

Reference has been made frequently to the fact that health visiting practice has changed in response to changing need and the Report outlined quite clearly (para. 54) the needs facing the community health services, some being related to the positive promotion of health and some to the provision of health care. It spelt out in some detail aspects of a preventive health care service, the health supervision of children under five and school children and the needs of handicapped and chronically sick, those at risk, the mentally disordered and elderly and also the need for the development of public understanding in support of community health measures and environmental hygiene and the need for health education (HMSO 1972).

As Clark suggested, it is the versatility of the health visitor which is her greatest strength and at the same time the greatest danger for the future (Clark 1973). Whatever the changes that may affect her skills, her function as spelt out in the Report of the Committee on Nursing is a clearly formulated challenge, and a comprehensive statement which provides a sense of direction for the future. For that reason para. 548 is quoted in full:

> family health sisters (i.e. health visitors) . . . will perform a range of functions in the areas of case-finding, support counselling and health education. They will visit the new mother and baby as soon as the special skills of the midwife are no longer required, and undertake supervision of all children both at home and at school, where they will be responsible for medical and hygiene inspections and screening tests, and participate in immunization programmes and teaching on health matters. They will have an important role in the provision of family planning advice. They

will provide health and nursing support for the chronic sick and handicapped in the community who do not require clinical nursing. In this work and in meeting the needs of those mentally ill and handicapped who are being cared for by nurses in the community they will cooperate with workers in the personal social services departments. They will help the elderly and their families to understand the normal physiology and psychology of old age and ensure that adequate support is provided to help the elderly remain independent. They will provide health education in the home and elsewhere on all relevant topics. In these and other spheres of activity they will play an important part in the positive promotion of health (HMSO 1972).

It is with this positive and stimulating challenge in mind that the student is invited to proceed with the health visitors course and to make full use of the remaining sections of this book.

SUMMARY

This chapter traces the development of health visiting as a profession in historical and social context and related to the growth of other caring professions. It shows how some of the early philosophy of health visiting is still relevant for today even though practice has moved in response to changing need and with new knowledge. The different phases of health visiting are described, showing clearly how health visitors while retaining their unique skills have adapted to current trends and needs, and are now recognized as being established in the wider nursing profession, with the promise of new horizons.

REFERENCES

Akester, J.M. & MacPhail, A.N. (1963) *Health Visiting in the Sixties* (based on a survey carried out in the City of Leeds). A *Nursing Times* publication. London: Macmillan.

Anderson, E. (1973) *The Role of the Nurse*, Project Series 2, 1, p. 10. London: Royal College of Nursing.

Buckoke, Y.E. & Irvine, D. (1971) Nursing in the community, a time for reform? *Nursing Times*, 67, 34 (26 August) Occasional Paper.

Chapman, C.M. (1974) Nurse education. *Nursing Times*, 70, 18 (2 May).

Clark, J. (1973) *A Family Visitor*, p. 11. London: Royal College of Nursing. *

Council for the Education and Training of Health Visitors (1967) *The Function of the Health Visitor*. London. *

Davis, C.F. et al. (1966) *The Nursing Profession*. New York: Wiley.

Department of Health and Social Security, Scottish Home and Health Department and the Welsh Office (1969) *Report of a Working Party on Management Structure in the Local Authority Nursing Services*. London: HMSO.

Dowling, W.C. (1963) Health visiting—expansion. *Health Visitor, 46*, 11, pp. 371–2 (November). *

Dowling, W.C. (1973*a*) Health visiting, the beginning, the missing link. *Health Visitor, 46*, 10, pp. 337–8 (October).

Dowling, W.C. (1973*b*) Health visiting—latter days. *Health Visitor, 46*, 12, pp. 410–12. *

Gilmore, M., Bruce, N. & Hunt, M. (1974) *The Work of the Nursing Team in General Practice*. London: Council for the Education and Training of Health Visitors.

Greenwood, E. (1967) Attributes of a profession: man, work and society. *Social Work, 2*, 45.

Hale, R., Loveland, M. & Owen, G.M. (1968) *The Principles and Practice of Health Visiting*, Chapter 1. London: Pergamon.

Health Visitors Association (1975) Health visiting in the seventies. Staffing of the health visiting and school nursing services. *Health Visitor, 48*, 9 (September). *

Hector, W. (1973) *Mrs Bedford Fenwick*. London: Royal College of Nursing.

Hill, C. (1971) The role conflicts of the new breed of health visitors. *Health Visitor, 44*, 120 (April).

HMSO (1943) *The Duties of the Health Visitor in the Present and Future Health Service. Report from a Joint Consultative Committee of Institutions Approved by the Minister of Health for the Training of Health Visitors and of Organisation of Health Visiting*. London: HMSO.

HMSO (1972) *Report of the Committee on Nursing*. Cmnd. 5115. London: HMSO. *

Hunt, M. (1972) The dilemma of identity in health visiting. *Nursing Times, 68*, 5 and 6 (3 and 10 February) Occasional Papers.

International Council of Nurses (1973) *International Nursing Review, 5*, 131.

Jefferys, M. (1965) The uncertain health visitor. *New Society, 14*, 4, pp. 16–18 (26 October).

Jupp, V. (1972) Professionalisation and new forms of nursing education. *International Journal of Nursing Studies, 9*, 19.

Loveland, M.K. (1971) The work of health visitors in urban and country areas. *Nursing Times, 67*, 22 (3 June).

McCleary, G.F. (1935*a*) *The Maternity and Child Welfare Movement*. London: King.

McCleary, G.F. (1935*b*) *The Early History of the Infant Welfare Movement*. London: H.K. Lewis.

McEwan, M. (1951) *Health Visiting*, 1st edn., p. 21. London: Faber & Faber.

McFarlane, J.K. (1970) Legacy for the seventies. *Nursing Times, 66*, 3, pp. 90–92 (15 January), pp. 113–14 (22 January).

MacQueen, I.A.G. (1962) From carbolic powder to social counsel. Health Visiting Centenary Lecture at Battersea College of Technology. *Nursing Times*, *58*, 866.

Marris, T. (1969) *The Work of Health Visitors in London*. Report no. 12. London: GLC Department of Planning and Transportation Research. *

Ministry of Health, Department of Health for Scotland and Ministry of Education (1956) *An Enquiry into Health Visiting on the Field of Work, Training and Recruitment of Health Visitors*. London: HMSO.

News Item (1962) *The Times* (28 August). In: Dowling, W.C. (1973).

Nightingale, F. (1892) *Letter to Mr Frederick Verney 1891*. (Reproduction of a printed report submitted to Buckingham County Council 1911 containing letters from Florence Nightingale on health visiting in rural districts, pp. 17–19.)

Nightingale, F. (1954) Sick Nursing and Health Visiting. A Paper read at the Chicago Exhibition 1893. In: *Selected Writings of Florence Nightingale*, ed. Lucy Ridgely Seymer, pp. 353–76. New York: Macmillan.

O'Connell, P. (1978) Health Visitor Education at University. *Royal College of Nursing Research Series*. London: Royal College of Nursing.

Prandy, K. (1965) *Professional Employees. A Study of Scientists and Engineers*. London: Faber & Faber.

Rienkemeyer, M.H. (1968) A nursing paradox. *Nursing Research*, *17* (January/February).

Rowntree, B.S. (1922) *Poverty: A Study of Town Life*. London: Longman.

Royal College of Nursing (1969) *The Future of Nursing in Relation to the Needs of the Community*. London.

Royal College of Nursing (1971) *The Role of the Health Visitor. Report of a Working Party on the Role of the Health Visitor Now and in a Changing National Health Service 1971*. London. *

Scott Wright, M. (1973) Nursing and the universities. *Nursing Times*, *69*, 7, pp. 222–7 (15 February).

FURTHER READING

Most of the useful texts for further reading in this area have already been cited as references and are marked with asterisks.

2. The Health Visitor Today

Grace M. Owen

THE SETTING IN WHICH THE HEALTH VISITOR WORKS

A health visitor is defined in the National Health Service (Qualifications of Health Visitors) Regulations 1972 as:

> a person employed by a local health authority to visit people in their homes or elsewhere for the purpose of giving advice as to the care of young children, persons suffering from illness, and expectant or nursing mothers, and as to the measures necessary to prevent the spread of infection (Council for the Education and Training of Health Visitors 1973).

This definition is obviously based on the Sections of the 1946 National Health Service Act which were repeated in the 1974 reorganization and it can be hoped that the wording will ultimately be revised as health visitors are now employed by district health authorities and it is also a somewhat limited definition in terms of recognition of the wide range of duties carried out by health visitors and the variations in skills practised.

The health visitor may be based in one of two different kinds of setting. She may cover a geographical area for her caseload with a recommended population limit of 3500 (Department of Health and Social Security 1972), in which case she is likely to work from an office located in a health centre of some kind or in some other area health authority premises. In this setting she will probably work with a small group of health visitors covering adjacent districts if she is in an urban area. Occasionally in more rural areas health visitors may work from their own homes.

Much more frequently these days, however, health visitors are to be found working in some kind of formal arrangement with general practitioner teams. This trend has been steadily increasing over the last two decades and now three different kinds of working patterns seem to have emerged.

Attachment Attachment is a formal arrangement by which the health visitor, although employed by the area health authority, is responsible for the health visiting services for the people on the list of a team of general practitioners. She does not have a clearly limited geographical area and may have an office based in the same premises as the practice unit. She works in close liaison with the other staff in the primary care team including the district nurse and midwife, practice nurse and social worker where they exist together.

Liaison Liaison is another formal arrangement which enables the health visitor and general practitioner to have a recognized and regular system of contact. The health visitor retains her own geographical area but communicates between the general practitioners and other health visitors concerning necessary visits in adjacent areas, acting as a liaison person.

Cooperation This is a less clearly defined kind of arrangement whereby health visitors see the doctors regularly for discussion, but may or may not maintain their own geographical areas, working from area health authority premises.

A survey of the work of the nursing team in general practice is the subject of the Council's first monograph (Gilmore et al. 1974)—essential reading for students wishing to get a realistic picture of working relationships in this setting.

Health visitors carry out their work, then, from a base or office in some kind of health centre or clinic, or a general practice unit, where they may also be contacted, receive clients, or give consultations by telephone, at certain recognized times during the day. From this base health visitors go out to visit families for whom they hold responsibilities, or visit child health clinics, schools, hospitals, or any other place where the clients may be found.

The health visitor is responsible to her employer, the district health authority, within the health service through the hierarchical nursing management structure. Health visitors are no longer responsible to medical officers, but may now seek their advice and supervision from nursing officers or senior nursing officers. There is a linear management relationship between health visitors, nursing and senior nursing officers and divisional and district nursing officers, and an advisory or monitoring relationship with the regional nursing officers. Generally speaking, since 1974, senior nursing officers and nursing officers have had responsibility for one discipline only, therefore health visitors could expect to be able to refer to senior staff who were themselves health visitors, especially with the grouping at divisional level being a functional one and community services being grouped together for this purpose. Under the 1980 Health Services Act, however, as the area level has been removed, there will be considerable restructuring at district and divisional level, and at the time of writing the position is not fully clear and may vary between districts.

THE ROLE AND FUNCTION OF THE HEALTH VISITOR

One of the earliest achievements of the Council arose in response to the lack of definition of the role and function of the health visitor, and the problems which had arisen from this have already been discussed in Chapter 1. A working group was set up to give priority to this problem, and their deliberations as set out in the Council's Third Report (CETHV 1967a) were subsequently published in a separate leaflet in 1967 (CETHV 1967b) which has been used widely.

The resulting statement was based on the International Definition of the World Health Organisation on the role and function of the public health nurse which reads:

> public health nursing is a special field of nursing which combines the skills of nursing, public health and some phases of social assistance. It functions as part of the total public health programme for the promotion of health, the improvement of conditions in the social and physical environment, rehabilitation and the prevention of illness and disability (World Health Organisation).

This statement was then related to the work of the health visitor in the United Kingdom and the five main areas of her work were defined.

> The health visitor is a nurse with post-registration qualification who provides a continuing service to families and individuals in the community. Her work has five main aspects:

1. The prevention of mental, physical and emotional ill health and its consequences.
2. Early detection of ill health and the surveillance of high risk groups.
3. Recognition and identification of need and mobilisation of appropriate resources where necessary.
4. Health teaching.
5. Provision of care; this will include support during periods of stress, and advice and guidance in cases of illness as well as in the care and management of children. The health visitor is not, however, actively engaged in technical nursing procedures (CETHV 1967*b*).

It was recognized that as a State Registered Nurse she came already equipped with certain knowledge and skills in the field of human biology, bacteriology, processes of disease and therapeutic methods. From obstetric nursing she had a knowledge of prenatal development, factors influencing subsequent child health; the care of mother and baby, and emotional factors relating to childbirth; and to these, the health visitors course added more preparation so that she came to her work in the community equipped with these skills (see Chapter 8). They are:

1. observational skills,
2. skills in developing interpersonal relationships,
3. skills in teaching individuals and groups,
4. skills in organization and planning in her own sphere.

These original statements were developed more fully in the Council's Fourth Report (1969) and published subsequently in a further leaflet, from which extensive extracts are quoted here because no discussion on the role and function of the health visitor can be complete without them, and to shorten them in any way would detract from their meaningfulness as a basis for this discussion.

The health visitor here is seen as providing a 'continuing health advisory service to families and individuals', her most usual means of contact being the visit to the family after the birth of a new baby, following the statutory birth notification.

Emphasis is placed firmly, first of all, on her role in terms of promotion of health through her contact with vulnerable groups in the community (see Chapter 10). Establishing priorities so that selective family visiting is based on need is the most usual practice, but the importance of contact with mothers and young children remains and must not be underestimated.

The health visitor, therefore, establishes contact with expectant mothers and visits all new babies within a defined area or, if she is working in the field of general practice, those born into families on the doctor's list. She provides systematic observation of children with particular reference to those under five years and a counselling service to their parents on the many facets of child development; in many areas she is also concerned in the health of the school child. The remainder of her caseload shows a varied picture. She not only follows up patients discharged from hospital to ensure that the necessary support is available, but is in contact with those awaiting admission. Other vulnerable groups with whom she is concerned are those families who themselves provide nursing care for one of their number—the physical and emotional strain this imposes can be extensive. The health visitor is also in contact with handicapped patients including the mentally subnormal, some of whom will be under the care of another statutory service. There will be need of support for some who have recently suffered bereavement, and referrals to and from other agencies, such as the social services departments for cooperation in care. The elderly are of special importance and the health visitor visits to assess need and to assist in mobilizing appropriate resources to improve conditions and increase independence wherever possible (CETHV 1973, p. 5).

The second main emphasis is placed on health teaching. Maintenance of health depends upon adequate knowledge being both available and acceptable, and in this connection the health visitor has a key role. It is one of her main functions to help individuals and groups make the best use of their resources to this end. Individual teaching is undertaken by all health visitors and those who discover they have an aptitude for group teaching have opportunities for developing further knowledge and skills. Work with groups is varied and extensive. The health visitor can be concerned with professional or lay audiences. Her sessions take place in health centres, clinics, the school classroom or group practice premises. Approach and methods vary from the promotion of small discussion groups to lectures for larger audiences. She may work with a planned syllabus, topics suggested by discussion groups, or participate in planning the incorporation of health teaching in a school curriculum as a whole (CETHV 1973).

Much of her work in terms of promotion of health is based on Caplan's (1961) concept of three different levels of prevention as a useful basis for consideration of the health visitors contribution to prevention.

Primary prevention is a community concept: to ensure healthy

development, we require certain physical, social and cultural resources—in short, a healthy environment. As the health visitor is
concerned with the promotion and maintenance of good health, it is
essential that she should be able to identify those features of the
environment which predispose toward ill health; she can then
consider to what extent she contributes to minimizing their influence. Her work provides the opportunity of seeing where community resources fall short or where the individual people with
whom she is in touch are unable to use them. As a field worker she is
in a good position to inform the appropriate authorities who are
responsible for community services about detrimental factors in
environment and services. Her records contribute to the establishment of knowledge on the state of health of the whole community
and on which health policy can be based.

Secondary prevention concerns the early detection of disease and the
treatment of conditions associated with particular stages in the cycle
of life. Although other workers, such as doctors, teachers and social
workers, are available to help through periods of illness and stress,
the health visitor can give anticipatory guidance or appropriate
practical help so that the person concerned makes a better adaptation to the situation. The general improvement in physical health
has allowed greater concentration on the emotional health of
children, and the Report of the Standing Medical Advisory Committee on Child Welfare Centres (HMSO 1967) refers to the health
visitor's particular contribution to this aspect of health. Her main
contribution lies in encouragement to the public to take advantage
of such schemes as are in current use, in allaying anxiety and in
ensuring that any abnormality is followed up. It does not necessarily
include carrying out the technical procedures involved.

Tertiary prevention is an aspect of aftercare concerned with containing and limiting the effects of a condition. The health visitor is
concerned in many circumstances which involve separation of the
individual from the family and support during the period of re-
integration is required. Satisfactory adjustment after a period of
stress is vital to the physical and mental health of the whole family.

The Council, however, is not the only voice to be heard when it
comes to making comment about the role of the health visitor. The
Report of the Royal College of Nursing Working Party (Royal
College of Nursing 1973) gave a very positive statement along much
the same lines as the extracts quoted earlier, but this time coming not
from a statutory body, but from a professional organization—an

indication of how health visitors saw their own role. This is a point of some significance as the definition of 'social role' concept implies an individual level of interaction. A social role refers to the expected behaviour associated with social position and it is individuals, not organizations, who play roles and occupy positions, and expected role behaviour is not necessarily identical with ideal role behaviour.

This Report is of interest because it identifies a specific set of 'core skills' for health visiting as distinct from other areas of nursing, again very similar to those outlined by the Council, and notes that it is not the skills which are unique but the particular combination of these skills. The Report also stresses the fact that the health visitor is a practitioner in her own right.

Another policy document of importance coming from health visitors themselves was the Health Visitors Association document, *Health Visiting in the Seventies* (Health Visitors Association 1975), once again setting out to define the proper function of the health visitor, as the basis of what the Association's members saw themselves as doing in ideal, or less than ideal, working conditions. This document should also be studied in order to appreciate its detailed implications, as it is only possible to comment here, and both professional organizations outlined in detail areas of work for health visitors in home visiting, particularly with expectant mothers, new births and under five-year-olds. School children, the elderly and families with special needs were also included. The health visitor was also seen as a consultant or coordinator and a health teacher and her priorities were spelled out within the above areas of work.

Perhaps one of the most important aspects to emerge from all these documents is the one that almost passes unnoticed because it is so implicit in the work of the health visitor—the fact that she is the one visitor to the home who may be there, not necessarily in response to recognized need, but on a routine visit or on a basis of selective visiting, and therefore is in an ideal position to carry out her functions in promotion of health, prevention of illness or anticipatory guidance. She is able to spot the potential crisis before it happens and therefore much of her work cannot be evaluated because in a sense the crisis 'doesn't happen'. Rehin (1972) refers to health visitors as 'essentially anonymous . . . a ubiquitous, silent minority', perhaps often unrecognized and underestimated, and suggests there is a need for health visitors to 'write their own script', or in other words to be more specific about their own professional practice.

THE IMAGE OF THE HEALTH VISITOR

Titmuss (1968) commented, 'professional people want their identity, role and functions to be known to others, for identity and specialization are linked to status'. The 'dilemma of identity', as described by Hunt, has already been discussed (Chapter 1) and Hunt (1972) goes on to suggest that this may lead to a somewhat diffuse public image, as indicated by the many different titles such as the 'welfare lady' or the 'clinic nurse', which are often heard. The title 'health visitor' does not necessarily describe any specific function that can be recognized by the general public and thus health visitors often tend to rely heavily on what they think is the public image of the nurse. Hunt recorded that one-half of the health visitors she interviewed felt that doctors and social workers held views of what a health visitor is and does, that were different from their own conception of their work. Sixty-four per cent of the health visitors also thought that their clients held quite different images of health visiting from their own. Hunt suggests that one of the difficulties is that most of the work done by health visitors is not really observed by anyone else, other than the client, so it is not easy for anyone to give a true evaluation or even description of what she does. Results are intangible and difficult to assess, and in addition to this, the client is not really the best person to assess the health visitor's efficiency objectively. Over 80 per cent of the health visitors felt they were accepted better by families because of their nursing background (Hunt 1972).

Rehin (1972) suggests that the health visitors' present dilemma is partly because they have reacted to and seen themselves as others see them, and certainly this suggestion would tie up with some of the reasons discussed in the historical context in Chapter 1. Rehin was particularly impressed with the vital functions that many health visitors were, in fact, performing, and conveys more than a veiled suggestion that other professionals would like to see health visitors in a more specific role of perhaps a different kind, in order to strengthen their own professional status. This is reinforced by the Health Visitors Association Manifesto which suggests many doctors and other voluntary organizations would be only too pleased to have health visitors working with them in specialities (Health Visitors Association 1975).

An interesting and positive approach by Pinder (1971) argues that the health visitor does in fact have a unique and key role, and what

she needs is recognition from employers and the public. The confusion lies not within health visiting, but in the current changes in
the nursing and social work structures.

Clark (1973) looked in some detail at the stereotypes of the health
visitor as held by clients, general practitioners and social workers;
and reduced them to three main elements.

1. Clientele was felt to be limited to mothers and young children
   —to the child with the family rather than family as a unit.
2. The health visitor's work was limited to maternal and child
   welfare, and her chief concern was with psychosocial aspects
   of health.
3. The health visitor's approach in her relationship with clients is
   didactic and authoritarian rather than non-judgemental and
   discussive.

The origins of the 'well baby nurse' image have already been
discussed in Chapter 1 and Clark maintains there is no clear
evidence to support the authoritarian approach which is probably
linked to the nurse image. In fact Singh and MacGuire (1971)
demonstrated that nurses differed from health visitors in occupational stereotypes in 9 out of 19 attributes. Health visitors were
perceived as more easy going, liberal and relaxed, objective and less
conforming among other things.

The Newsons' study in Nottingham (1965) gives a very interesting
and salutory example of a situation where mothers had certain ideas
of what health visitors expected of them and this influenced the kind
of information that they gave in situations relating to infant care and
feeding. The mothers' images of the health visitors here could have
differed widely from reality.

Clark goes on to note the general practitioners' tendency to
regard the health visitor as authoritarian and interfering and also
to note the well-documented evidence that social workers tend to
regard her as limited to dealing with physical problems and concentrating on the child rather than the family as a whole. Health
visitors do in fact have a more total approach to care than is often
realized, in that they see it as impracticable to separate emotional
and social needs from physical care, whereas other professionals
tend to see health visitors as dealing mainly with physical aspects of
care or those 'deemed to require health education' (Clark 1973).
With all these conflicting images and expectations existing between
other professionals and clients it is important to establish what the

health visitor really does do. The positive definitions on her statutory position for employment, place of work, also her role and function as outlined by the Council and two main professional organizations, have been clearly stated, but the student will be seeking more information on what the health visitor actually does with her time. Students will have opportunities for visiting with health visitors, and field work teachers, but may well ask whether their approach to health visiting is usual, or whether the area presents different problems, or the emphasis, placed on certain aspects of work, is typical of all areas.

WHAT THE HEALTH VISITOR DOES

Here our first reference must once again be to the Report of the Health Visitors Association (1975), a document which includes a descriptive account of health visiting based on a sample survey of opinion from members of the Association. While it cannot be doubted that this represents a substantial and typical volume of opinion, it should be observed that not all health visitors belong to the Association.

The document comments on the high degree of support for the Council's five aims, as set out earlier in this chapter, but notes that health visitors observed some difficulties in translating these into day-to-day situations. The title of health visitor, it is suggested, is relevant—the health content of her work is obvious, and the description of 'visitor' a very apt one, as much of her work is done in homes, at the invitation of a member of the family and she has no legal right of entry. These characteristics have a special value in maintaining the relationships basic to health visiting, but also give rise to some of the ambiguities already observed.

Any account given by health visitors of their work tends to relate it to the human life cycle and this is perhaps a convenient way of outlining what the health visitor does in a descriptive way (see Chapters 10 and 11).

Expectant Mothers
The antenatal period is an important one for making contact with expectant mothers at a time when the well-being of mother and child are important and the client is very receptive to health education. The relationship built up in this period is valuable when it comes to visiting the new baby.

New Births

New births are generally accepted as an essential part of health visitor's work, as the notification of all births gives her the opportunity to call on every family when a baby is born.

> At this first visit the health visitor will observe the physical, mental and social condition of the family while giving advice on the physical and emotional needs of the baby and control of its environment. She may also explain the relevant services available in the vicinity, drawing attention to the value of attendance at child health clinics and to the importance of immunization and, if appropriate, she may discuss family planning. At the same time she will be assessing any social needs, remaining constantly alert to the possibility of puerperal depression, child abuse or inadequate parentcraft. Support and encouragement with breast-feeding and advice on postnatal exercises and examinations may also be appropriate.
>
> On the basis of this first visit, information about the birth and any relevant facts available, the health visitor will assess how soon she should visit again (Health Visitors Association 1975, p. 330).

This question of assessing the need for a return visit is a very vital one because much of the value of the health visitor's work depends on building up a relationship with people and noting potential areas of need as the family grows or situations develop. It will be noted later on that many health visitors regard 'routine visiting' as a possibility only under average working conditions and it tends to lapse when staff shortages occur. Routine visiting is described below.

> Health visitors make a first or initial visit to every family with a new baby. Thereafter, if the health visitor has too heavy a case-load, she may only visit again for some special purpose.
>
> When her case-load is not unreasonable, a health visitor will make periodic visits to all families with young children, whether or not she knows of any special reason for doing so. This is routine visiting and when it is not possible the health visitor is not able to perform her most important function of regular checking of normal development in order to recognize early and, happily, prevent or mitigate deviations from normality (Health Visitors Association 1975, p. 326).

This must be seen in the context of 'selective visiting'—something which most health visitors practise normally, as they establish priorities on the basis of their judgement of need in relation to time available and the nature of the case-load and resources available. Even the most skilled health visitors may decide a family does not need visiting, when 'routine visiting' could well have revealed some unsuspected problems.

One to Five Years of Age

Routine visiting is particularly important in terms of the next group, the 1–5 year age group where health visitors are responsible for regular visiting and find many opportunities for teaching and guidance in both physical and emotional development of the child in the most important formative years of life. Only if a good working relationship exists can health visitors expect to be able to effectively communicate their understanding of the need for a child to have a warm stable relationship with a parent figure, and to help mothers in understanding the phases of development.

Other Groups

The other groups described in the document include school children, adults, particularly in terms of aftercare, and long or short-term illness, and also elderly people and families with special needs of different kinds.

Priorities in Health Visiting

The document (Health Visitors Association 1975) also gives a useful discussion on priorities which is included here because it goes a long way towards showing the student how health visitors see themselves working in ideal circumstances or, as unfortunately happens, in less than ideal situations of staff shortage, and thus emphasizes the importance of maintaining resources in order to maintain standards.

As the headings indicate, three levels of priority have been set. The first for the unfortunate health visitors working in those situations of almost desperate staff shortage which regrettably pertain in a few areas particularly in London and some other large cities. The second level probably applies to most of the rest of the country where the shortage is by no means so severe but most health visitors carry more than even the far-from ideal case-load recommended by the DHSS. Finally at the third level comes all the additional work which health visitors are trained and equipped to do and which would be so valuable if ever there are enough health visitors everywhere to permit of small enough case-loads for them all.

1. Recommended selection of work for health visitors working within severe staff shortages
    Urgent home visiting, i.e. to new births; actual or suspected cases of non-accidental injury to children; in response to requests from families; to handicapped children and to children in the 'observation' category who have failed to attend; to newly reported TB cases; to antenatal mothers especially primiparae.

Urgent referrals from general practitioners and hospitals which are properly within the health visitor's province.
Efficient record-keeping.
Involvement in the training of student health visitors.
Child health clinics.

2. Recommended additional work for health visitors working under only average pressure
Routine visiting of all children up to school age.
Visits to all antenatal mothers.
Supportive visits, e.g. to discharged patients and the bereaved.
Follow-up of immunization failures, new arrivals etc.
Health teaching to groups of adults and in schools.
Full liaison with hospitals and professional colleagues.
Involvement in the training of medical students, student nurses and social work students.

3. Recommended additions for health visitors who may one day have really small case-loads
Routine visiting of all children up to school leaving age, with time to attend to the needs of all members of the family.
Support for all families under stress from, e.g. psychiatric problems, chronic illness, handicap.
Counselling and health education at family planning and cytology sessions and other appropriate clinics.
Paediatric developmental testing at home of non-clinic attenders.
Visits to play groups and nurseries.
Involvement in research projects.
Regular visits to schools and hospital wards (Health Visitors Association 1975, p. 327).

A new edition of this document *Health Visiting in the Eighties* (Health Visitors Association 1980) reinforces these priorities with one addition under 2:

Paediatric development testing at home of non-clinic attenders.

It also sets health visiting in the context of the 'vast hierarchical structure of nursing management', and highlights some of the problems for the health visitor, as an independent practitioner within this structure. There is also some detailed discussion on the role of the health visitor within the context of the primary care team. The report concentrates on the re-definition of true fundamentals of health visiting—concluding that health visiting needs no defending—as the 'unique development of the British public health service, it has been, and still is, envied and emulated throughout the world' (Health Visitors Association 1980).

Other examples of major contributions to factual evidence on what health visitors 'do' can be found in surveys such as Clark's *A Family Visitor* (1973), and The Marris Report on health visiting in the London boroughs (1969).

Orr's study, *Health Visiting in Focus* (1980), gives a consumer's perspective on the health visitor's role. Clark's review *What do Health Visitors do?* (1981) gives a summary of all health visiting-related studies carried out between 1960 and 1980 and is a valuable source of reference for students and all health visitors. In order to illustrate their contribution in this context the student would do well to read these studies in some detail as they make an interesting profile of the nature of the work done. They must be seen, however, in the context of the difficulties described by the authors and others (Owen 1972) in terms of evaluation and definition of what health visitors see themselves doing. An example of this occurs in the Marris Report where no classification for 'health education' is given under 'techniques used'. This is probably because health visitors unconsciously assumed all their work to be health education and consequently gave it no place in analysis, only to find eventually they needed it as a specific classification.

Points of interest that emerge from both surveys include the high incidence of topics relating to child management and diet and visits to mothers with young children. Clark records over 70 per cent of visits were made to households with a young child under five, and approximately two-thirds of these to households with a baby under one year. Another interesting feature was that in 72·1 per cent of the families visited the health visitor was thought to be the only health or social agency visiting—a very revealing point in terms of her potential value. More than two-thirds of the visits were initiated by the health visitor herself, 14 per cent by the client and about 4 per cent by the general practitioner. One in five of all visits was to a household which had a person over 65 years of age (Clark 1972).

Although different classifications were used in the Marris Report, similar inferences can be drawn. The actual proportion of 'people served' relating to mothers with young children not at school emerges at roughly two-thirds, and over two-thirds of time is spent with these groups in home visiting.

Again similar comparisons can be made in terms of topics handled in discussion, Clark recording 51 different topic headings and Marris 38.

Clark concludes that the health visitor's clientele still consists largely of families with young children. However, her findings do not show the health visitor as concerned primarily with the child, but as having a wider interest in the family as a unit; and it is also interesting to note the high incidence of topics dealing with psychosocial aspects of health. She also observes that health visitors detect and actually deal with a large number of social problems during the course of home visiting and their work includes a large component of 'social care'. This of course is an area where there could be overlap of function with social workers, but again it must be seen in the context of the fact that in 70 per cent of the families visited the health visitor was the only visitor there and had it not been for her presence many of these situations may have gone unnoticed or become major crises, or even have resolved themselves! Her study could find no evidence to support the stereotype of an authoritarian didactic type of visitor.

In the Marris Report also a close inspection of the statistical data given reveals how much of her work is in the nature of anticipatory guidance and as such defies evaluation.

THE HEALTH VISITOR, AN AGENT FOR SOCIAL CONTROL·OR SOCIAL CHANGE

Discussion on these Reports should present the student with some indication of a general picture of what health visitors are doing today, also what they *think* they are doing, what others *see* them as doing, and perhaps what other professionals would *like* them to be doing. The limitations of these Reports as evidence, however, must be recognized, as they relate to opinions, or to data restricted to specific areas only in the country. However, taken together, they do present a useful documentary and profile, and a basis for further research. A question which often arises in discussion, but as yet has only produced opinionated comments, is the extent to which the health visitor acts as an agent of social control, or social change. More thought has been given to the role of the social worker in this context, particularly in relation to subjects such as social deviance, or even to the medical profession, often criticized for possessing a body of knowledge about health and disease and surrounding itself with a protective mystique which enables control of procedures, to set standards, define illness, or determine the function of other professional groups in society (Cox & Mead 1975). It may well be asked whether health visiting fits into the Parsons' *structural functionalist* approach (1951) as helping to alleviate disease in society, or is it concerned with perpetuating or establishing 'middle-class' values in relation to health behaviour or child-rearing practices? Other questions may well relate to the role of the health visitor as a health educator, having certain manipulative skills, in persuading people to adopt certain courses of behaviour in relation to health.

These are all questions which the student may well be invited to discuss during a health visitors course, and questions which help in gaining a balanced perspective and approach to the work to be done.

A fitting definition with which to conclude this chapter is found in the Council's publication *An Investigation into the Principles of Health Visiting* (1977).

> The professional practice of health visiting consists of planned activities aimed at the promotion of health and prevention of ill-health. It thereby contributes substantially to individual and social well-being, by focusing attention at various times on either an individual, a social group or community. It has three unique functions.
>
> 1. Identifying and fulfilling self-declared and recognised as well as unacknowledged and unrecognised health needs of individuals and social groups.
>
> 2. Providing a generalist health agent service in an era of increasing specialisation in the health care available to individuals and communities.
>
> 3. Monitoring simultaneously the health needs and demands of individuals and communities; contributing to the fulfillment of those needs; and facilitating appropriate care and service by other professional health care groups.

This implies that the health visiting service shall be provided for all age groups but that primary consideration should be for child health in the context of family life.

Some factors, however, stand out from the foregoing discussion in these two chapters. First of all it is apparent that health visiting practice has changed in response to changing social and individual need over the years, and obviously still is responsive to need. The extent to which present changes may influence future developments will be discussed in Chapter 12, but it is sufficient to note here that the present administrative structure with its emphasis on integration is providing the health visitor with a greater challenge than ever before in establishing her identity in one aspect of her role—that of liaison and communication.

Secondly, it is also apparent that current economic constraints are compelling the policy makers to think carefully about allocation of resources, and at last the wisdom of spending money on prevention is breaking through. This, coupled with the increasing trend to place more responsibility for health management on the individual, recognizing that there is a limit to the extent to which the services can support the nation's demands, is giving the health visitor new opportunities for health education in terms of promoting health (HMSO 1976).

There are many other interesting new trends, such as the current enthusiasm for breast-feeding, which may well indicate changed emphasis for the health visitor in her work, making different kinds of demands on her time and skills.

Finally, throughout these two chapters inevitably some discussion has focused on the doubts, anxieties and dilemmas surrounding the role and function of the health visitor. It is to be hoped that the student may by now appreciate the origins and reasons for some of these uncertainties, and recognize some of the pressures which arise from the demands of other professionals or desires of the consumers themselves. Also, hopefully, it is possible to see, in some of the actual evidence building up, what the health visitor *does* do. This, together with recent positive statements from the Council and professional bodies, should go a long way towards clarifying issues and establishing a positive identity which exists even if in the very uniqueness of the combination of skills the health visitor provides.

The health visitor is now firmly established within the administrative structure, the need is there and the education and training available today should go a long way towards equipping her for that need.

SUMMARY

The setting in which health visitors work is described, also their role and function in this setting, and the concepts of promotion of health and prevention of illness are seen as central to the work, and also to health teaching. Attempts have been made to describe what the health visitor does and to identify her unique skills and contribution to society and some of these attempts are discussed, showing the nature of her work and some of the difficulties inherent in trying to define or evaluate health visiting practice. It is, however, possible to identify some areas of priority and to assess those areas where need arises most frequently and is being met.

REFERENCES

An Investigation into the Principles of Health Visiting (1977) London: Council for the Education and Training of Health Visitors.

Caplan, G. (1961) *An Approach to Community Mental Health*. London: Tavistock Publications. *

CETHV (1967a) *Third Report*. London.

CETHV (1967b) *The Function of the Health Visitor*. London.

CETHV (1969) *Fourth Report*. London

CETHV (1973) *The Health Visitor, Functions and Implications for Training*. London.

Clark, J. (1972) What do health visitors do? *Nursing Times*, *68*, 30 (27 July).

Clark, J. (1973) *A Family Visitor*. London: Royal College of Nursing. *

Clark, J. (1981) *What do Health Visitors do?* London: Royal College of Nursing Research Series.

Cox, C. & Mead, A. (1975) *A Sociology of Medical Practice*. London: Collier MacMillan.

Department of Health and Social Security (1972) *Local Authority Nursing Staff*. Circular no. 72. London.

Gilmore, M., Bruce, N. & Hunt, M. (1974) *The Work of the Nursing Team in General Practice*. London: Council for the Education and Training of Health Visitors. *

Health Visitors Association (1975) Health visiting in the seventies. Staffing of the health visiting and school nursing services. *Health Visitor*, *48*, 9 (September). *

Health Visitors Association (1980) *Health visiting in the 80s*. London.

HMSO (1967) *The Report of the Standing Medical Advisory Committee on Child Welfare Centres*. London.

HMSO (1976) *Prevention and Health: Everybody's Business. A Reassessment of Public and Personal Health. A Consultative Document*. London. *

Hunt, M. (1972) The dilemma of identity in health visiting. *Nursing Times*, *68*, 5 and 6 (3 and 10 February). Occasional Papers.

Marris, J. (1969) *The Work of Health Visitors in London*. Report no. 12. London: GLC Department of Planning and Transportation Research.

Newson, J. and E. (1965) *Patterns of Infant Care*. Harmondsworth: Pelican.

Orr, J. (1980) *Health Visiting in Focus*. London: Royal College of Nursing Research Series.

Owen, G.M. (1972) Book review on the work of health visitors in London. *Nursing Times*, *68*, 7 (17 February).

Parsons, T. (1951) *The Social System*. New York: Free Press.

Pinder, J.E. (1971) A reply to the role conflicts of the new breed of health visitor. *Health Visitor*, *44*, 6 (June).

Rehin, G.F. (1972) The point and purpose of the health visitor. *Nursing Times*, *68*, 11 (16 March).

Robinson, J. (1982) *An Evaluation of Health Visiting*. London: Council for the Education and Training of Health Visitors.

Royal College of Nursing (1973) *Report of the Working Party on the Role of the Health Visitor*. London. *

Singh, A.J. & MacGuire, J.M. (1971) Occupational values and stereotypes in a group of trained nurses. *Nursing Times*, 67, 42 pp. 165–8 (21 October). Occasional Papers.

Titmuss, R. (1968) *Commitment to Welfare*. London: Allen & Unwin.

World Health Organisation *Technical Report no. 167*. Geneva.

FURTHER READING

The books in the reference list marked with an asterisk are useful basic material for general reading.

II. The Education and Training of the Health Visitor

3. The Health Visitors Course

Grace M. Owen

THE ESTABLISHMENT OF THE COUNCIL FOR THE EDUCATION AND TRAINING OF HEALTH VISITORS

The events leading up to the establishment of the first Council for the Training of Health Visitors were outlined in Chapter 1. The Health Visitor and Social Workers (Training) Act (1962), set up two councils with a joint secretary and chairman for health visiting and social work. In Section 2 of the Act the role of the Council for the Training of Health Visitors was clearly defined as follows:

> to promote the training of health visitors by seeking to secure suitable facilities for the training of persons intending to become health visitors, by approving courses as suitable to be attended by such persons, and by seeking to attract persons to such courses.

The Council also had authority to provide and secure provision of courses for further training and arrangement of exams and an additional remit to carry out, or assist others to carry out, research (Council for the Education and Training of Health Visitors 1966).

The National Health Service (Qualifications of Health Visitors) Regulations, 1964 (para. 2a) made provision for the Council's Certificate to become a condition for employment to practise as a health visitor in the United Kingdom.

Thus, from its inauguration, the Council was to play a dynamic role in the provision of preparation or 'training' of health visitors, and in shaping the 'new breed' of health visitors (CETHV 1966). At that time there were 29 training schools in the United Kingdom in a wide variety of situations, in universities, colleges of advanced technology and technical colleges, while some were organized within local health authorities. Facilities for students also showed a wide variation, some being excellent and others very limited. The Council immediately set itself three fundamental issues to deal with.

The syllabus for training health visitors.
The need to change practical experience.
The need to reorganize the examination system.

Many factors had to be taken into consideration, not least the wide range of duties required of qualified health visitors. It was also necessary to produce a flexible syllabus including recognition of recent extensions of knowledge in medical and behavioural and social sciences, and the relevance of these studies to health visiting. It is a significant measure of the success of that first Council's deliberations that the five main areas of study outlined have remained basic to the course until the time of writing this chapter. They are:

1. the development of the individual,
2. the individual in the group,
3. the development of social policy,
4. social aspects of health and disease,
5. principles and practice of health visiting.

The original objectives of the syllabus as approved by the Council in 1964, to come into operation in 1965, were set out in a leaflet giving the background. The syllabus was designed to:

1. sharpen the student's capacity to perceive early deviations from normal,
2. give knowledge of various statutory and voluntary agencies,
3. provide practice in the working out of a programme of help for the individual,
4. prepare her to select the method of health education likely to be the most successful (CETHV 1965).

The need for increased depth in fieldwork experience was recognized and provision was made for the appointment of fieldwork instructors to work closely with the training centres in providing the students with teaching in the community.

Two important new features were introduced with the 1964 syllabus; firstly, the course was to be lengthened to one calendar year, which allowed for a period of approximately 11 to 12 weeks fieldwork experience under supervision, immediately following the written examinations. The second innovation was that each centre should submit its own course for approval, and conduct its own examination appointing its own internal examiners, together with an external examiner approved by the Council. This has become a significant and important feature, as each centre, while providing the required basic 'common core' of the course as outlined in the syllabus, has been able to develop and retain its own identity. It has certain advantages in that while minimal standards are maintained in all courses, the facilities of the educational establishment or local area health authority may be fully utilized to bring certain extra strengths to a particular course, and thus avoid producing stereotyped health visitors.

The newly formed Council had an additional responsibility for the recruitment of health visitors, seeking provision for new centres throughout the United Kingdom, and for stimulating the provision for training health visitor tutors. The recommended ratio of 1 qualified tutor to every 15 students meant that 20 more tutors were required immediately to staff existing schools.

The First Report of the Council included comment on the consideration given to admitting men into health visiting, noting the unique contribution they could make, and reference was made also to the establishment of a group to consider research.

In just two years the Council had demonstrated its ability to move swiftly towards a fresh approach to health visitor training. The new concepts were communicated to the training centres by a team of professional advisors under the leadership of the first Chief Professional Advisor, Miss Elaine Wilkie. The First Report was evidence of the influence the Council was to have in future years.

One valuable method of communication maintained by the Council has been the production and distribution of attractive and informative leaflets, many of which will be used as sources of reference in this book, and also the issue of regular news bulletins to training schools, giving reports on progress and indicating current trends in objectives in training. By the time the Council's Third Report was issued in 1967 (CETHV 1967a) the role and function of the health visitor had been clarified (see Chapter 2) and the Fourth Report in 1969 amplified this and set out the training objectives (see p. 59).

The next report of the Council was not issued until 1975 and this covered five eventful years of change in local government and the health and social services administration, and also the publication of the Report of the Committee on Nursing (HMSO 1972). During this period the Local Authority Social Services Act (1970) had allowed for the enlargement and separation of the joint Councils with independent chairmen and new titles. The inclusion of the word 'education' in the title of both Councils was greatly appreciated by the professions as it had long been recognized that there must be a balance between education and training in preparation for health visiting or social work.

THE ROLE OF THE COUNCIL IN RELATION TO THE EDUCATION AND TRAINING OF HEALTH VISITORS

The Third and Fourth Reports of the Council had indicated the philosophy which guided its policy and which had become established and implemented over the years. There was a continuation of the trend to site all courses within higher and further education establishments, with a consequent broadening of the range of academic staff involved in teaching, and an increase in the numbers of qualified tutors in colleges. This has, as noted in the Fifth Report, considerably enlarged the horizons for health visitor training. Many from other academic disciplines have shown increasing interest in teaching on these courses and in making a valuable contribution to the planning and organization of courses and examination procedures. The Council's faith in the competence of educational establishments to interpret the broad outlines of the syllabus and maintain good standards in the examination appeared to have been justified, when the system was reviewed in 1969–70. The Council has retained its policy of flexibility in approach to interpretation of the syllabus and examination pattern, and also towards the need for the availability of modified courses for individuals or groups of students with certain specific experience or qualifications.

The Fifth Report also commented on the improvement, if slow, in the quality of fieldwork teaching following the introduction in 1967 of a 30-day course of preparation for fieldwork instructors. Much discussion has taken place over the years concerning the need for change in this area, but progress was delayed partly while awaiting a statement of intent to implement the proposals of the Report of the Committee on Nursing.

One further achievement during these years was the setting up of two obstetric courses especially organized for men who wished to become health visitors, and in 1973 the first two groups of men completed this training.

Other areas where the Council has linked its policy with education and training include the promotion of interprofessional cooperation and the establishment of new courses, and initiation of refresher courses. The Council has organized a variety of interdisciplinary conferences and encouraged interdisciplinary experiments within training courses.

All this indicates that the Council has played a very active and dynamic role since its inception, establishing a pattern of relationships with training centres, which enables maintenance of basic standards of preparation for health visiting yet allows for flexibility within the system in a way which enables courses to take advantage of local facilities and expertise and to develop an experimental approach in a constant search for improvement, and progress.

Progress since 1962 and the Changing Role of the Health Visitor Tutor

At the time the Council was set up there were 29 Training Centres in the United Kingdom offering approximately 800 places for students, and by the time the Fifth Report was issued in 1975 there were 57 centres accepting over 1350 students annually. In 1981 there were 49 centres listed, with a total of 1333 students registered in the UK, and 10 of these were male students. These figures include modified, degree and experimental course students. Figure 2a demonstrates the growth rate between 1964 and 1973 and an interesting prediction published in 1974 of growth rate based on forecast population growth. The *actual* growth rate between 1974 and 1981 shows a very different picture, and a considerable shortfall from the optimum requirement forecast in 1974. A number of factors may be responsible for the shortfall, not least the current constraints in financial provision of health authorities, and review of places in certain educational establishments where resources are reduced (Figure 2b).

The Fifth Report of 1974 and current figures from CETHV Returns (1982 January) show that while the number of single women students remained virtually constant, between 1968 and 1974 the number of married students had almost doubled in that time. There was little change in these proportions in figures published in 1981/2. This is not simply a reflection of the increased popularity of marriage, but clearly an increase over the early years in

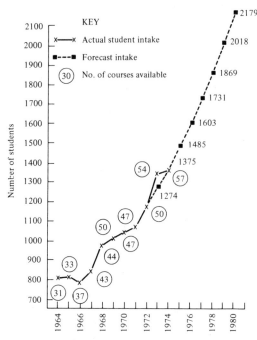

Fig. 2a. Growth rate of the number of health visitor courses and student intake. Based on the forecast population growth rate of 1:3500 the optimum number of health visitors would not be achieved until July 1981 (CETHV 1975, p.12)

Table 1. Marital status of health students, post-registration only (CETHV 1975).

	Married	Single
1968	429	463
1969	491	436
1970	515	444
1971	553	419
1972	609	457
1973	799	443

the number of married women recruited; and is particularly evident in the 'over 40' age group.

Other interesting factors shown in the 1981/2 figures (CETHV) show that significantly more than half of students recruited are State Certified Midwives, and approximately one-quarter obtain required

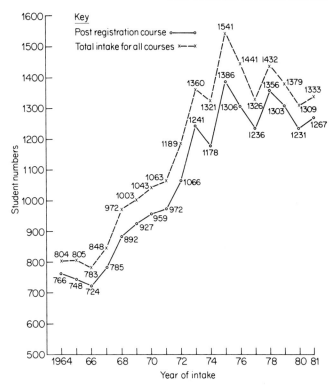

Fig. 2b. Actual intake of health visitor students (all courses since 1964). (Source: Health Visitors Student Analysis 1981/2, CETHV Records Dept. Jan. 1982.)

obstetric experience outside general training. A breakdown of the age structure on one-year full time courses in the UK, shows that 32.8% of the intake of students are between 25 and 29 years of age and 36.6% are between 35 and 40 years.

After 1962 there was an increasing trend for courses to move from the local health authority situation into further and higher education establishments, and this was not without its effect on the role of the health visitor tutor. At one time most tutors were very much occupied with course administration and tutorial work in the health visiting field, and supervision of fieldwork placements. Increasingly health visitor tutors are finding themselves involved in the more general aspects of work in the educational establishment and involved in planning and developing other courses in related areas of work.

Many have developed their own subject areas of expertise in

specialities related to health visiting and teach on a wide variety of courses. An unpublished survey carried out by members of a Standing Conference for Health Visitor Training Centres in the South East Region (1971) showed that the health visitor tutors present had some involvement in a range of over 20 different kinds of courses including such groups as nursery nurses, social work or health education courses, teacher training or nursing degree courses. Many tutors are heavily involved in the general life of their own departments and several have achieved the status of becoming head of department or division. This has considerably changed the pattern of life for some tutors and has not been without its difficulties as they have pioneered in fields where no precedents have been set. At the same time, however, it has advantages in that health visitor tutors are able to hold major responsibilities in their own specialities of work in addition to those on the health visitors course. This broadens horizons, and allows opportunities to expand in research and experimental courses or short courses, in an educational setting. In addition, many tutors have made a contribution of value as they bring new dimensions of expertise and skill into the life of the college concerned. Their primary role, of course, remains that of overall planning, organization and supervision of the health visitors course, which involves a considerable load of specific teaching and tutorial work, fieldwork organization and communication and personal student counselling. Since 1962 the qualified health visitor tutor has played an increasingly important role in the progress and planning of courses and the general recognition of health visiting in educational establishments.

One other point worthy of comment over the years, which emerged in the Fifth Report, was the particularly low examination failure rate. Between 1968 and 1974 the pass rate varied between 90.46 per cent and 93.96 per cent, and this often raises questions of various kinds, although it could, of course, reflect an efficient selection system. Many other factors could be involved, such as the students' high motivation, and the fact that they are already to some extent preselected, having successfully completed one professional qualification. It should, however, be recognized that there is a possibility as on any professional course that students are only selected for the course if they appear to be acceptable to the selectors in college and community, thus perpetuating the present professional image, and possibly eliminating those who might contribute too much innovatory thought or change.

THE HEALTH VISITORS COURSE

Philosophy, Aims and Objectives

It was noted earlier that the profession received with appreciation the inclusion of the concept of education within the title of the Council. A Conference of the Association of Integrated and Degree Courses in Nursing in 1975 examined the theme 'Nursing—an Education or a Training?' and a wide variety of definitions on these two terms were set out by speakers, in support of differences, or alternatively maintaining that the two are inseparable in a professional preparation.

Education, it was suggested, may be broadly defined as a systematic instruction in the acquisition of knowledge in preparation for life in general. It includes the acquisition of skills, development of knowledge and potential of the individual (Association of Integrated and Degree Courses in Nursing 1975), which implies a response in terms of behavioural change on the part of the individual during the learning processes. Training, however, is more closely concerned with preparing the individual for efficiency in a specific field of activity. For members of a profession this is complicated by the need for control over preparation, training and qualification to practise within certain defined limits.

Training, then, is largely concerned with *how* an activity is performed, and education more generally concerned with *why* things are done as they are. Chapman (1974) points out the necessity for both these approaches in professional preparation, and McFarlane (1970) notes that education and training are tools which contribute to the efficient use of manpower.

An appreciation of the use of these terms is an essential prerequisite for understanding the philosophy of the course preparing for the practice of health visiting. A close study of the Council's *Guide to the Syllabus for Training* (CETHV 1972) shows that insights are required into the theories underlying both human behaviour and the social influences affecting the individual. A considerable amount of factual information is available to the student in relation to these areas of study, also relating to the contemporary social services and social aspects of health and disease and the principles of health visiting. Even if the content of the course should change over the years, the basic principles and their interpretation remain a fundamental necessity for insights into health visiting practice.

The Council's leaflet on the function of the health visitor, first introduced in 1967 (CETHV 1967*b*), noted that the health visitor brought to her work in the community:

observational skills,
skills in developing interpersonal relationships,
skills in teaching individual groups,
skills in organization and planning in her own sphere.

Some of these skills are already established as a result of nursing training and education. An extended version of this leaflet published in 1973 (CETHV 1973) developed this discussion to show how the function of the health visitor had implications for the objectives in education and training. The leaflet outlined the aims of the one-year training for health visiting as follows.

1. To develop that skill in establishing interpersonal relationships, which will provide a basis for constructive work with families and individuals.
2. To sharpen the student's perception of early deviation from normal.
3. To give a knowledge of various statutory and voluntary agencies which may act in any particular family situation.
4. To provide practice in working out with families and individuals, programmes of help where these are required.
5. To illustrate and practise methods of health education and to help develop a critical attitude in their use.

It will be noticed that this was an extension of the original aims as stated in the first leaflet issued. It was suggested that the course was 'designed to develop a quality of perception, sensitivity to need and a capacity for the organization of care which has its earlier origins in nurse training' (CETHV 1973), and it is important to recognize that the present health visitor course is constructed on the basis of the existing nurse training. Emphasis is also given to the importance of the practical application of principles learned in the classroom and the role of the fieldwork teacher in this situation.

It is apparent that the aims and objectives as outlined here cannot be achieved by acquisition of knowledge and factual information, or by fieldwork alone. For some students the change of emphasis from curative nursing care, to preventive aspects and the promotion of health, may involve considerable processes of attitude change which can give rise to certain stresses at various stages of the course. This, of necessity, calls for the application of educational principles in planning the course and in the careful selection of teaching methods used and indicates the need for the health visitor tutor to be available in a supportive and counselling role at all times. The course is therefore arranged with this in mind and there is usually a logical progression working from and building on the student's existing knowledge and experience. Often the 'normal' and 'routine' aspects of work are dealt with first, moving on to the more complex ideas and problematic areas later in the course. It is recognized that theory and practice must be correlated and fieldwork teachers are kept well informed of the student's progress in theoretical work and also of the requirements of the course in terms of the timing of the introduction of experience and taking responsibility.

The Course Planning and Organization

The general pattern of the course as established in the 1960s was to offer a balance of approximately two-thirds based in an educational establishment and one-third in the community with the fieldwork teacher. This principle is still applied in a variety of different ways, some colleges using the pattern of several weeks 'block placement' for fieldwork experience, while others prefer the method of 'concurrent' or more continuous placement.

The former method (when students spend two or three weeks based entirely in the community with a fieldwork teacher) enables students to gain a general total picture of the work of the health visitor more easily and allows for a build up of relationships with colleagues and clients demanding less frequent reorientation to different aspects of the course. It does have its disadvantages, however, in that it cuts across the opportunities for students to share lecturing courses with other students on different courses. The value of this sharing of lectures is debatable, however, as while in theory it economizes in staff resources and should help students to mix, in actual practice it is very difficult to organize administratively and in fact students do not mix any more readily or exchange ideas in the lecture situation. The second method of concurrent placement involves one or two days each week in the community. If this is used, care must be taken to provide the student with opportunities to see the entire range of work by varying the days from week to week. This method, however, does allow for more regular visiting of families. Often a combination of both methods is used to provide the advantages of each.

The close integration of theory and practice is maintained by regular meetings between the course tutors, fieldwork teachers, and community nursing officers, to maintain good communication and understanding of the course philosophy and progression. The health visitor tutor is constantly seeking to help students to relate academic studies to the realities of health visiting.

Some modifications in the course pattern have been made on the basis of experience and, as it stands at the time of writing, students take Part I of the examination at the end of the academic year, and on successful completion of this proceed to their period of approximately 11 weeks supervised practice, after which they complete Part II of the examination, which is an oral discussion on the health visiting studies presented. In principle, Part I of the examination consists of written papers or course work relating to the five sections of the syllabus. Different colleges may have slightly different interpretations of this, but many use the kind of examination question which requires an application of theory to practice. Examples may be seen at the end of some chapters. During the year students also prepare a neighbourhood study of the area in which they are based for experience and also health visiting studies which are presented for examination at the end of the academic year on the basis of the Part II examination. The number of health visiting studies required for presentation for examination has been four, but it is likely that the Council may recommend a reduction in the near future. In fact a number of colleges are already operating alternative schemes, and where students are presenting projects they may only be required to prepare two or three studies. On successful completion of the course the student applies to the Council for a certificate to practise as a health visitor.

It would not be a useful exercise to break down the course content and examination system any further here, as the content of the syllabus may be found in the Council's leaflet, and each course has its own way of interpreting the syllabus on the lines already described. Also the Council allows for experimentation of new ideas, and changes are under consideration for the examination system with the aim of decreasing the load in terms of written papers.

Some courses have additional requirements such as the presentation of projects, which are considered a valuable teaching tool.

Much controversy has raged around the desirability of lengthening the course by varying periods from one term, to making it a two-year course. However, the advantages have to be set against the constraints in terms of economic resources available in the health and welfare sector and also changes must be considered in the light of possible changes in nursing education, which could ultimately influence the plan and content of the health visitors course.

Methods Used on the Course

Most courses make use of a wide range of teaching methods and approaches to study, including the formal lecture for some major subjects where factual teaching of a specialist nature is required. Some courses use the seminar method quite extensively, where one or two students prepare papers on a specific topic and the remainder of the group contribute to the discussion. Small groups or individual tutorials are also used frequently, particularly where attitude change is required, or where practical application of theoretical studies is required.

Students are usually required to undertake a considerable amount of private study, especially in preparation for written work such as essays and seminar papers and while this may generate a certain amount of pressure, it is in these situations where the student is personally involved in the process of enquiry and organization of material that learning takes place most effectively.

Although many students feel more secure when they can take well-structured notes or receive 'handouts', a good deal of time is set aside for informal discussion, to allow for critical analysis of new concepts and ideas. Students who have been used to 'note-taking' methods may fear they are wasting time in the more unstructured group situation, but it is important to recognize that when the group is led by a skilled tutor, the dynamic situation within the group is a valuable one for situations requiring a change of attitude or acceptance of new ideas.

Considerable use is made of material available on tape, in films or produced on video tape, and other methods such as role play and project presentation have their place in learning new skills. Team teaching is often used where staff from several different disciplines participate in seminars. The use of organized written work, projects and health visiting studies are discussed in more detail later in the chapter.

It is essential that the course should provide a continuous learning experience for the student, together with opportunities to acquire specific new skills. Students, tutors, fieldwork teachers and other academic staff are all involved together in the process and every student embarking on the course may do so with confidence that the programme is based on a well-tried and well-structured framework, knowing that there are experienced tutorial staff available to give guidance in all aspects of the course.

The Student's Approach to the Course

The foregoing discussion may be of interest in giving a total picture of the training but every potential student will be wanting to ask questions about her own personal approach to the course in terms of the kind of demands it will make on time, energy and intellectual ability and concerning the best methods of study to adopt. Some of the areas of conflict include the intensive reading required, the adjustment to new ideas and approaches to study, or even adjustment to life in an educational setting, where there is an atmosphere of academic freedom for students to work out their own priorities and to follow their own interests.

It is usual for students to apply to one or more colleges of their own choice and also to a health authority for financial secondment. Selection is carried out either separately or jointly by the educational establishment and the prospective employer, usually by means of interviews and often a written test. On receiving an offer of a place in the college, students may well receive a list of books for pre-course reading, or other helpful instructions for preparation. It is always advisable to follow any such suggestions as the course is very intensive once it starts and any preliminary work is useful.

Those who have not studied for many years could find one of the small handbooks on approach to study would give helpful advice, such as *A Student's Guide to Efficient Study* by D. James.

For the early weeks of the course, students are often advised to read widely and generally, and to absorb new ideas and explore the range of source material available to get a general feeling of what the course is about. After that, more specific requirements in the nature of preparing essays or seminar papers will guide the student into particular aspects of study and by the second term the areas needing more intensive study become very clearly defined. The third term is generally one of consolidation, and the student will experience the satisfaction of seeing various aspects of the course 'slotting into place' within the total situation.

Most students find it helpful to organize their time by working out a plan that suits their personal domestic situation and allows for regular disciplined study. It is generally wise to break up any longer periods of time available for study into shorter sessions of about three-quarters to one hour, and it often helps to have some brief spell of physical activity between sessions, such as taking the dog for a walk or preparing a meal. Most mature students, however, establish their own personal 'rhythm' that they find most suitable. The most important thing is to have a plan and follow it, bearing in mind the factors that make for fatigue and boredom, and to allow for proper use of leisure breaks.

The use of reading material The lengthy book lists presented to students at the beginning of some courses can be very daunting but it is reassuring to know that generally speaking it is possible to be selective in approach to reading and it is helpful to have some idea how to go about this.

Basically, students will need to use three different kinds of books or reading material.

1. The smaller, cheaper kind of paperbacks which can be read relatively easily, purchased, and kept for reference, or marked with the student's own notes. Examples can be seen in some of the community studies used in sociology or the smaller collections of articles (e.g. *The Sociology of Modern Britain*, Butterworth & Wier 1970).

2. The longer, and often expensive type of textbook, a 'reader', which is often recommended for reference purposes and most likely to be borrowed from the library. Occasionally lecturers will suggest one basic text in their subject and will advise on the choice, but more often they prefer students to read more generally.

3. Journals and current research publications, which can again be found in most libraries and will provide students with up-to-date knowledge on specialist areas of study or controversial issues.

It is important to discuss the books that course tutors consider to be basic or essential reading before spending money on expensive books and to acquire the art of reading selectively and not necessarily reading every book from cover to cover. Some students find it useful to work in groups for purchasing or reading books and writing synopses for their colleagues, but while short cuts may be helpful, there is no actual substitute for personal study.

One useful practice is to keep some kind of organized record system for reading completed. For some students an alphabetical card index system is adequate, simply to record the author, title, publisher, and a brief synopsis of the content or major issues discussed. Other students may prefer to make a more detailed précis of the book or article and keep it in a loose-leaf filing system for future reference. Whatever method is used it is a good idea to have a systematic approach from the start and build it up, as it will serve a useful purpose throughout a professional career and save considerable time hunting for material at a later date.

Most subjects studied on the health visitors course require general reading, to allow for assimilation of ideas and theoretical approaches which can be explored more fully in group discussion situations. There are, however, some areas where certain basic factual knowledge must be acquired, such as in understanding the principles of infant-feeding or the stages of normal child development or the routine procedure to be carried out at a first visit to a new baby. It is vital in such cases that students have access to and know how to use the fundamental knowledge required. Again James' book has helpful suggestions on note taking and memorizing.

Written work during the course The kind and quantity of written work required from students will vary from course to course, but inevitably it will be part of the total programme. Its purpose is twofold—partly to give the student some aims and objectives in planning reading aimed at specific topics, thinking through the subject and then reorganizing the material. This in itself is an aid to learning. Secondly, it is an exercise in itself in organizing and reproducing factual material, or expressing ideas in an orderly way and relating theory to reality in health visiting. This is quite a useful exercise in developing skills in record keeping and report writing and ultimately preparation for examination questions. In addition, it helps with reinforcement in the learning processes.

Early in the course students often tend to read in breadth and write more lengthy essays, but as the course proceeds it is necessary to acquire a more disciplined approach to producing the kind of answer that could be required in an examination question or essay, which can be written in 45 minutes or one hour. Many students lose marks because of failure to read a question properly or to answer it fully, and for students who have not been studying for some time the following example may be of use.

Question:
Discuss the relationship between home background and educational achievement in Britain today. To what extent does this topic interest the health visitor?

When marking questions of this kind it is usual for the tutor to give equal weighting to both parts of the question because application is as important as the understanding of theory for the health visitor, therefore both parts of the question must be answered fully. It may help to underline the operative words before planning the answer in order to ensure a properly constructed essay. Always look for the instructions such as 'discuss', 'outline', 'describe' or 'relate', as this will indicate the nature of approach required. For example, discussion necessitates putting forward several different schools of thought or assembling several different aspects of factual material and weighing up the differences, and any opinions or evidence quoted should always be backed up by the source. For example, a statement of fact on the above question could read as follows.

> Bernstein's studies on language development (1970) have demonstrated a strong relationship between social class factors and language development, which also has an ultimate bearing on educational achievement . . .

(In writing essays during the course it is helpful to record all sources of reference, for later revision.)

The second part of the above question allows the student plenty of scope for relating the theoretical studies to practice and using her own observations and including illustrations from her own area of fieldwork experience.

Seminar papers require a similar approach but must be written remembering that they have to be presented, and in a limited time. There should be a general statement of introduction to the topic, some discussion on the range of ideas or information available, and the conclusion may raise some vital issues or questions for further discussion, as the other members of the group should come prepared to contribute.

Preparation of projects This always involves a certain amount of activity, personal enquiry, or reading in a specific subject area, often chosen because of its particular interest for the student. Sometimes students follow an individual project, or alternatively contribute one section of a group project. A project is a valuable opportunity for learning—the student acquires a depth of knowledge in a specific topic and learns methods of discovery, enquiry, and organization of material. The discipline of selecting and presenting material is a useful exercise, and the value of the project is considerably increased if students have an opportunity to present and discuss their work with others in the group, who often learn from it as well. Sometimes it is easy to get overwhelmed with material and therefore important to get the terms of reference sorted out early on, and not to be sidetracked. Any original enquiry must be small and manageable so that it does not take too large a proportion of the students' time and energy. As with reading, a card index system for recording references is useful and may save time. When writing up the project for presentation it is usual to give a general introduction to the area to be studied, followed by discussion or relevant literature and an explanation of the method and plan to be followed. Any original investigation should then be recorded, and results discussed in the context of subjects studied. The source material should be carefully documented with appropriate references throughout the text, and a bibliography at the end.

The neighbourhood and health visiting studies Neighbourhood and health visiting studies were introduced with the new syllabus in 1965 and are a general requirement for all courses, with minor modifications in the number, or method of presentation. The health visiting studies are preceded by a short 'neighbourhood study' written about the area where the student has been visiting the families recorded. According to the Council's *Guidelines* (1970), this study should include a consideration of 'sociological factors . . . and could include such matters as industry and occupation, amenities and services available . . . and community dynamics'. Unfortunately, students usually begin neighbourhood studies early in the course before they have had an opportunity to develop a sociological perspective on their approach and it is very easy for the study to become a historical saga on the area, or a list of services provided, or an account of schools, hospitals and housing.

The phrase 'community dynamics' in the *Guidelines* is a key factor in making the exercise come alive for the student. The neighbourhood study is basically about the *people* who live there, how they *interact* with each other and with *groups* in the *community* and how they respond to the *social pressures*, or react to the *environment* in which they live. One problem is the definition of the 'neighbourhood' and the student needs to have this clarified early on because there is quite a difference in writing a study on a small town or an area covered by a general practice team or simply a self-contained housing estate or a group of streets within an area.

While it is useful to encourage the student to find out about the services available in the neighbourhood visited, she needs to relate the provisions to the needs of the people—and the way in which they use the services. It is often helpful for students to read one of the community studies which describes an area similar to the one being visited; for example Rosser and Harris's Study on Swansea (1965) for a student visiting in a Welsh urban area; Kerr's Study on Ship Street (1958) for a student working in a port or dockland area, could help to bring a new dimension into the approach, and give the student some insight into the kind of factors to be observed. In writing up the study, some reference can be made to such studies for comparison.

The neighbourhood needs to be seen and written up as a *dynamic entity* rather than a list of events or facts. For example, if the area under consideration is a newly developing housing estate, it is important to know where the people come from and how their *social class* background or *age distribution* compares with the *national statistics*. This is relevant because it can affect the kind of services needed—and the way in which the services are used and that is particularly interesting to health visitors.

It should be possible to discuss the effects of housing and transport facilities in relation to neurosis, family ties, or loneliness, for example. The kind of patterns of behaviour in relation to health and child-rearing is of interest, or the incidence of disease or health risks due to occupation may be discussed as they can indicate areas of special need for health education or provision for a vulnerable group.

This is the kind of 'interaction picture' which the student should be seeking to make the study come to life and to be meaningful in relation to the families she is visiting within that neighbourhood.

The Council's *Guidelines* also give very detailed assistance for preparation of the health visiting studies, their aims and methods of assessment. Students often find difficulty in knowing just how much to record and once again the emphasis often tends to be placed on detailed factual information on the family history and health record, which, although essential aspects, are relatively straightforward. It is not quite as easy to record the actual visiting in a way which demonstrates the student's developing ability to assess and handle situations, or make relevant observations. It is generally felt to be more valuable for the student in the learning situation to record each visit separately rather than writing a 'case history' type of report. This gives an opportunity for the student to think through the aims and objectives before each visit, to report on observations made, assessment of the situation and action taken, and to attempt to evaluate the outcome of the visit, making recommendations for future reference.

One aspect of particular importance is the student's appraisal of her own performance and evaluation of the visit. Students often feel they must present studies according to some stereotyped style and this tends to inhibit their ability to make observations on their own reactions to situations, or assessment of need, and subsequent action taken. As the studies proceed one would expect to see evidence of the student's skills, in assessment of response to situations, growing and developing, and recorded as she acquires ability to identify the skills of health visiting.

Some indication of a structured approach to visiting is valuable, setting out the objectives, recording the observations made, actions taken and at the end, identifying achievements and noting future action necessary. This kind of framework, however, allows the student considerable scope for enlarging on aspects of the visit which were important to her in the learning situation, or to indicate areas where she felt unable to handle things adequately, and to record any subsequent discussion with her fieldwork teacher.

Some attempt to evaluate her progress in establishing relationships with the family and an assessment of the family's progress and development are therefore useful evaluations at the end of each study.

There are also certain areas where the student needs to demonstrate an awareness of the need for organized assessment on the basis of factual knowledge, for example, when writing a report on a first visit made to a new baby where it is important to spell out the observations made and note any deviation from normal. Some examples where detailed information should be recorded relate to infant-feeding and weaning, immunization, physical development or use of the social services. In general, examiners will be looking for the following.

1. Ability to approach work in an organized way and to record relevant factors accurately.
2. An awareness of the need to establish relationships and assessment of progress in this respect.
3. Demonstration of observation of the normal and recognition of deviation from the normal.
4. Some indication of methods of communication used and understanding of approach needed, and any action taken.

5. Identification of progress in developing health visiting skills.
6. An objective appraisal of achievements and remaining areas of need.

Some recognition of the link between the neighbourhood study and health visiting studies is also useful.

The health visiting studies are used as a basis for the Part II examination allowing for opportunity to enlarge upon any area or make a more critical appraisal of the work done, in retrospect.

Fieldwork experience 'The provision of good fieldwork training is the cornerstone of all professional education.' This statement in the Council's Fifth Report (CETHV 1975) is an indication of the importance attached to the placement of the student with a field-work teacher during the academic year of her course. Generally one or two students are attached to one fieldwork teacher, although some recent experiments have been established attaching students to groups of fieldwork teachers to provide a more comprehensive and coordinated form of experience. It was concluded that a great deal more research needed to be carried out in this area.

The fieldwork teacher is a qualified and experienced health visitor who has completed a special course to prepare her for this additional role. She carries a caseload of her own and provides the student with opportunities for observation and development and extension of her skills in health visiting (CETHV 1974). At first the student accompanies the fieldwork teacher on visits, learning through observation of professional skills, discussing and analysing after the visit is over. The student is constantly learning how to formulate objectives and to assess situations and decide on methods of communication and courses of action, in the real-life situation. Once confidence is gained the student assumes some responsibility for visiting, particularly with the families she is to study. Opportunities are available to plan work and discuss progress with the fieldwork teacher who is available for reference and consultation whenever necessary.

As well as acquiring health visiting skills in practice, the student has the opportunity to reinforce knowledge gained in the classroom, to meet with and observe other professionals at work, to gain experience in health education, and to learn about the mobilization of services available.

The fieldwork teacher liaises directly with the health visitor tutor when required and takes a personal interest in the student's progress on the course. Her role is set out quite clearly in the Council's leaflet (1974), which students would do well to read.

The period of supervised practice following the Part I exam allows the student to carry a small caseload and work under the guidance of a senior health visitor who is available for consultation. This period gives an opportunity for the consolidation of skills and to gain confidence in practice leading up to the second part of the examination.

EVALUATION OF THE HEALTH VISITORS COURSE

At the time of writing, very little work has been done on evaluating the health visitor's course as a successful method of preparing students for the role of the health visitor. This is partly due to the fact that as yet there is a lack of adequate criteria available for assessment of skills and evaluation of performance, and there is no clearly defined profile of health visiting as a role. In addition to this it presents an enormous task to attempt to assess the value of a course of this kind because there are so many variables involved, which are constantly changing.

One small study carried out by Loveland (1971) on the health visitor's course at Surrey University demonstrated that the students prepared on that particular course appeared to be adequately prepared for the work they were required to do in urban and country areas. In addition the Council itself carried out a small survey on the range of experience available for health visitor students and found that in the main students were appreciative of the contribution made by fieldwork teachers.

A study by Dingwall (1976) presented observations made during a one-year study of health visitor students based on a particular school, with fieldwork in different kinds of area. Naturalistic research methods were used which involved detailed observation of events as they occurred. While this research has thrown up some interesting questions for further investigation, it must be remembered that it only involved one school and therefore cannot be assumed typical of all courses. Of necessity, therefore, there are certain gaps in the observations made where situations involved confidentiality and this missing component could be a very important aspect of training.

It is difficult to draw any conclusions which help in actual evaluation of courses from studies of this kind. One interesting observation emerges related to the acceptance by the students of the 'credibility' of the experts in certain fields, such as their health visitor tutors or medical lecturers, and the difficulties some experienced in accepting lecturers from some other disciplines. Questions were raised about certain assumptions held by students and this is understandable when it is remembered that the course offers an educational experience which is likely to include a critical analysis of one's previous ideas and attitudes.

One other area that this research seems to highlight is the strength of the tutors' influence and the nature of the course in the socializing process of producing a professional worker. Dingwall notes that innovatory thinking in schools of health visiting can have relatively little impact on health visiting practice without corresponding reforms in work situations, and this emphasizes the need for colleges to be more involved with in-service training. While the constraints imposed by the 'public' image of the nurse/health visitor and the structure in which she works have already been noted as important, it is also encouraging to read Anderson's comment (1973) that 'where role discrepancies are identified nursing leaders can help decide what direction nursing should take and what changes can be made. . .'. Lamond's discussion (1974) on Moore's theory (1969) is also of interest in this context and Lamond noted the importance of a strong degree of consensus and 'consistently interpreted value system' within a profession to maintain internal control of its own destiny.

While these studies do not give us any firm answers about the value of our present system of training and education, they do indicate the strength and importance of the role of the tutor and fieldwork teachers and the influences of the course in terms of transmitting and maintaining the values and the objectives of health visiting as a profession.

CURRENT TRENDS IN COUNCIL'S ACTIVITIES

Other interesting details of the formative years of the Council's growth can be found in a personal account by the Council's first Director (Wilkie 1979). The work of the Council in more recent years has included a focus on several major areas of current professional interest, such as the preparation of courses for school nurses, and the European situation, and accounts of these and other activities can be found in the Quarterly Bulletins published by the Council.

A Report from a working party set up to look at the criteria for the nature of the health visitors course, with a view to producing guidelines for a new syllabus, put forward comment on content and proposals for a new course curriculum and structure in 1982, for consideration.

The Council is also taking steps to establish its research remit and has shown its support for the concept of further education for health visitors in a Report which outlines the facilities available for continuing education (CETHV 1981). Currently, the officers of the Council are very closely involved with the setting up of the new machinery, under the new statutory bodies, and the next few years will see many changes in the administrative structures.

The remainder of this section will be concerned with discussion and interpretation of various aspects of the health visitors syllabus. It should be remembered that in no way do these chapters offer a potted version of the subjects under review, but the aim is to help students understand the relevance of the studies and to find for themselves ways in which they can interpret the theoretical approaches offered. It is also hoped that some assistance may be found for students meeting problematic areas.

Again, it is stressed that for certain aspects of the course, knowledge is constantly changing and these areas have been deliberately omitted, but students may find references to appropriate journals helpful. Emphasis has been placed on a general approach to major areas of study in a way that may help students to gain a comprehensive appreciation of the course as a whole and to make the most of what can be a challenging and exciting year of study.

SUMMARY

This chapter reviews the work of the Council in its earlier years, and describes its role in setting up the current pattern of education for health visitors. The course structure is then outlined, with detailed discussion on various aspects of the course, to assist students in their approach to study and in their general appreciation of the whole pattern of training. The chapter concludes with reference to fieldwork, and to the current role of the Council in continuing education and planning for the future.

REFERENCES

Anderson, E.R. (1973) *The Role of the Nurse*, p. 10. RCN Research Project. London: Royal College of Nursing.

Association of Integrated and Degree Courses in Nursing (1975) *Report on Third Annual Conference* (Unpublished report).

Bernstein, B.B. (1970) Education cannot compensate for society. *New Society*, *38* (26 February).

Chapman, C. (1974) Nurse education. *Nursing Times*, *70*, 18, p. 680 (2 May).

Council for the Education and Training of Health Visitors (CETHV) (1965) *Background to the Syllabus of Training*. London.

CETHV (1966) *First Report 1962–1964*. London.

CETHV (1967a) *Third Report*. London.

CETHV (1967b) *The Function of the Health Visitor*. London.

CETHV (1969) *Fourth Report. The Health Visitor, her Function and its Implications for Training*. London.

CETHV (1970) *Guidelines for Health Visiting Studies*. London.

CETHV (1972) *Guide to the Syllabus of Training*. London.

CETHV (1973) *The Health Visitor, Functions and Implications for Training*. London.

CETHV (1974) *The Role of the Fieldwork Teacher*. London. *

CETHV (1975) *Fifth Report 1969–1974*. London.

CETHV (1981) *Report on Continuing Education for Health Visitors*. London.

CETHV (1982) *Report of the Working Party on Curriculum Development*, Part II. London.

Dingwall, R. (1976) The social organisation of health visitor training. *Nursing Times*, *72*, 7, 8, 9 and 10 (19 and 26 February, 4 and 11 March). Occasional Papers.

HMSO (1972) *The Report of the Committee on Nursing*. Cmnd. 5115. London. *

Kerr, M. (1958) *The People of Ship Street*. London: Routledge & Kegan Paul.

Lamond, N. (1974) *Becoming a Nurse*, pp. 3–4. RCN Research Series. London: Royal College of Nursing.

Loveland, M.K. (1971) The work of health visitors in an urban and country area. *Nursing Times*, *67*, 22 (3 June).

McFarlane, J.K. (1970) Legacy for the seventies. *Nursing Times*, *66*, 3 (15 January).

Moore, W.E. (1969) Occupation and socialization. In: *Handbook of Socialization: Theory and Research*, ed. D.A. Goslin. Chicago: Rand McNally.

Rosser, C. & Harris, C. (1965) *The Family and Social Change*. London: Routledge & Kegan Paul.

Standing Conference of Health Visitor Training Centres (1971) *The Role of Health Visitor Tutors* (Unpublished survey).

Wilkie, E.E. (1979) *The History of the Council for the Education and Training of Health Visitors*. London: CETHV.

FURTHER READING
The books in the reference list marked with an asterisk are also useful for more general reading.

Borger, R. & Seaborne, A.E.M. (1966) *The Psychology of Learning*. Harmondsworth: Penguin.

Butterworth, E. & Weir, D. (1970) *The Sociology of Modern Britain*, pp. 169–177. London: Fontana.

Clark, J. & Henderson, J. (1983) *Community Health*. Edinburgh: Churchill Livingstone.

Hunter, I.M.L. (1957) *Memory, Fact and Fallacy*. Harmondsworth: Penguin.

James, D. (1967) *A Student's Guide to Efficient Study*. London: Pergamon.

Journals
Nursing Times
Nursing Mirror
Health Visitor
Health Visitor and Midwife
CETHV Quarterly Bulletin, Education and Training Council Information

4. Psychological Insights

Susan Freeman

There is a need for a grounding in psychological theory as a background to health visiting practice. Health visiting has always been a notoriously difficult area to define, because as a profession it has constantly needed to adapt to the changing health needs of the community. However, there would seem little doubt that the basic aims of the job have remained much as they always were in prevention of ill-health and promotion of health (Chapter 1).

Caplan has set out a definition of prevention which can serve as a useful yardstick against which to consider health visiting activities. He divides prevention into three categories (Caplan 1961).

1. Primary prevention which is action designed to prevent the occurrence of a problem, e.g. immunization.
2. Secondary prevention, i.e. the early detection of illness or deviation from normal where treatment may cure or control, e.g. routine developmental assessment of young children.
3. Tertiary prevention—aftercare concerned with containing and alleviating an established condition, e.g. helping an individual and family adjust to illness or incapacity (see p. 38).

Practically all proper health visiting activities should fall into one or other of these categories, but one could argue that to be truly preventive one should aim for the 'primary' area, which includes basic health education. In order to prevent ill-health, the health visitor attempts to use health education as a means of influencing people to change from 'unhealthy' to 'healthy' behaviour. She uses direct teaching of subjects relevant to mental or physical health, both in groups and on a one-to-one basis. She also tries to influence behaviour indirectly by the use of counselling techniques, in order to encourage individuals to solve their own problems and reach their own decisions.

Therefore, it is essential that the skills used in health visiting should be based on a sound knowledge of normal and abnormal behaviour. A few gifted people have that enviable knowledge of 'what makes people tick' by experience of a lifetime of working with others, but this must inevitably involve trial and error learning in an area where mistakes cannot easily be rectified. This method of learning may have a certain limited application, but it does not build up a professional body of knowledge, and is almost impossible to teach to others. For these reasons basic psychology is used as just one of the subjects to be learned by the health visitor needing to develop expertise in preventive health education.

A study of the behavioural sciences and in particular of certain branches of psychology contributes to many aspects of the health visitor's work. Learning theory, for example, helps in observing the normal phases of a child's progress, and with her knowledge of developmental psychology, enables her to assist parents to be supportive and accepting of their children during the various stages of growth. Social psychology offers a basis for understanding human behaviour and social interaction within groups of all kinds, and brings insights which assist in establishing human relationships.

Developmental psychology is perhaps the most relevant aspect, giving a basis for understanding the child's needs for emotional growth during the formative years. The health visitor is in a highly privileged position here, having access to families and being able to assist in this crucial period. Insights thus gained into human behaviour also help in many crisis situations, such as handicap, bereavement or sudden change, which can occur in any family.

Educational psychology and communication theories contribute to the understanding of the growth of skills in health education. Thus all these aspects of psychology provide a useful theoretical basis—sometimes the theories are conflicting and confusing to a new student unable to grasp their relevance, but with experience and the guidance of tutors and field staff it will emerge that these theories provide a foundation for insight and understanding rather than a prescription for action.

A potted psychology course would not be appropriate in a chapter such as this, but some instances of how psychological theory relates to the health visitor's work may encourage the reader to understand its importance and perhaps to reappraise background knowledge. It is so easy when coping with day-to-day problems to forget to up-date one's own knowledge of recent findings. Psychology is a new science and owing to the difficulties involved in studying human behaviour in its 'natural' setting, research projects inevitably take a long time to complete. The multiplicity of human situations has meant that there has also been a tendency to divide the science into different disciplines, so that there are experts working in such varied fields as clinical, developmental, social, experimental, industrial and educational psychology.

Some examples from learning theory For instance, two of the men most responsible for popularizing the science of psychology were Sigmund Freud and Ivan Pavlov and yet their fields of study were completely different. Freud pioneered the study of personality and founded psychoanalysis (Stafford-Clark 1967). He emphasized the importance of the *libido* (sexual drive) in our actions, and considered that gratification or frustration of this energy source determined eventual behaviour. Others working in the same field usually placed the emphasis on different aspects of the personality. Adler felt the most important need was a feeling of superiority; Fromm stressed avoidance of insecurity (Brown 1961). G.W. Allport, on the other hand, began the study of personality *traits*, which he considered were partly inherited and partly moulded by the environment (Allport 1937). More recently, psychologists have attempted to formulate personality inventories to isolate these traits and measure one personality against another. Eysenck, for example, considers that each individual can be tested to assess levels of stability/instability and extraversion/introversion to give a characteristic profile for comparison with others (Eysenck 1947). Cattell (1950) attempts a similar task, but with 16 or more traits. These theories, however, are still somewhat controversial, since there is a distinct danger of *stereotyping* people into groups, rather than emphasizing each person's uniqueness.

The other famous pioneer, Ivan Pavlov, worked mainly on the psychology of learning. His original work forms part of a whole school of thought in educational psychology called the *Associationists*. This group contends that all learning is a habit, formed after responding to a stimulus (Foss 1966).

Pavlov and, later, Thorndike and Skinner based most of their theories on animal experimentation. Pavlov used dogs to demonstrate his famous *conditioned response* to different signals. He noticed that when food was offered to the animal it salivated before taking food into its mouth, showing that the sight as well as the taste of the food had produced the response. He then rang a bell or turned on a light just before the food was produced and the animal soon learned to associate the light or bell with food. Pavlov was then able to demonstrate the salivating response to the bell or light alone. By *reinforcing* the stimulus with a reward, a substitution had been made and the same response was made to both stimuli. Thorndike and Skinner followed up Pavlov's work by studying *operant conditioning* or *trial and error learning* in animals. They placed the cat or rat in a situation where random activities eventually produced a reward. For instance, the animal would be placed in a box with a lever which when pressed delivered food. Eventually the animal pressed the lever by accident, and it was found that the length of time taken to release the food gradually became shorter as the animal learned to repeat the activity which had produced the reward (Borger & Seaborne 1966; Foss 1966).

These original experiments have led to further work on *shaping* of behaviour, where specific behaviour patterns are desired. By rewarding the desired response and ignoring all others, animals have been taught quite complicated activities.

The other main school of learning psychologists is known as the Gestalt (or whole) school (Ellis 1938). Psychologists of this school feel that animals or people prefer to see problems in organized relationships and attempt to understand the solution rather than hoping to hit upon the answer by trial and error. Wolfgang Kohler (1957) used chimpanzees to substantiate the Gestalt theory. He placed them in situations where food was available but the way to obtain it was not immediately obvious. For example, a piece of fruit was positioned behind bars out of reach of the chimpanzee, a couple of long sticks slightly nearer and a short stick near enough to pick up. At first, the animal tried to reach the fruit with the short stick, but when that failed he spent some time gazing at the problem. Eventually he took the small stick and used it to manoeuvre the longest stick towards him with which he obtained the fruit. Once he had decided upon the solution, the activity was performed as a continuous whole. This ability to see solutions to problems is known as *insight* and if the solution comes as a flash of inspiration it has been called the 'aha' experience.

To try to put some psychological concepts into perspective we will imagine how they apply to some of the everyday situations encountered by the health visitor.

PSYCHOLOGY AND HEALTH VISITING

Starting a New Job

All of us at some time in our lives have had to start a new job, and our thoughts have inevitably tended to centre upon our own feelings and anxieties in unfamiliar surroundings. But how many of us really consider the impact of a stranger on a working group? Many health visitors in the past have worked largely in isolation and the problems of integrating themselves into a team of workers have not really arisen. Now, however, the trend is towards health care as a team effort and the health visitor may find she has to apply the group psychology she has learned in theory, in order to understand the best way of being accepted into her new team.

It is useful to consider the concepts which might be useful to her. She should, perhaps, remember that she is entering a secondary group where she will be seen, especially at first, largely in terms of her professional capabilities. She will be judged by the amount of expertise she brings to her *role* as a health visitor within that group, unlike her *primary* group (family, close friends) where personal qualities tend to assume greater importance. Individual idiosyncracies, such as unpunctuality or scruffiness, may be frowned upon within the secondary group, where her role is seen to include good time-keeping and neatness, whereas they may be treated with tolerant amusement within her primary group. This is not to say, of course, that members of the secondary group may not eventually be included in the primary group, but this usually occurs only after information of a more personal nature has been exchanged.

It is also useful to remember that, as a rule, a newcomer to a group starts at the bottom of the *status* ladder and has to work his way up by fulfilling his role in an accepted way. He may of course, possess a certain amount of status already by virtue of his known qualifications or previous experience, but there is still likely to be some wariness amongst his colleagues until he has proved his worth.

It is also important that the *norms* of accepted behaviour in the group should not be violated too soon by the newcomer. In an already established group the bounds of behaviour, such as the use of first names, tend to be fairly clearly defined and a newcomer overstepping these bounds is rapidly corrected or rejected. One might argue that norms of which one disapproved should be commented upon, but if, for example, a new health visitor were to immediately pronounce her disapproval of the smoke-filled atmosphere in the office, before establishing a certain status within the group, she would be likely to alienate herself from her fellow workers, no matter how justifiable her complaint. Once she has been accepted as a worthy member of the group, her opinions are more likely to be accepted (Merei 1949).

Being able to balance the need for unity of the group, whilst maintaining her own individuality is an important attribute of the health visitor, since it will indicate her sensitivity to other people's feelings (empathy) and an ability to adjust her reactions accordingly.

In a group where all the individuals have this ability, morale is likely to be high, with good cooperation between members and an efficient *communications* system. Influences upon such a system are numerous, but it is sufficient to say that the language used must be clearly understood so that sender and receiver reduce misinterpretations to the minimum. In this way, frustrations are reduced and morale maintained. Further discussion on groups and communications can be found in Chapter 11, in the context of group work and health education.

Organization of Work

The health visitor is a practitioner in her own right, and is expected to organize her work in such a way as to reconcile the demands of her training and the constraints placed upon her by limitations such as accommodation, size of practice population or available ancillary help.

She will presumably have formulated a *concept* (generalized group of ideas) of 'health visiting' in her mind during her training and will try to avoid activities which conflict with it. She may, however, encounter situations which do not entirely concur with the image of a health visitor which she has built up in her mind and the concept will have to be adapted with experience.

If she is unable to fulfil the obligations of the job as she sees them, because of her own shortcomings or influences beyond her control, she may find she cannot gain *job satisfaction* and will therefore experience *role strain*. The health visitor should remind herself during the course of her work that many of the physical or mental ills exhibited by her clients may be aggravated by role strain. Many of them are having to endure boring or uncongenial work simply for the sake of a wage packet at the end of the week, or are housewives with no outside interests who find domesticity unstimulating.

The health visitor has, one assumes, displayed qualities which should enable her to gain satisfaction from her job. During her training she is expected to demonstrate her ability to form good relationships with clients and colleagues, to have a good command of language and the written word, and to be sufficiently intelligent to be able to apply her previous knowledge to problems which might confront her.

A health visitor who is unable to put herself into other people's shoes and understand how they feel about everyday occurrences will find the job impossible, no matter how extensive her theoretical psychological knowledge. She will probably spend most of her working day in a state of latent annoyance at the inability of her clients to solve problems which to her appear mere trifles, and their perverseness at not accepting the readymade solutions with which she presents them.

She may find that the same feelings surface in her dealings with her colleagues if she has not used her health visitor training to examine her own motives and attitudes and to constantly question her own actions.

We have already mentioned how people are thought to prefer solving problems by seeing them as a whole (Ellis 1938), and how the chimpanzee appeared to be using insight to overcome his difficulty (Kohler 1957). But why should the chimpanzee, rather than say, the pigeon, be able to use such a technique? Is it because he is more intelligent? As soon as the word intelligence is used we find difficulty in defining what is meant by the word. The only way it appears to be possible to assess intelligence is by testing the reasoning ability of the individual, or in other words, the ability to see relationships between sets of information to solve problems. In fact the whole area of intelligence assessment is a contentious one in which many aspects of bias need to be eliminated. Many tests used in the early days were distinctly biased towards good verbal ability, which does not necessarily equate with intelligence. For this reason it was found that those first tests favoured children from 'middle-class' homes where books and language were more extensively used.

A parallel can be drawn with the health visitor about to decide how to tackle the problems confronting her in her first job. Although many of the situations she encounters will be new to her, she will have her nursing and health visitor training to help her to reason a solution to each problem as it arises. If, however, one were to confront someone from a completely different discipline, such as a mathematician or a linguist, with the same problems, one could not expect either of them to achieve the same results, since their background, experience and language would be of little help to them (Borger & Seaborne 1966).

Home Visiting

A large and important part of the health visitor's day is taken up with home visiting. She may be helping a young mother to cope with a new baby, discussing the development of the pre-school child, following up a school child with learning difficulties, listening to a mentally disturbed adult, or assessing the health of an old person, but whatever activity she happens to be engaged in, she will need to recognize the uniqueness of each individual *personality*, and the influences which have affected its development. The word personality is used to mean all the various characteristics such as sociability, generosity, and aggressiveness which have formed as the person has matured.

The presence of these characteristics is due to two general areas of influence upon the individual, namely, heredity and environment. There has been much speculation amongst psychologists as to which is the more important—some arguing firmly for heredity as the overriding influence and others the converse—but the truth probably lies somewhere between the two (James 1968). As long as the health visitor is aware of these influences, she can help to promote an understanding of how personality develops. There is little she can do to ameliorate the effects of heredity upon personality, since genetic counselling is still in its infancy and concentrates mainly on preventing such detectable chromosomal abnormalities as Down's syndrome.

However, she can hope to educate parents about the importance of environmental influences upon the development of young children. Many of the parents with whom she works will not have escaped physical or emotional deprivation in childhood and may well be in danger of repeating the pattern with their own children. If so it is vital that these parents be given extra help to understand the effect of the home background upon the child's personality.

The health visitor's role in the formative years The significance of influences in the formative years has long been recognized by health visitors who appreciate their unique position as family visitor at this crucial time. There is now, however, an increasing awareness of current research emerging on the effects of intrauterine influences on the fetus during pregnancy and the effects of birth trauma. The work of Janov (1977) and Lake (1982) recognizes what is known as the maternal–fetal distress syndrome, and that acute anxiety in the mother, for example, can predispose to anxiety neuroses in later years. Some find the evidence on birth trauma somewhat more convincing as it begins to accumulate, although much of this work arouses controversy as yet (Segal & Yaharaes 1981). It does, however, emphasize the importance of the health visitor's role in preventive aspects, in terms of being available to expectant mothers to assist in alleviating anxiety where possible and to help to promote a positive attitude to birth. In addition, the knowledge that there has been a traumatic birth can help in the management of the infant in the early days, particularly where the baby cries incessantly (Verney & Kelly 1982).

More widely recognized is the accumulated evidence concerning mother–child relationships. Much of Bowlby's early work (1972) on deprivation was misinterpreted, but recent studies still support his central themes, although Rutter (1981), who explores their validity, questions their value. The work of Winnicott (see Davis & Wallbridge 1982) and others (e.g. Argyle 1973) tends to indicate that these early experiences may have far-reaching effects, which can be seen in disturbed children and adults. Of particular interest to health visitors is Winnicott's theory of the un-integrated child, as he emphasizes the importance of holding the infant in early days, and of the 'good-enough mother'. Harlow's work (1961) also highlights the significance of the infant–mother bonding process, while other studies bring attention to the value of tactile and visual contact in early days.

A health visitor could find a frustrating situation, where an infant is expressing important needs, crying incessantly, vomiting or failing to thrive, but where the mother herself is too disturbed or deprived to meet the needs, even with guidance and support. It is essential then to secure the help and understanding of others in the family where possible—particularly the father—to help in a critical period. Distress signals from the baby or mother are vital at this time and the health visitor can be alert to potential problems in her preventive role.

However controversial the evidence, or conflicting the theories in this area of psychology, the importance of early relationships cannot be ignored, and some writers are beginning to think it has some relevance in terms of present-day violence among young people.

A particularly interesting theory amongst psychologists studying young children is the concept of *readiness*. It states that at certain points as the child matures it is ready to achieve new skills. For instance, it is not ready to walk until around one year old, when its muscles and nervous system are sufficiently well developed. Similarly, bladder control is not gained until towards the end of the second year. According to psychologists, the same concept can be applied to more intellectual skills such as reading and writing, but in addition it has been stated that if these points of readiness are missed and the skills which should have been learned are not acquired, then they are never properly attained later on. The last is a point to be argued, but there is no doubt that if a skill such as reading is not learned at around the mental age of seven (chronological age may be misleading) it becomes a much harder task if tackled later in life (James 1968; see also Chapter 9).

In addition, emotional needs such as receiving love and affection must be satisfied from the beginning, or the reciprocal ability in the child will not develop. The child who has been deprived of love may well reach adulthood unable to maintain a stable, loving relationship with another human being. There is also the danger of course of the mother–child relationship being interrupted by a separation such as admission to hospital of either mother or child. In this case, even where the child has received constant love and affection, if separation occurs during the critical early years, short- or long-term damage may be done to his emotional development (Sears et al. 1966).

We have emphasized the importance of the environment upon the child's development because it is the area where the health visitor is most likely to have some influence, but she should not forget to consider the possibility of hereditary factors on personality. Such simple attributes as physical stature, colour of skin, or a facial birthmark may have a distinct bearing on the way the individual sees himself fitting into society and therefore how his personality is shaped. It is difficult to say whether differences of temperament such as docility or aggressiveness are purely inherited, or are also the result of attitudes copied from parents, but physical variations such as a slightly under- or overactive thyroid or a high or low basal metabolic rate can affect the way we act, and may well be familial traits.

The health visitor will spend a large proportion of her visiting time with mothers and pre-school age children. This would seem to be the proper balance, since neglect of these early years can, as has been mentioned, have long-lasting detrimental effects and no amount of work later on can redress the balance. She must be the expert within the primary health care team, on normal child development, and should understand the ways in which it can be impaired.

Socialization Argyle (1973) points out that human beings are reared in families on which they are heavily dependent and from which they learn their social behaviour. He points out that the majority of the most pressing social problems are concerned with human relationships, and connected with a breakdown in communications and interaction.

Socialization is therefore a vital aspect of the developing relationships within the family. By example the child learns how to live in harmony with other people, starting with his parents and siblings. Gradually his sphere of experience widens and if the attitudes and behaviour of his parents have been consistent and in tune with the society in which they live, he should be able to integrate reasonably smoothly into his ever-widening circle of acquaintances. Problems may arise if the initial socializing process carried out by his parents is at variance with his immediate social group. If for instance his parents attempt to instil into him middle-class values and attitudes when he lives in a working-class area and mixes with the children of working-class parents, he is likely to find difficulty in gaining acceptance amongst both children and parents. As he gets older his desire to be accepted within the group will strengthen and he will probably either adapt his behaviour and speech to conform to the group, or withdraw from it. Many mothers become extremely upset when they find their well-brought-up little boy or girl has adopted inappropriate attitudes or language. If, however, parents understand the reasons for the behaviour there is a chance that they will be more able to accept it. Many resourceful children develop two almost distinct forms of behaviour—one for home and one for their friends—but too much of a division may cause a conflict of loyalties in the child and problems may result.

It is relevant at this point to refer back to the concept of readiness which was mentioned earlier, since the health visitor frequently uses this concept to help parents to adjust their expectations of the child. Some parents, especially those who are anxious that their child should 'do well', begin to expect too much of him, to the detriment of his personality development. It is perfectly laudable for parents to encourage a child in whatever skill he might be attempting to acquire, but if they constantly urge him to do things for which he is not ready (such as drawing a house before learning to scribble) his sense of achievement when he does eventually master these activities will have been stifled by his own frustration and his parents' disappointment at the length of time he spends learning one task. It may mean that because he can never please his parents he stops trying altogether or, conversely, spends all his time working towards his next goal and never enjoying the task itself.

An important aspect of the socialization process is that of conscience formation. As with most areas of psychological research, theories are mostly tentative, due to the lack of empirical evidence. However, studies seem to indicate that different methods of child-rearing can affect the strength of the self-critical faculty in the child (Sears et al. 1966; Secord & Backman 1966).

The most important factor appears to be the way that the parents discipline the child. Forms of punishment such as physical or verbal assault tend to be less effective than methods like explaining or verbal disapproval at producing a high level of self-control in the child. The former method concentrates the child's thoughts on external factors stemming from his behaviour (such as punishment) whereas the latter focuses on his own intentions and the general principles of conduct relevant to his behaviour. His feelings of self-criticism are unpleasant and he is likely to alter his behaviour in order to feel better, assuming that he is willing to sacrifice the 'rewards' of the original action (e.g. stealing).

The development of high moral standards and behaviour in an individual, as opposed to the absence of one or both factors, appears from recent work to depend on good cognitive and emotional support of the child by the parents. In other words, the child is encouraged to understand the consequences of his own actions and to develop his capacity for self-judgement, while the parents resist the temptation to use love-withdrawal as a means of manipulating the child's behaviour. Secord and Backman (1966) conclude that conscience formation is a joint function of the development of a warm relationship with a parent and the use of love-oriented discipline.

The pioneer Jean Piaget felt that moral judgement in children is subject to distinct age differences. Since then Kohlberg (1963) has redefined these stages as follows.

Level I. Pre-moral level
1. Punishment and obedience orientation, i.e. obey rules to avoid punishment.
2. Naive instrumental hedonism, i.e. conform to obtain rewards and have favours returned.

Level II. Morality of conventional rule conformity
3. Good boy/girl morality of maintaining good relations and approval of others, i.e. conform to avoid disapproval and dislike by others.
4. Authority maintaining morality, i.e. conform to avoid censure by legitimate authority and the resulting guilt.

Level III. Morality of self-accepted moral principles
5. Morality of contract and democratically accepted law, i.e. conform to maintain the respect of the impartial spectator, judging in terms of community welfare.
6. Morality of individual principles of conscience, i.e. conform to avoid self-condemnation.

The role of play The health visitor is in an excellent position during the child's first few years to educate parents as to the milestones they should expect him to reach as he matures. She can advise them on suitable play materials and new experiences which he should be allowed to meet appropriate to his age.

Play has a significant part in the child's development, as it is during play he learns much about human relationships, roles and expectations. Through play he also develops his physical and intellectual skills, given appropriate materials, space and stimulation. Play has an additional value in its therapeutic function, and a discerning parent or health visitor may see a child working through his fears and apprehensions during his games. He can be reassured and encouraged once his fear has been expressed. The make-believe aspects of play allow the child to anticipate, through fantasy, some potentially frightening experiences, such as hospitalization, and so prepare himself (Rodin 1983). Play, of course, has an intrinsic value for its own sake in bringing sheer delight and pleasure to children and individuals of all ages (Kellner Pringle 1975).

The health visitor will, of course, be on the look-out for any child who does not appear to be progressing as he should, since some children may need channelling into special education or remedial therapy. However, she may be able to prevent a child from falling behind by being aware of those parents who tend to understimulate their children in order that they might be encouraged to widen their experiences both in and out of the home.

A moving account of an emotionally lost child who found himself can be found in *Dibs — In Search of Self*, a delightful story which can help students to appreciate the nature of emotional development and play therapy (Axline 1981).

The school child Although the health visitor's main sphere of influence tends to be in the age group of children under five, there is no doubt that a great deal of health education can be continued once the child reaches school age. A happy and stable pre-school period will have prepared him for the growing responsibilities of maturity and his home influence will continue to be the overriding factor in his social and psychological development. However, there are bound to be some problems with school or leisure activities which cause anxiety to parents, so the health visitor should not appear to be abandoning them as soon as the child reaches school age.

When the child first enters school, the health visitor may be the only person who has known him both at home and at school, and can be a reassuring sight in strange surroundings. If she maintains good relationships with teachers and works closely with school doctor and nurse, she can be a valuable link between school and home. Behaviour problems which seem inexplicable to the teacher can often be understood when discussed in confidence with someone who knows the home background. Many children become the victims of a vicious circle of deprivation at home and at school. If they belong to a family where little encouragement is given for their efforts, they are likely to seek attention at school. If this attention takes the form of disruptive behaviour, the teacher is less likely to give the extra encouragement needed by such children, since they will soon be classified in the 'tearaway' group with whom they can most readily identify.

The growing problem of illegitimacy means that an increasing proportion of mothers are young and inexperienced, with no idea of the psychological and social problems which rearing a child alone can present. The health visitor may be the only source of practical and psychological support for a particularly vulnerable group of mothers and children or for the one-parent family. She should also recognize that abortion is not necessarily less traumatic to a woman than giving birth to an illegitimate child. In many ways, a pregnancy gives time to think about the reasons why it occurred and how best to come to terms with the problems. Abortion, however, may be undertaken in haste with no real counselling for the girl or woman concerned. Doctors and psychologists have frequently stated that for some women abortion without counselling can be pointless, since the problem that caused the pregnancy in the first place has not been resolved. The difficulty may range from a simple ignorance of contraceptive methods, to an unconscious desire for a child to replace a lack of love in childhood, but whatever the reason, a sympathetic health visitor who understands the possible motives can act as an unbiased sounding-board to a girl who must make her own decision about her own and the baby's future.

Psychiatric and emotional problems Learning about the normal development of the personality means that abnormalities are easier to understand and the health visitor with a basic knowledge of psychiatry acquired during her nursing and health visiting training often finds mental illness or emotional disturbance less worrying when able to relate to the normal. It is unlikely that the health visitor would need to specialize in working with the mentally ill, as this would seem to be the prerogative of the psychiatric community nurse and social worker. However, since such a large proportion of the population needs treatment for mental illness of some sort, or suffers from mild anxiety problems, it is inevitable that as a member of a primary health care team, clients with psychiatric difficulties will be referred to the health visitor. As with any other problematic area of work, the health visitor should be prepared to examine her own attitudes towards mental illness and, if necessary, to keep up to date with her knowledge. She can then help to counteract the fearful attitudes brought about by ignorance and enable her clients to understand some of the reasons for mental illness and the various treatments available. A large number of psychiatric disorders are thought to be due to physical malfunction of some kind and although much of the research along these lines is not conclusive, it may help relatives to accept the illness better if the difficult behaviour which seems to be directed at them can be seen as a symptom of illness as genuine as high blood pressure or temperature.

Once stress and strain are accepted as just another cause of illness, clients may be more willing to talk about their problems—and possibly reach some solution—rather than display physical symptoms of an underlying psychological cause.

The aged Probably the second largest age group with whom the health visitor works is that of over-retirement age. Her visits to the elderly will usually include a general assessment of physical and mental health, in order to help prevent deterioration in the quality of life, by helping to maintain mobility, social contact and nutrition for example. Study of the psychological development of childhood and early adulthood will have concentrated mainly upon the effects of maturation on the personality, but once into middle and old age the most noticeable changes will be those wrought by ageing rather than growth.

The limitations placed upon the individual by increasing age may themselves be the cause of frustration and consequent personality distortion. Lapses of memory and some slowing down of the learning processes are just examples of the mental deterioration that follows degeneration of nerve cells. The more obvious physical manifestations of age such as loss of muscle power, visual acuity and hearing all contribute to the individual's declining powers, and considerable adjustments need to be made in the way he sees his role in society. If life's achievements do not seem to compensate for the loss, these adjustments may be difficult to make.

Some elderly people may not recognize the extent to which their powers have deteriorated or attempt to ignore their failing sight or lack of mobility by trying to do just as much as they always did. The health visitor should be able to recognize those psychological manifestations of ageing, such as failure of recent memory, which must be accepted and which need practical aids such as shopping lists, address books and diaries to cope with them. In contrast, she should also realize the existence of problems such as mental confusion which may only be the temporary results of poor fluid intake or chest infection, where high levels of circulating toxins or low oxygen supply to the brain can be completely reversed and the problem resolved. Narrowed arteries cannot be widened but at least the nutrients and gases circulating in the blood can be kept at their optimum level.

The importance of maintaining skills and abilities acquired in former years is perhaps worth mentioning at this point. In spite of all that has been said about failing powers, their significance can be minimal in the person who is willing to adapt his life-style to a certain extent, but does not assume that ageing inevitably means giving up all the pleasures of life. It is foolhardy to expect to be able to suddenly overtax a body or mind which has not been regularly exercised, but physical, sexual and intellectual abilities can all be enjoyed well into old age if preparation has been good.

When working with the elderly, the health visitor will realize the greater likelihood of crises such as the death of a loved one, severe illness, or loneliness occurring, and she should be on the look-out for newly emerging psychological problems. She should be particularly aware of the abnormal reactions which can distort normal occurrences such as bereavement. If she is aware of the normal grieving process including the feelings of numbness, guilt, and anger, she will be more able to assess the extent to which these emotions have become prolonged or excessive. Old people with little family support, whose partners have died, are particularly at risk of failing health and in fact many die themselves within a year of the loss.

The Clinic

Although the clinic should never be thought to be a substitute for the home visit, it can be a valuable means of maintaining contact with clients, especially now that working with general practitioners has presented so many more opportunities for health education in the middle and older age groups. Apart from the regular child health clinic where mothers can bring their children for medical checks, developmental assessment and general advice, many GP's surgeries are expanding to include enuretic, obesity, well-woman, coronary prevention and geriatric clinics, frequently run by the health visitor with medical support where necessary.

Inevitably the people who respond to invitations to attend such sessions cannot represent the whole of the population at risk, since they are the statistician's nightmare—the volunteers. However, if careful thought is given to the motives, anxieties, social and health problems of the target group, the clinic can be designed to meet their needs and elicit a good response. If they feel that the people running the clinic really care about them and if the clinic itself is relevant to them, they are more likely to make use of it. This is not to say of course that an immediate response should be expected, especially where a clinic depends upon the health visitor getting to know her clients and being able to show an interest in them individually.

At the child health clinic, for instance, it may be some time before a whole new generation of mothers recognize the counselling role that the health visitor takes in addition to her concern with the health of the child. As has been mentioned, a person's mental health has a vital bearing upon his or her general well-being, and although physical progress of the child must not be neglected, family relationships are almost more important to progress, and time should be given for mothers to discuss any problems that arise.

The health visitor should recognize the existence of counselling expertise and make efforts to develop her skills in listening and responding in such a way that clients can be encouraged towards their own decision-making and problem-solving. It is useless to present a client with a ready-made answer to a problem, until she has had the opportunity to see how it arose and what her alternative courses of action might be. Even when a direct opinion is sought it is sometimes better to find out what lines of thought prompted the question before responding. Here, the principles of counselling (see Chapter 8) will assist in developing skills.

Apart from the one-to-one consultation, the clinic can also form a valuable source of social contact. The health visitor will frequently recognize the symptoms of social isolation in clients of all ages, but particularly amongst mothers of young children and the elderly who are confined to the house for large parts of the day. Informal contact with others in similar circumstances can often serve to prevent recourse to drugs to alleviate depression. New mothers are particularly at risk of postnatal depression if isolation is an added factor, and the health visitor who gets to know her clients is able to recognize changes in behaviour which might indicate psychological problems. Once again, one of her most important roles is permeating knowledge about health and removing fear of the unknown.

Teaching
Although placed under a separate heading, the division is a somewhat arbitrary one, since teaching is an integral part of health education. However, it is useful to consider where group teaching in particular can be of value and what learning principles are involved (see Chapter 11).

Instances of the health education needs of young people have been mentioned, but of course many health visitors find health education in schools particularly rewarding and much valuable work can be done to prepare the parents of the future for some of the decisions they will have to make. Knowledge about conception, pregnancy, childbirth, contraception, child development and family life all helps young people to make informed decisions about their future, instead of learning by trial and all too frequent error.

Group teaching can often be extremely valuable in the surgery or clinic when a topic of interest to several people, such as 'Problems of the two-year-old' or 'Combating obesity', can be covered more effectively. In addition to the health visitor's time being used more efficiently, the contact and support of members of a group can be useful educationally as well as socially. It has been shown that changes in behaviour are more likely to take place if the decision to make the change is taken by a group rather than by the individual alone. If the desired change is one which will prove difficult, such as a dietary revolution for the obese, the pressures of the group are likely to be a useful addition to variable self-discipline (Lewin 1947).

Learning can be defined as a relatively permanent change in behaviour that occurs as the result of practice. By understanding the processes which are taking place in the learning situation, the teacher is more able to produce the change in behaviour that is desired. There are bound to be variations in the teacher and the subject which affect the amount of learning that takes place. The teacher's personality, expertise, enthusiasm for her subject, and its presentation all have a great bearing on the effectiveness of the lesson, but assuming these factors have all been properly dealt with, what aspects of the learner will affect what learning actually takes place?

No matter how expert the teacher, there are occasions when very little change in behaviour is seen. She may have spent hours deciding on the teaching method to use and becoming expert in her subject, but have forgotten to consider the *motivation* of the learners. There is little point in spending valuable preparation and teaching time on a subject that none of the learners feels is relevant to him. Even if the teacher is absolutely certain of its value to them, she has still got to convince them of the fact, perhaps by having a preliminary discussion on why that particular subject is being taught, before launching straight into the lesson. It is much easier to understand the motives of the members of a group if time is spent getting to know them. If, for instance, one were teaching about the effects of cigarette smoking, it may be necessary to take a completely different approach to the subject with different age groups. A group of middle-aged men may be very susceptible to facts about their increased risk of heart disease and bronchitis, whereas teenagers may be swayed more by the financial constraints it places upon them.

So, let us now assume that the group can see the importance of the subject and is keen to learn. What other factors must we consider? The problem of defining intelligence has already been mentioned, and it is not sufficient to say that people who are more intelligent learn better, since there are so many different processes involved. Memory, concentration, attention, speed of perception, word fluency, and reasoning all vary with intelligence, so there is little doubt that the teaching method will need to be adapted to suit different groups.

Perception is the process by which stimuli from our surroundings are formed by the brain into pictures, including not only what we see, but what we hear, feel, smell, and taste. If one could imagine two people in exactly the same circumstances, receiving the same stimuli from their environment, one would expect that the *percept* (or picture) that each forms in his brain would be identical. In fact the form these percepts take will depend on variations within the individual. Eyesight and hearing will affect the clarity of the picture, but past experience will also dictate which of the numerous signals to accept or reject. For instance, a country dweller unused to noisy traffic and brightly lit shop windows would find great difficulty in deciding which of the flood of strange stimuli were important, whereas the city dweller would selectively ignore most of them, unless something was brought to his *attention*. This ability of the brain to selectively reject some stimuli is particularly important for the teacher to remember, since a lesson conducted in one boring tone of voice, with no change of activity may cause the learner's attention to wander. This is even more likely if the learner is of low intelligence and motivation. Even the most intelligent learner finds *concentration* difficult for more than 20 minutes at a stretch and may find much of the information is lost during short naps called *micro-sleeps*.

It has been shown that people remember more of a given set of information when it is perceived in short bursts rather than long sessions. In addition, a complete change of activity, or even better a short rest following each period of learning, will greatly improve the chances of the material being retained. It is useful for the teacher to realize that *memory* consists of several different characteristics. *Recognition* occurs when we are confronted with an object or situation which seems familiar to us. It is usually much easier to recognize a person we have met before than to *recall* everything about him when someone says, 'Do you remember Fred Bloggs?' (James 1968).

Some teachers are inclined to make their jobs more difficult by expecting their learners to be able to recall everything that is taught, when all that is needed is an ability to recognize a situation as familiar to be able to deal with it. It is also useful for students to realize that *relearning* is much easier than learning something new. Even if a student thinks he has completely forgotten something once learned, he will find the learning time reduced when he tackles the task a second time.

PSYCHOLOGY AND THE HEALTH VISITOR

This chapter would not be complete without some specific comment on the value of the study of psychology to the health visitor in understanding herself and her own personal reactions to her work and interaction with people. It is helpful to recognize that the health visitor too has her own needs, motives and attitudes. For example, Maslow's description of a hierarchy of human needs (Krech et al. 1962) can be useful in giving insights into one's own reactions to very simple things such as hunger and fatigue or to more complex situations such as status, prestige and job satisfaction. Understanding such situations is often the first step towards the solution of problems and many of these aspects of psychology are often included in management courses for senior personnel. Similarly, an awareness of the causes and effects of frustration, fear or anxiety may help the health visitor come to terms with any personal difficulties encountered in relationships with colleagues or clients. Once such reactions are understood and accepted within oneself it is more possible to help other people effectively. (See James 1968, Chapter 13 for a useful discussion on this topic.)

A chapter such as this can only hope to show a limited number of ways in which a knowledge of psychological theory can help the health visitor. But perhaps these few instances are enough to enable the health visitor to realize how difficult her job would be without a basis of psychology. So often, the things people say and do bear little resemblance to the real motives behind their actions and therefore it is vital that the health visitor has a professional and knowledgeable attitude towards the problems of human interaction which she will inevitably meet. She may occasionally be subject to bursts of aggression from unhappy and frustrated clients who have no one upon whom to vent their anger. By accepting such anger without resentment as an indication of the person's state of mind she may be privileged to help her client to come to terms with her problems. The concept of stress is currently of interest in our present day, and has implications for much family life and health, in adjusting to rapid social change in our society. Menzies' study (1970) on defence mechanisms in nurses is also an interesting psychological study which throws light on some personal attitudes students may find themselves examining in the course. Understanding the nature of baffling human behaviour is the first step towards improving relationships and relieving stress.

If she adds to all this her knowledge of how heredity, maturation and the environment affect the growth of each individual, the health visitor should be able to make a substantial contribution to health and happiness during the course of her work.

SUMMARY

In this chapter the reader is introduced to the relevance of the behavioural sciences to health visiting practice. Some theories and terminologies used are discussed as a preliminary to highlighting areas of practice where the theories are particularly relevant. The place and organization of work, the home visit and the clinic are used as focal points to show how theory can give a foundation for the acquisition of understanding and insight. The role of the health visitor in helping to establish emotional stability in family life is discussed and the need to lay the foundations for healthy happy living, and to assist in adjusting to social problems.

QUESTIONS FOR ESSAY OR DISCUSSION

1. What procedures may be used to assess the psychological development of a child from birth to the age of five years? Discuss their value.
2. Discuss some of the work done on attachment and separation in childhood. What implications does this have for the work of the health visitor?
3. Discuss the psychology of ageing. What implications does this have for the care of the aged in the community?
4. What is the significance of play in relation to the development of the young child? Discuss this in the context of your work as a health visitor.
5. 'Too much emphasis has been laid on maternal deprivation and its effects on socialization.' Discuss this statement.

6. Outline some of the theories of learning and discuss their relevance to your work as a health visitor.
7. Discuss some of the processes through which behaviour changes. Show how this can be applied to health visiting.
8. Outline the evidence on the relationships existing between social class and language development. How can the health visitor be of assistance where a child is disadvantaged in this respect?
9. 'Adolescence—a period of great turmoil and little security.' To what extent is this statement valid?
10. Discuss the value of an understanding of psychology in relation to health visiting practice.

REFERENCES

Allport, G.W. (1937) *Personality: A Psychological Interpretation*. London: Constable.

Argyle, M. (1973) *Social Interaction*. London: Tavistock.

Axline, Virginia (1981) *Dibs — In Search of Self*. Harmondsworth: Pelican.

Borger, R. & Seaborne, A.E.M. (1966) *The Psychology of Learning*, Chapter 4. Harmondsworth: Pelican.

Bowlby, J. (1972) *Attachment*. Harmondsworth: Pelican.

Brown, J.A.C. (1961) *Freud and the Post-Freudians*. Harmondsworth: Pelican.

Caplan, G. (1961) *An Approach to Community Mental Health*. London: Tavistock.

Cattell, R.B. (1950) *An Introduction to Personality Study*. London: Hutchinson.

Davis, M. & Wallbridge, D. (1982) *Boundary and Space — An Introduction to the Work of D.W. Winnicott*. Karnac.

Ellis, W.D. (1938) *A Source Book of Gestalt Psychology*. New York: Harcourt Brace.

Eysenck, H.J. (1947) *Dimensions of Personality*. London: Routledge & Kegan Paul.

Foss, B.M. (ed.) (1966) *New Horizons in Psychology*. Harmondsworth: Pelican.

Harlow, H.F. (1961) In: *Determinants of Infant Behaviour*, ed. B.M. Foss, Vol. 1. London: Methuen.

Janov, A.J. (1977) *The Feeling Child*. Tunbridge Wells: Abacus.

James, D. (1968) *Introduction to Psychology*, Chapter 13. London: Constable.

Kellner Pringle, M. (1975) *The Needs of Children*. London: Hutchinson.

Kohlberg, L. (1963) The development of children's orientations towards a moral code. *Vita Humana*, p. 6.

Kohler, W. (1957) *The Mentality of Apes*. Harmondsworth: Pelican.

Krech, D., Crutchfield, R.S. & Ballachey, E.L. (1962) *The Individual in Society*, Chapter 3, New York: McGraw-Hill.

Lake, F. (1982) *With Respect*, Chapter 7. London: Darton, Longman & Todd.

Lewin, K. (1947) Frontiers in group dynamics. *Human Relations*, *1*, 5.

Menzies, I. (1970) *The Functioning of Social Systems as a Defence against Anxiety*. London: Tavistock.

Merei, F. (1949) Group leadership and institutionalization. *Human Relations*, 2, 23.

Rodin, J. (1983) *Will this Hurt?* London: Royal College of Nursing.

Rutter, M. (1981) *Maternal Deprivation Re-assessed.* Harmondsworth: Penguin Education.

Sears, R., Macoby, E. & Levin, H. (1966) *Patterns of Child Rearing.* London: Harper & Row.

Secord, P.F. & Backman, C.W. (1966) *Problems in Social Psychology.* New York: McGraw-Hill.

Segal, J. & Yaharaes, H. (1981) *A Child's Journey.* Harmondsworth: Penguin Education.

Stafford-Clark, D. (1967) *What Freud Really Said.* Harmondsworth: Penguin.

Verney, T. & Kelly, J. (1982) *The Secret Life of the Unborn Child.* London: Sphere.

FURTHER READING

Argyle, M. (1967) *The Psychology of Interpersonal Behaviour.* Harmondsworth: Penguin.

Borger, R. & Seaborne, A.E.M. (1966) *The Psychology of Learning.* Harmondsworth: Penguin. A basic reference book for health visitors.

Bowlby, J. (1965) *Child Care and the Growth of Love.* Harmondsworth: Penguin.

Bowlby, J. (1971) *Attachment and Loss.* Harmondsworth: Penguin.

Bromley, D.B. (1966) *The Psychology of Human Ageing.* Harmondsworth: Penguin. Useful for students particularly interested in this field in depth.

Elkin, F. (1960) *The Child and Society.* New York: Random House. A useful introduction to socialization.

Foss, B. (1975) *New Perspectives in Child Development.* Harmondsworth: Penguin Education.

James, D.E. (1968) *Introduction to Psychology (for Teachers, Nurses and other Social Workers).* London: Constable. A useful basic text for health visitor students.

Krech, D., Crutchfield, R.S. & Ballachey, E.L. (1962) *The Individual in Society.* New York: McGraw-Hill. A useful general text for students wishing to study in greater depth.

Millar, S. (1968) *The Psychology of Play.* Harmondsworth: Penguin.

Mussen, P.H. (1965) *The Normal Development of the Child.* New York: Prentice Hall. A useful general text on developmental psychology.

Sprott, W.J.H. (1951) *Human Groups.* Harmondsworth: Penguin.

Vernon, M.D. (1962) *The Psychology of Perception.* Harmondsworth: Penguin.

Winnicott, D.W. (1964) *The Child, the Family and the Outside World.* Harmondsworth: Penguin.

Winnicott, D.W. (1980) *Playing and Reality.* Harmondsworth: Pelican.

World Health Organisation (1962) *Deprivation and Maternal Care.* Public Health Paper 14. Geneva. Gives a useful summary of work done in this area until 1962.

5. The Sociological Perspective

Grace M. Owen

In 1965 the Council for the Training of Health Visitors introduced its new syllabus which included as the second section 'The Individual in the Group'. This meant that for the first time all training schools in the United Kingdom would be including sociology as one of the main subject areas of the course. Previously a few colleges had been offering sociological studies of some kind within the curriculum and many health visitors were dubious about the wisdom of introducing an academic discipline of such a complex nature into an applied professional course. Over the years, however, as more health visitors have been introduced to sociological studies, they have become much more appreciative of a discipline which has opened up many new horizons and new approaches to the study of man in society, in a way that gave new insight into age old problems.

A problem for health visitor students when the subject was first introduced arose from the difficulty of teaching a complex discipline in a meaningful way within a one-year course. It is not usually sensible to refer to 'difficulties' when first introducing a new subject, for fear of putting people off, but it has been found from experience of teaching this subject that it is far more satisfactory to 'grasp the nettle' firmly and deal first with some of the aspects which cause problems for students, as many of them prove to be easily dispersed. Also as more sociologists have become familiar with health visitors through teaching on their courses and tutors have become more experienced at helping with interpretation and application, many of the earlier suspicions and prejudices have fallen away.

For this reason this chapter will look first at some explanations and definitions of terminologies used, before investigating specific areas of subject matter. Obviously not all sociologists will teach from the same topic areas, but perhaps the areas used here will be common to many courses and will serve to illustrate how the subject matter can be used and the kind of insights that can be gained into health visiting situations.

INTRODUCING SOCIOLOGY

Reading Sociology

One of the most daunting aspects for sociology students is the wide range of reading material available, often expressing divergent points of view. Students need considerable guidance in learning to be selective in reading, both in terms of books borrowed or purchased, and also chapters selected within a book. Lecturers are often reluctant to suggest single textbooks or books offering a 'potted version' of sociology, as this is not likely to help students to gain a true sociological perspective. However, once the student has some idea what sociology is all about, it is often helpful to take a specific topic, with which the student is already familiar to some extent, or a particular study such as *Patterns of Infant Care in an Urban Community* (Newson J. & E. 1965) and use it to illustrate some of the concepts and theories used by sociologists. This way sociology becomes meaningful and purposeful and therefore more interesting and worthwhile. Alternatively a basic reader, such as *Sociology of Modern Britain* by Butterworth and Weir (1970) gives a comprehensive view of a wide range of topics, presented in a form that is both accessible and readable for students who are studying on a course which allows limited reading time.

The Use of Sociological Jargon

Another aspect which often presents difficulties is sociological jargon and it is thus important to spend a little time early on in the course coming to terms with terminology, otherwise whole areas of the subject matter can remain unintelligible for far too long. Any scientific discipline usually has a certain amount of its own jargon, as one of the 'tools' for classification and definition. Just as the professional person in the medical and nursing world makes extensive use of jargon which is often unintelligible and even threatening to the layman, so the sociologist may fail to be understood by the doctor or nurse. Sociologists tend to use words that are descriptive in another sense of things in everyday life, such as a 'random sample', or a social 'institution', but they have a different interpretation for the sociologist. As Berger (1966) points out, however, it is just because we are well acquainted with so many of the terms used that our perception of them is imprecise and erroneous. Both tutor and student need to come to a mutual agreement on the importance of understanding the terminology at an early stage in the course. Some explanatory texts, such as Chapter 1 in Cotgrove's *The Science of Society* (1967) or the use of Duncan Mitchell's *Dictionary of Sociology* (1968) can be quite helpful in the early days.

Expectations Unfulfilled

Sometimes students become disappointed or disillusioned with sociology because they come to it looking for solutions to the problems of society and expecting either answers to their questions or some new knowledge that can be applied directly to their work, and their expectations are not realized. Thus they feel they are wasting their time on a somewhat nebulous subject when there is so much informative material waiting to be absorbed, which gives them greater security in doing their job, while sociology raises awkward questions and provides few direct answers. As Berger (1966) says, 'People who like to avoid shocking discoveries, or have no curiosity about human beings, should stay away from sociology'.

What is Sociology?

Many sociologists have attempted to define sociology; some would call it a study of the individual in society and others would say it is a 'science of society'. A great deal of argument has revolved around this question of whether it is a science or not. The sociologist is certainly concerned with a study of individuals and their behaviour and relationships with others in groups and with the forces that shape this behaviour, *not* however in the way the psychologist studies behaviour. The sociologist is much more concerned with the *structure* and fabric of the *society* within which *individuals* and *groups* are set and the *social forces* that generate *interaction, social pressures* and *social change* within that society.

In a way it is easier to say what sociology is not, than to define what it is. Berger (1966) outlines some of the widely held misconceptions about sociology. One common mistake is to identify sociology with social work and social reform. *Social work* is a kind of professional practice in society and *social reform* is an attempt to put *social policy* into action to produce social change. Sociology has no claim to do either of these things, but is much more of an attempt to understand what the structure of the situation is and what causes certain events. Sociology may offer *explanations* and *insights* and attempt to offer *predictions*; it may analyse situations, but not prescribe a course of action following the analysis. Although sociology leads to understanding rather than practice, it is an understanding that can be recommended to people such as social workers and nurses (and naturally to health visitors). In fact it can be 'recommended to anyone whose goals involve the manipulation of men' (Berger 1966). This kind of understanding can influence our attitudes and increase our effectiveness in helping the people with whom we are concerned.

For example, it can help health visitors to understand why children in some working-class families tend to leave school early and go into work that offers no apparent prospects, when they might have the ability to move into higher education where the long-term prospects could be more attractive. While sociology may help to understand the reasons for inequality of opportunity in education, it does not say what action could be taken to change the situation, decide whether any action should be taken or whether things should be left as they are. These are not sociological responsibilities.

Another commonly held image of the sociologist is that of a 'gatherer of statistics' about human behaviour (Berger 1966). Sociologists do in fact collect *data*, because as a science sociology must seek to provide accurate information about the members of society and their behaviour. The sociologist does attempt to classify data and evolve tools for use in research, but there is more involved. 'Statistical data by themselves do not make sociology. They become sociology only when they are sociologically interpreted, put in a theoretical frame of reference that is sociological . . . the interpretation is broader than the data.'

Studies on family life in Bethnal Green, *Family and Kinship in East London* (Young & Wilmott 1957) and others using similar methods to study family life in Swansea, *The Family and Social Change* (Rosser & Harris 1965), have both included some accurate documentation of statistical material but in such a way that the material in each study can be compared with others. They have moreover gone further than that. Rosser and Harris (1965), for example, examine in detail the nature of the function of the family in contemporary society in Swansea. Using a *functional* theoretical approach to assist in the interpretation of data, they were able to conclude that kinship was still as strong a social force in Swansea as it was in Bethnal Green, at the time of the studies. In this way reliable information was provided on a subject which is all too often judged on the basis of inaccurate assumptions and impressions.

One other misconception sometimes apparent is that the sociologist is a 'detached sardonic observer, and a cold manipulator of men' (Berger 1966). To some extent the research worker must remain detached in order to be objective and unbiased in observation. However, this does not mean he is not concerned or does not care about people, their feelings and their welfare.

The sociologist is disciplined in his approach to studying society, within a clearly defined frame of reference, struggling to maintain a *'value-free'* and objective approach. He may be equally concerned, for example, in his attempt to document and interpret the facts about the position of the elderly in society, as the doctor is in treating their sickness, or the health visitor in maintaining their health. He is occupied in his scientific approach with collection and *classification* of information, *explanation* and *interpretation*, and within certain limits, *prediction*, and in order to do this he needs to use tools, *theories* and *methods* specifically devised for the task.

It is not always easy to differentiate clearly between sociology and the other social sciences which include sciences dealing with the human individual, such as psychology, social psychology, social policy and administration, economics and anthropology. Psychology is concerned with the individual and his behaviour and sociology with man's social behaviour, but often drawing upon other disciplines which may contribute to an understanding of society. The subject matter of sociology covers a very wide scope and it would be impossible to include all areas on a health visitors course. Probably the aspects most often studied are related to the social structure of, say, modern Britain which includes the various *social institutions*, social *stratification*, social *processes* and social *change* and gives opportunities for introducing other perspectives on theories and methods, comparative studies and social problems.

Having thus attempted to define what sociology is, we may well ask now what its relevance is for health visiting.

Why Study Sociology?

A number of writers have attempted to explain the value of sociology for the health visitor's training. Most emphasize the point already made that it increases the health visitor's understanding of the society in which she works, but does not attempt to prescribe action for solutions (Owen 1968). Barber (1968) describes it as a means of communication in the sense that it offers an understanding of groups and different *cultures* and therefore helps in establishing social contact. It may well also help students to overcome any rigidity or authoritarianism in approach which could have been acquired during the fairly traditional framework of the hospital setting and could be very important in helping to establish suitable attitudes and developing a sense of maturity and a readiness to question their own value systems where necessary. Chivers (1969) makes the point that sociological investigation helps in determining 'what is obvious and true from what is obvious but untrue' and this is why so often students may feel and complain that it is 'just common sense'. Although it does not give us the answers to problems, it may well help in directing away from one course of action and suggest the possibility of seeking other courses.

North (1975) stresses the value of relevant knowledge of the 'shape' or structure of society and understanding of how it works.

This 'understanding' acquired from an acquaintance with sociology can thus bring an extra dimension to the health visitor's approach to her work; hence the title of this chapter. For some it may prove a difficult, complex or even nebulous subject to study. For others it may be a traumatic process to have some of their attitudes and value systems destroyed and re-established. But at the same time, given a course with well-chosen topics and tutorial time to discuss and assimilate new ideas and a careful introduction to jargon, it can prove a highly stimulating and rewarding subject helping the student to gain a critical and analytical approach to her work.

SOCIOLOGY IN THE HEALTH VISITORS COURSE

Health visitors work primarily in the context of families and small groups in towns, cities or rural areas and are therefore interested in such topics as the relationship between family background and educational achievement, or cultural differences in child-rearing patterns, because this has a direct application to their work.

We now move on to examine some of these aspects of sociology which could be included in any health visitors course, always remembering that this chapter does not attempt to offer a brief course in sociology, but rather to select from a wide range a few topics that are basic to understanding the subject, or that can be used to illustrate how sociology can be used to gain a sociological perspective for health visiting. The fact that areas chosen are those of considerable interest for health visitors, makes the approach more meaningful and worthwhile for study.

In the process of studying these topics students may well be introduced to theoretical approaches used or various other aspects of sociology and different lecturers are likely to select those areas in which they themselves have most expertise. This selection looks at a few of the basic theories and concepts used, attempting to give an understanding of the jargon and showing how these topics can give a sociological perspective to health visiting.

Terminology

There are terms in frequent use in most sociological literature which tend to be very much interrelated and therefore some appreciation of their meaning is essential for the student.

Concepts are useful tools used by sociologists to help in distinguishing the context of some of the more abstract ideas, or in symbolizing the *variables*, and are essential for communication. One of the key concepts in common use is that of the *social system*, particularly as some sociologists use a *systems approach* to their study of society. A social system denotes a 'basic unit of two or more individuals, directly or indirectly interacting in a bounded situation' (Duncan Mitchell 1968). It can include small or large groups or whole societies, these usually being referred to as open systems because they are interdependent with other systems, and often act with reference to them. The major *structural* components are organizations which cluster around and relate to the major *functions* which must be carried on for society to exist. For example, there are kinship systems, political, economical and legal systems and educational systems all of which have many related subsystems, such as the school which is a subsystem of education. These systems are all linked or held together by the fabric of society, the structural patterns of relationships including recognized *norms*, *values* and *beliefs*, and *roles*. The total pattern is often referred to as the '*social structure*'.

The collections of norms, values and customs surrounding major systems are known as *social institutions*, for example the social institution of marriage and family life is related to the kinship system. These sets of norms and values give individuals patterns of expectations in relation to behaviour within society. Life would become intolerable without some awareness of the kind of behaviour expected in everyday life. In Great Britain we expect to queue for buses, pay for our food with money, drive on the left side of the road, or respect other people's property; other forms of behaviour in these situations may be regarded to a greater or lesser extent as some form of deviance.

Actions, feelings and thoughts are generated by these expectations in accordance with an individual's position in society and these are referred to as *'role' expectations*. There are, for example, family roles, such as mother, uncle or grandfather, or occupational roles such as manager, teacher, shop assistant or foreman, each role carrying its own set of recognized expectations.

For health visitors it is relevant to build up the concept of a social system with discussion around the kinship systems and the social institutions of the family and marriage, and the role relationships of members of the family, or the role of women in society. The roles and values surrounding these institutions can be observed in the variety of community studies on life in Britain. The family and kinship, however, cannot be viewed as a 'closed' system because it is affected by the nature of the economic and industrial systems—the factors governing occupation and income—and these in turn will most probably have been influenced by the families' educational background and achievement, which influence the kind of job obtained. The behaviour patterns of families and individuals in groups all go to make up the 'culture of a society'.

Where material possessions such as cars, televisions and refrigerators are highly valued in a society individuals will be motivated to want them and motivation necessitates a means of achieving the goals, as Cotgrove (1967) explains so clearly. These are all matters of interest for the everyday work of the health visitor, and this kind of sociological perspective can form a useful backcloth against which new insights can be gained and used in helping individuals to change where change is needed. It is also possible to acquire a wider vision of people as 'products' of a social system, understanding the pressures of expectations, culture patterns and peer groups that influence the shaping of an individual's personality, attitudes and goals; this is the *socialization* process which is fundamental to the health visitor's understanding of factors influencing child development.

Theories and Methods

Health visitors may sometimes find themselves participating in a survey or sociological investigation, or may be involved in the many community studies or reports on health statistics. Any of these may well stimulate an interest in gaining an appreciation of research method. Methodology, however, includes much more than understanding the use of basic research techniques. The nature of the relationship between theory and empirical research discussed by Cotgrove (1967) and already noted, shows how a theoretical approach enables the formulation of a *hypothesis* and provides a disciplined framework for collection and interpretation of data. Bottomore (1962) in his description discusses various methods used in sociological enquiry including the *historical* and *comparative* approaches and the uses of *functional* and *evolutionary* theories. He also examines the extent to which prediction is possible in sociology. Unlike some of the more exact sciences, sociology presents many variables that cannot be controlled or excluded in research and may be influenced by the unpredictability of human nature and the processes of social change with the passage of time. It is possible, however, to discover trends and indicate probabilities.

Some courses in sociology may approach the introduction to theories and methods historically, as many aspects of contemporary theory have their origins in the work of the earlier sociologists, such as Durkheim, Comte, Weber, or Marx, and this makes a logical foundation for understanding present-day approaches.

Finally, no discussion on theories and methods should pass without some reference to the use of *models*, as they are increasingly popular as an aid to scientific methods, and a step in theory building. Inkeles (1964) gives a useful explanation of their use and value. A model may be constructed in such a way as to allow a systematic description of all the variables and the relationships between them, thus providing a framework within which initial ideas can be tested in the process of theory building. An example of a model that could be used in the sociological approach to studying nursing education is shown in Chapter 1 (p. 27). This can be used to look at the forces that have shaped the growth of nursing education and indicate some of the pressures and constraints. Some areas of the model we may know very little about, while in others, such as resources available and manpower provision, there may be accurate factual information available. The model helps to ensure that all possible variables are taken into consideration when planning and policy making, and also allows for examination of areas where further research is needed. It could be modified or expanded to examine the interrelationships between the variables, such as the changes of welfare provision and effects of these on the role of professionals. This shows how a sociological perspective can give a more complete or total approach to studying professional education for the nurse and health visitor.

This brief introduction to terminology and methods of approach gives a foundation from which it is possible to move with greater awareness to look at more specific topics.

TOPICS IN SOCIOLOGY OF SPECIFIC INTEREST TO THE HEALTH VISITOR

There are several topic areas particularly useful for health visitors; their discussion here, however, is not intended as a substitute for further reading, but rather to demonstrate the interrelationships between the topics, and the ways in which they add a wider dimension to health visiting and also to act as a useful guide and stimulant to further study in a wider field.

The Family and the Kinship System

An obvious starting point and a subject fundamental to the work of all health visitors is the family and kinship system as it covers an introduction to kinship structures and variations in other cultures as well as the United Kingdom, including marriage institutions and family relationships, and extending into differences in child-rearing patterns and the process of socialization. It has to be seen in the context of social class and cultural variations, population structure and the processes of social change. The interrelationships will become apparent as these aspects and other social institutions are studied. A useful introduction may be found in Farmer's book (1970) *The Family* or Fletcher's (1962) *The Family and Marriage*, both of which set the family in the context outlined above.

It is interesting to consider the variations in family life and patterns in different parts of this country, and also in different subcultures, especially in the light of changes over the last century. Sometimes students query the value of reading studies written some years previously, as they are hoping to find descriptions of life as it exists today to help them in their work. However, these studies take time to complete and it is valuable to see the characteristics of families in previous decades and discover the various aspects of change, or to note where traditional customs and patterns are so strongly established that they die hard. Examples can be seen in the Swansea (Rosser & Harris 1965) and Bethnal Green (Young & Wilmott 1957) studies which show how kinship still exerted a powerful force in traditonal working-class areas and that the extended family ties still existed, if in modified form, in the 1960s, although some family ties have weakened and many are changing.

The situation may have changed even more up to the present time, but a close study of this kind of investigation can help the student to define the kind of patterns of behaviour to observe and the likelihood of their existence in certain types of area. Fletcher (1962) describes the main functions of the family in society and maintains that the essential ones still exist, although they may be carried out differently and in some ways more satisfactorily, although some sociologists dispute this. The McGregors (1957) suggest that the increase in the divorce rate does not necessarily indicate a decline in the stability and importance of the family as a social institution.

A currently topical subject related to family studies is the role of women in society. This has some important implications for roles and relationships in the family, especially for the care of the very young and the elderly or sick in society. Hannah Gavron (1960) provides a useful historical background to changes which have taken place in the last 150 years in the rights of women and, subsequently, in the feminine role, which is closely allied with the employment situation. Concern has frequently been expressed by health visitors and others about the effects of mothers working on the care of young children and some sources indicate that about one-third of working mothers have children under five who could be receiving substandard care (Farmer 1970, Chapter 5). It is important, however, not to attribute causal relationships where they do not exist, and to determine the main factors involved in order to avoid making generalizations.

Some American studies indicate that the important feature is the quality and continuity of care given. Where the care is substandard, there are frequently other variables involved, such as fathers who have unstable working patterns, or children who receive inconsistent patterns of discipline. There is some evidence in this country that children of working mothers on the whole do better than average at school, tend to have better material living standards, and have mothers who make good use of clinics and welfare services. Some parents claim enrichment of family relationships and a more democratic approach to family life, with little to support the suggestions of neglect. Farmer's discussion (1970) on this topic may be helpful to students seeking to acquire an informed approach to the subject. The important feature, it appears, is to ensure that mothers are aware of the value of a close and consistent relationship with children in the very early days of life, and the need for the quality and continuity of care to be maintained if and when they need to go to work. The health visitor may well be in a position to assist a mother to assess the need to work and to help her consider all these aspects of the situation. If she decides she must work, the health visitor can help her make the necessary safeguards, so that she may enjoy her work free of feelings of guilt.

Studies on family life also show differentiation of sex roles, comparative styles of life and child-rearing patterns. Most health visitors will be familiar with the Newsons' work in Nottingham (1965), and Klein's *Samples from Three Cultures* (1965). Such studies help to establish realistic expectations of behaviour and indicate factors which could be resistant to change and are relevant to the primary socialization of the child. Elkin's book (1960) gives a helpful approach to the student seeking to differentiate between the sociological and psychological theories of socialization and gives some insight into the role of the family as an agent of socialization. This again is a topic of fundamental importance and needs to be studied in relation to the work of psychologists (World Health Organisation 1962), and the theories of identification and conscience formation (see Chapter 4).

Obviously this discussion is not intended to be comprehensive but rather to indicate the value of further reading. Where reading time is limited, any method of study which can give a broader perspective can be helpful. It is quite useful to use the community studies as a basis for seminar work, as they demonstrate the relationships between sociological theory and real life. Individual students may take responsibility for producing a brief account of one study to initiate discussion, and then copies of the paper may be made available to others in the group. This will ensure that all students acquire a general acquaintance with a variety of studies, though some will have a closer familiarity with a specific topic than others. In addition, all students will become acquainted with the methods of using these studies. Important things to look for include the following.

1. Methods of approach and research techniques used.
2. Aims and objectives.
3. Interesting aspects for health visitors.
4. Conclusions and comparisons with other studies.

Frankenburg's *Communities In Britain* (1966) is quite useful for helping students to appreciate the value of these studies in a theoretical context and Mary Farmer's conclusion (1970) offers some thoughts on the links with social policy. Within the context of studying the family cultural differences, brief reference should be made to the position of immigrant families, although students may well wish to spend some time on this area. They may be very concerned with the problems of immigrant families particularly in relation to housing, health, education or communication difficulties.

Sociologists are interested in studying the problems of integration or conflict within societies, prejudice and cultural differences, and the interaction and adaptation that take place.

The process of integration is an interesting one as certain patterns emerge. Immigrants enter a host society quite often low on the social scale and as they become established there may be some upward social mobility as they acquire the skills necessary for gaining better jobs. There are three possible results in terms of acceptance in a host society.

1. *Total assimilation.* The immigrants adapt, are accepted, intermarry and tend to disappear.
2. *Integration.* The host society accepts the new groups who retain their different customs and agree to differ on some aspects such as child-rearing patterns.
3. *The transitory phase.* Here the immigrants are accommodated and this is the most likely course of events in Britain. The testing points have often turned out to be culture and intermarriage.

The health visitor may be helped to understand the origin of some of the problems encountered, and awareness and acceptance of these cultural, communication and possible religious differences are particularly important where health education is concerned. An understanding of the process of integration involves more than just an awareness of the facts.

Urbanization

A topic closely linked with any study of family life in Britain, where now 70 per cent of the population live in cities, is urbanization. It must be recognized that it involves a wider concept than just a consideration of the effects of living in urban conurbations. Wirth (1938) proposes that urbanization is a 'way of life' and that cities exert certain social influences on the life of the people, which are greater than the ratio of urban to rural population would suggest.

> The city is not only the dwelling place of modern man but also the initiating and controlling centre of economic, political and cultural life that has drawn the most remote communities of the world into its orbit (Wirth 1938).

Peter Mann (1965) emphasizes the need to look at the relationship between the people and their environment, the aspects of social organization and the way of thinking so typical of urban life. He outlines some theoretical approaches to the study of urban and rural life.

In his interpretation of Burgess' theory of concentric zones, as applied to some British conurbations, Mann provides a fascinating perspective for any health visitor who has worked in a city. He also develops the concepts of *community* and *neighbourhood*, highlighting the main characteristics in terms of relationships between people in groups and in a geographical area, and makes a further comparison between urban and rural communities.

The health visitor student preparing a neighbourhood study should find this approach helpful in overcoming some of the difficulties outlined in Chapter 3, and will also discover some starting points for considering the interaction between people and the neighbourhood in which they live, and the effects of local characteristics. An important new dimension will emerge that helps to avoid the 'flat' kind of descriptive study which fails to take into account the dynamic aspects of the real-life situation.

Social Class and Social Stratification

Inevitably students raise so many questions about the concept of *social class* that it is sensible to introduce the topic for discussion fairly early in the course as it is frequently involved in consideration of the social institutions. This subject often generates heated discussion, particularly when it is realized that the criteria used for classification are not considered very reliable ones. It is helpful to distinguish the

differences between *social stratification* and *social class* and to introduce the subject by looking at some earlier forms of stratification
such as feudalism or the caste system, to demonstrate the different
kinds of criteria used in the various theoretical approaches.
Sergeant (1971) points out that Weber used the notion of *social
prestige* and *status* to establish a basis for classification while many
other sociologists have used occupation, income, education, or
power.

The selection of readings introduced by Butterworth and Weir
(1970) could provide a rationale for understanding the use of social
class as a tool for studying various aspects of health and vital
statistics, assessing health problems, or the need for a particular
approach in health education. Arie's paper *Class Differences in Life
Chances* (1970) is a good illustration of the value of understanding
class differentials for the health visitor.

Another study of social class variations useful for health visitors
relates to the differences in norms, values and beliefs. Goldthorpe
and Lockwood (1963) describe the differences between the
working-class and middle-class perspective in terms of acceptance of
authority. Klein (1965) gives a fascinating account of life styles and
family networks, outlining the four major areas of difference.

1. The ability to abstract in general terms from the concrete actual
   situation.
2. The ability to perceive the world as an ordered universe in which
   rational action is rewarded.
3. The ability to plan ahead.
4. The ability to exercise self-control.

These behavioural patterns are particularly significant for health
visitors who need to be sensitive to their existence in all teaching
situations with families and groups. The ability to plan ahead, for
example, is basic for a housewife planning a long-term family
budget, while lack of it may well be one reason for failure to manage
on a limited income.

Lawson (1968) describes how these four areas of difference are also
relevant to educational achievement. It should begin to become
apparent to the student after becoming familiar with a few of these
topics just how much they are interrelated, and how difficult it is to
study them in isolation.

Education
Wherever a system of social stratification exists, it is likely that there

will be corresponding patterns of differences in the education system. Health visitors being familiar as they are with the strong links between family life, culture, school and environment will appreciate that Britain is no exception, and therefore should find this an absorbing topic.

Sociologists may approach the study of education differently. Some see it as an agent for *social control*, others as a means of intiating *social change*. As the former it transmits norms and values, and in some primitive societies the family may well be the main agency concerned. Education is often seen as maintaining a balance of power between social control and social change, transmitting the culture or reinforcing and reflecting the existing situation. There is some dilemma over the relationship between education and social change, as to whether the labour market creates a demand for a certain kind of education which dominates the system and so initiates change, or whether the system provides a specific type of education that ultimately stimulates changes in technology and industry.

The historical development of the educational system in Britain offers numerous examples of the strength of differences existing among the educational, religious, and political systems and the constraints and pressures of economic situations and technological progress.

The main topic of interest, however, revolves round the question of *equality of opportunity* in education and its relationship with *educational achievement*. As health visitors are often involved in discussions with parents and teachers about the progress of children in school or asked for advice about careers guidance, familiarity with the evidence in this area is essential. Most of the research falls into one of two main areas: the influence of family background or of the school environment. Lawson's summary of findings (1968) shows that factors such as the size of family, overcrowding, parental attitudes and occupation are all related variables, while the kind of school, its organization and techniques of teaching also affect progress.

For health visitors, however, the greatest significance lies in Bernstein's work (1970) on the linguistic deprivation of the working-class child in relation to educational achievement. He describes the effects of restricted vocabulary and sentence construction in the early and formative years of life and relates them to the development of thought processes and reasoning. Language, however, is not the only factor involved. The working-class child tends to have a less formally organized family structure, while the middle-class child grows up in the context of a relationship that provides a dynamic interaction which is part of the socialization process and provides a direct link for the middle-class milieu of the school and does not conflict with the values of the home. The working-class child may well have a limited verbal expression of feelings and perception and an environment that may well be in conflict with the formal educational system.

This area of investigation is still in progress and health visitors will be awaiting further developments with interest, well aware that they are visiting families during these crucial formative years of life for the child. With their knowledge of some of the determinants of linguistic deprivation, health visitors may then be prepared to assist mothers in appreciating the value of the complementary effects of things such as pre-school play groups.

One other area of current controversy in our present educational system, the value of which parents may wish to discuss with the health visitor, is the provision of comprehensive schools. The ideal of comprehensive education has been slowly gaining popularity since the 1950s, many hoping that it would remove some of the existing inequalities of opportunity. The major reports on education over the last two decades show that the middle-class child has distinct advantages over the working-class child in terms of successful achievement—if, that is, this means gaining entry into the higher educational system.

While some of the anomalies, such as the selection at the age of 11, have been removed and certain advantages, such as a wider choice of subjects for all children, have been established, many inequalities still exist. In fact the question concerning the possibility of reaching *equality* of opportunity is open to discussion. Julien Ford (1969) takes a critical look at the evidence on both sides and shows the extent to which comprehensive schools have been successful and also some of the anomalies which still exist or have been re-created.

Other studies demonstrate the importance of parental attitudes to education for the child and open up possible areas for seeking ways in which deprivation and disadvantage may be overcome (Marsden & Jackson 1962).

Current Sociological Concerns

There are many current issues upon which a sociological prospective is important for health visitors. The effects of the influences of modern technology on the 'symmetrical family' are described by Young and Wilmott (1975), with particular reference to important topics such as work and leisure. Butterworth and Weir (1972) provide useful readings also on these issues and include such topics as crime, drug taking, strikes and unemployment, and problems relating to minority groups. The situation in relation to these issues is constantly changing and the health visitor needs to be aware of the trends and the possible effects on family life and health.

Medical Sociology and Health Care
Medical sociology has become an increasingly popular subject over the last few years and many courses will include some introduction to this area of study. The conceptual bases for health and illness are of interest to health visitors, as these are relative concepts and often determined by different cultural values. Perception of health and illness is influenced by family and cultural attitudes and by the dissemination of health information in society, and a variety of other life experiences. Twaddle and Hessler (1977) suggest that health and sickness are socially defined, and the concept of the 'sick role' is a transitory one and may be determined by an individual's personal decision, and it alters expectations of his behaviour, particularly in relation to his availability for work. Some forms of deviant behaviour may be classified as illness in some societies and not in others. Medicine may be viewed as an agent of social control, and here the sociology of the professional is an interesting area of study— particularly the effects of professional socialization.

The health visitor's understanding of this area of sociology is of particular value, in establishing work priorities, or planning for health education and in helping individuals with their own attitudes towards health and illness (Patrick & Scambler 1982).

The topics in this chapter are among those most frequently discussed in sociology courses and an attempt has been made here to show a method of approach for health visitor students which could assist in developing a sociological perspective and retaining a curiosity and fascination for the subject which will stimulate further reading. Space does not allow further exposition of other social institutions such as politics, religion, and economics, all of which are relevant in influencing the quality of life and behaviour patterns. Occupation is another topic which generates interest, particularly when seen in the context of organizational theory and bureaucracy and may well intrigue health visitors moving on to management posts, or interested in professional development (Chapters 1 and 2).

Concepts such as *social deviance* and *stigma* which are linked with a study of social problems in drug dependency and mental illness raise interesting questions for discussion, and may well assist students in gaining a broader attitude in their approach to these areas of work.

The interesting thing about sociology is that whatever kind of area health visitors work in, or whatever aspect of their skills they are interested in developing more fully, sociology offers some new dimensions of thought. It may well raise unanswered questions but may also open up new courses of enquiry, new ideas for research, new ways of approaching problems and also provide an ever-intriguing background for the work of health visitors.

SUMMARY

This chapter introduces the student to the complex subject of sociology, in an attempt to demonstrate its relevance for health visiting. After some explanations of terminology, and the various approaches used, some specific areas are discussed with particular relevance to health visiting practice. The family, urbanization, education and medical sociology are selected as examples and some areas for further reading are indicated throughout the text.

QUESTIONS FOR ESSAY OR DISCUSSION

1. 'Industrialization has stripped the family of its functions.' Discuss this statement with reference to the role of the family in Britain today.
2. Discuss any social survey or community study with which you are familiar and show how it has contributed to your understanding of your work as a health visitor.
3. Discuss the sociological concept of 'total institutions'. How useful is it in the study of some organizations and their effects on people?
4. Discuss the ways in which some occupations achieve professional status. Relate this to your own profession.
5. What social factors can be said to influence educational achievement?
6. Discuss the similarities and differences of primary and secondary socialization in an occupation or profession.
7. To what extent has the changing role of women in society affected the family life in Britain over the last century?
8. To what extent can 'equality of opportunity' be said to exist in the educational system in Britain today? Why is this of interest to the health visitor?

9. Discuss the factors affecting the fertility rate in Britain during the last 100 years.
10. Discuss the relationship between social class and child-rearing practices in Britain. Illustrate your answer with examples from any community studies you have read.
11. 'Deviance is socially created and therefore demands social remedies.' Discuss this statement.
12. Discuss the social role of religion in contemporary Britain.
13. Examine the role of the family as an agent of socialization in Britain today. Why is this of interest to health visitors?
14. 'Urbanism is a way of life.' To what extent is this true of Britain today?

REFERENCES

Arie, T. (1970) Class differences in life chances. In: *The Sociology of Modern Britain*, ed. E. Butterworth & D. Weir, pp. 213–18. London: Fontana.

Barber, C.R. (1968) The role of sociology in the curriculum of the health visitor course. *Health Visitor*, *41*, 4, pp. 183–5 (April).

Berger, P.L. (1966) *Invitation to Sociology*. Harmondsworth: Penguin. *

Bernstein, B. (1970) Education cannot compensate for society. *New Society*, *387*, 344 (26 February).

Bottomore, T.B. (1962) *Sociology*, Chapter 3. London: Allen & Unwin.

Butterworth, E. & Weir, D. (1970) *The Sociology of Modern Britain*. London: Fontana. *

Butterworth, E. & Weir, D. (1972) *Social Problems of Modern Britain*. London: Fontana.

Chivers, J.S. (1969) Sociology for health visitors. *Nursing Times*, *64*, 4, 5 and 6 (23 and 30 January, 6 February). Occasional Papers.

Cotgrove, S. (1967) *The Science of Society*. London: Allen & Unwin. *

Council for the Education and Training of Health Visitors (1970) *Guide to the Syllabus of Training*. London.

Duncan Mitchell, G. (1968) *A Dictionary of Sociology*. London: Routledge & Kegan Paul.

Elkin, F. (1960) *The Child and Society*. Montreal: Random House.

Farmer, M. (1970) *The Family*. Harlow: Longman. *

Fletcher, R. (1962) *The Family and Marriage*. Harmondsworth: Penguin. *

Ford, J. (1969) *Social Class and the Comprehensive School*. London: Routledge & Kegan Paul.

Frankenburg, R. (1966) *Communities in Britain*. Harmondsworth: Penguin. *

Gavron, H. (1960) *The Captive Wife*. London: Routledge & Kegan Paul. *

Goldthorpe, J.H. & Lockwood, D. (1963) Affluence and the British class structure. *Sociological Review*, *11*, 2.

Inkeles, A. (1964) *What is Sociology?* New Jersey: Prentice Hall.

Klein, J. (1965) *Samples from Three Cultures*, Vol. 1. London: Routledge & Kegan Paul. *

Lawson, D. (1968) *Social Class, Language and Education*. London: Routledge & Kegan Paul. *

McGregor, O. & R. (1957) *Divorce in England*. London: Heinemann.

Mann, P. (1965) *An Approach to Urban Sociology*. London: Routledge & Kegan Paul. *

Marsden, D. & Jackson, B. (1962) *Education and the Working Class*. Harmondsworth: Penguin.

Newson, J. & E. (1965) *Patterns of Infant Care in an Urban Community*. Harmondsworth: Penguin.

North, M. (1975) Why sociology? *Health Visitor*, *48*, 4, pp. 113–14. (April).

Owen, G.M. (1968) The health visitor in the social context. *Midwife and Health Visitor Journal*, *6*, 10, 11 and 12 (October, November and December).

Patrick, D. & Scambler, G. (1982) *Sociology as Applied to Medicine*. London: Baillière Tindall.

Rosser, C. & Harris, C. (1965) *The Family and Social Change*. London: Routledge & Kegan Paul.

Sergeant, G. (1971) *A Textbook of Sociology*. London: Macmillan.

Twaddle, A.C. & Hessler, R.M. (1977) *A Sociology of Health*. St Louis: Mosby.

Wirth, L. (1938) Urbanism as a way of life. *American Journal of Sociology*, *44* (July).

World Health Organisation (1962) Public Health Paper No. 14. Geneva.

Young, M. & Wilmott, P. (1957) *Family and Kinship in East London*. London: Routledge & Kegan Paul.

Young, M. & Wilmott, P. (1975) *The Symmetrical Family*. Harmondsworth: Penguin.

FURTHER READING

Books in the reference list that are marked with an asterisk are also useful basic reading.

Berger, P. & B. (1972) *Sociology, A Biographical Approach*. Harmondsworth: Penguin.

Bott, E. (1957) *The Family and Social Network*. London: Tavistock.

Brothers, J. (1971) *Religious Institutions*. Harlow: Longman.

Butterworth, E. & Weir, D. (1972) *Social Problems in Modern Britain*. London: Fontana.

Butterworth, E. & Weir, D. (1973) *Man and Work in Modern Britain*. London: Fontana.

Clarke, J. & Henderson, J. (1983) *Community Health*. Edinburgh: Churchill Livingstone.

Cox, C. & Mead, A. (1975) *A Sociology of Medical Practice*. London: Collier MacMillan.

Douglas, J.W.B. (1964) *The Home and the School*. St Albans: Granada.

Hill, C. (1970) *Immigration and Integration*. London: Pergamon.

Jones, G. (1970) *The Political Structure*. Harlow: Longman.

Jones, G. (1973) *Rural Life*. Harlow: Longman.

Jones, K. & Jones, P. (1975) *Sociology in Medicine*. E.U. Press.

Kelsall, R.K. (1967) *Population*. Harlow: Longman.

Kerr, M. (1958) *People of Ship Street*. London: Routledge & Kegan Paul.

King, R. (1971) *Education*. Harlow: Longman.

Martin, D. (1967) *A Sociology of English Religion*. London: Heinemann.

Musgrove, P.W. (1971) *The Economic Structure*. Harlow: Longman.

Newson, J. & E. (1978) *Seven Years Old in the Home Environment*. Harmondsworth: Pelican.

Pahl, R.E. (ed.) (1967) *Urban Sociology in Great Britain*. Readings in Sociology. London: Pergamon.

Pahl, R.E. (1970) *Patterns of Urban Life*. Harlow: Longman.

Raynor, J. (1969) *The Middle Class*. Harlow: Longman.

Rex, J. & Moore, R. (1967) *Race Community and Conflict*. Oxford: Oxford University Press.

Roberts, K. (1976) *Leisure*. Social Structure of Modern Britain Series. Harlow: Longman.

Rose, G. (1968) *The Working Class*. Harlow: Longman.

Ross, D. & Simpson, T. (1968) *All Our Future*. London: Peter Davis.

Smith, A. (1976) *Social Change*. Aspects of Modern Sociology. Harlow: Longman.

Townsend, P. (1963) *The Family Life of Old People*. Harmondsworth: Penguin.

Wilmott, P. & Young, M. (1959) *Family and Class in a London Suburb*. Harmondsworth: Penguin.

Wright-Mills, C. (1959) *The Sociological Imagination*. Harmondsworth: Penguin.

Yudkin, S. & Holme, A. (1963) *Working Mothers and Their Children*. London: Michael Joseph.

6. The Administrative Framework of the Health and Social Services

Jean Gaffin

Health visitors do not work in isolation but as members of the community health team, in the front line of the National Health Service, just one of the social services. Because health visitors work within the community, cooperation and liaison with members of the local authority social service department (such as the home help organizer or the local social workers), are part of the job. Health visitors work with individuals and families who may have problems, such as inadequate housing or poverty, where an understanding of the local authority's housing department's functions and the scope of the social security scheme will be relevant to helping the client. An understanding of the way in which the social services develop and are organized is thus an important aspect of the knowledge a health visitor needs to do the job effectively.

There are, however, other reasons why health visitors need an understanding of the administrative framework of the social services. Knowing what resources are available in the community is most important, but health visitors are also members of an occupational group with its own professional association. As such, they can present factual knowledge to local and central government in order to argue for improved provisions for groups they see as having unmet needs. Such arguments need to be made with an understanding of competing claims on available resources if they are to be successful. Individuals and families with problems tend to see those problems in isolation: the collective knowledge of the health visitor can therefore be of real value to those making decisions about the future of the social services.

Health visitors are also citizens in a democratic country, who vote, pay taxes and complain about their rate bills. With the knowledge of needs and provision their job gives them, health visitors who join pressure groups, neighbourhood groups or political parties have a particularly important role to play in such associations. We all bring to a study of social policy our own values and opinions. Knowing that a long-haired teenager is living 'off the state', we may have a different attitude towards him if he is a student than if he is unemployed. By studying the administrative framework of the social services and the social policies that lie behind them, we can understand ourselves a little more, as well as becoming more effective as citizens, within our professional associations and in relation to those we seek to help.

SOCIAL POLICY AND THE SOCIAL SERVICES

To understand what social policy is, how it is made and how it is likely to develop, helps the health visitor to understand the changes in her own working environment as well as changes in her client's situation. If it is decided that heating allowances are to be more easily obtained by the elderly, the health visitor will worry less about the possibility of hypothermia. If the local authority in whose area she works changes the criteria for the allocation of places in a day nursery, she may find it more difficult to help the categories of family now excluded.

Social policy is difficult to define. 'It is not a technical term with an exact meaning,' explains Marshall (1970) who takes it 'to refer to the policy of governments with regard to action having a direct impact on the welfare of the citizens by providing them with services or income.' These 'services or income' are usually taken to be social security, education, health services, personal social services and housing.

Social policy is closely related to *economic policy*. For example, rapid inflation and high unemployment cause hardship and stress to many families with whom the health visitor is involved—and perhaps to her own family too. Social policy is often constrained by economic policy. From 1976 this constraint was clear: the Government's economic strategy involved reduced public expenditure. One way of distinguishing economic and social action is to think of the way in which the health visitor offers her services to her clients, with no thought of anything given back in exchange. When shopping, she expects to pay for goods received. The social exchange is unilateral, the economic exchange is not. It is necessary to remember that social policy is not necessarily benevolent. Hitler's Germany had policies towards gypsies and mental defectives that would not be condoned today. The psychiatric services in Russia may at times be used against critics of that society.

Social policy is about how much *welfare* the State should provide, how it should be paid for, who should get it and how. Titmuss (1974) gives us three models of social policy in order to explain the functions of social policy. Introducing these he says, 'The purpose of model-building is not to admire the architecture of the building, but to help us see some order in all the disorder and confusion of facts, systems and choices concerning certain areas of our economic and social life'. He calls his first model the 'residual welfare model' of social policy. It is based on the idea of two natural channels through which individual needs are met: the private market (e.g. a job), and the family. Only when these break down should *social services* become involved in meeting need. Those who agree with the ideas behind this model might argue, for example, that children should be financially responsible for their parents. The second model is called by Titmuss the 'industrial achievement performance model'. He describes it as 'holding that social needs should be met on the basis of merit, work performance and productivity'. Supporters of this model would object to the fact that in some circumstances unemployed workers may be able to claim more in social security benefits than they might earn at work. The third model is called the 'institutional redistributive model'. It is based on ideas of *social equality*, including within it ideas about the *redistribution of resources*, with services being provided outside the private market on the *principle of need*.

These models are, then, useful in helping us to sort out our ideas about the job that social policy is trying to do. Supporters of the first and third models have approaches to social policy often known as *selectivist* for the residual model supporters and *universalist* for the institutional model supporters. The selectivist favours a test of the means of those seeking help to ensure resources are not 'wasted' in the sense of being devoted to those who do not need them. Universalists are keen to see services provided as of right, without a means test.

Family Income Supplement is a selectivist social security benefit and Family Allowance virtually universal. We are now seeing a trend towards selecting groups in need. This avoids the *stigma* of asking people to find out about a benefit, come forward and identify themselves as poor and then fill out a form. Instead benefits such as the pension for the over-80s or the mobility allowance for the disabled are based on categories of need and so bestow benefits selectively but without the stigma associated with individual tests of need. The problem remains of making even these benefits known and ensuring all claim entitlement.

The discussion on these different attitudes to welfare and their links with the political left and right, helps us to understand why some aspects of social policy are stressed by one government, and some by another. At an individual level, some may feel the biggest problem of the social services is abuse, perhaps by claiming social security benefits under false pretences (HMSO 1973). Others may be much more concerned at the way in which means-tested benefits are not claimed by those who need them. *The Times* reported in October 1975 that 1 500 000 families were not claiming social security benefits they were entitled to.

The Development of the Social Services
Differing attitudes to the social services reflecting as they do the different interests of various groups within society partly explain the way the services have developed and are developing in Britain. Detailed case studies may help us to understand current changes in specific parts of the social service network and Donnison and his colleagues (1975) examine the strands which help explain how the social services develop. First we need to look at Donnison's definition of the social services as this throws light on his historical analysis. He defines them as:

> not an optional extra or an unproductive frill tacked on to the economy as a charitable afterthought; they are an integral and (in some form or other) a necessary part of an urban, industrial society—forms of collective provision which are required to meet the needs of a changing economy, to protect its citizens and to assure a market for its products. They are developed, differentiated and developed again in accordance with the changing aspirations of those who work in them and those whom they serve (Donnison et al. 1975).

Donnison says the study of the development of social policies reveals many tangled strands—he describes five. The first strand is the *need to provide the environment* necessary for industrial development. The industrial revolution made increasingly clear-cut distinctions between those who worked and those who did not and as the young and the old were gradually excluded from the labour market, the poverty cycle which afflicted children, their parents and the aged was intensified. As new towns developed to house the labour needed by factories, industry needed an environment which included police forces, medical services and housing, initially company provided or supported. Donnison says this strand can still be seen in the way companies offer benefits such as help towards house purchase, or subsidized canteens to improve productivity, reduce absenteeism and help recruitment.

A second strand Donnison introduces is *defence of the nation* against military and economic rivals. The poor physical health of men called upon to fight in the Boer War led to an Interdepartmental Committee on Physical Deterioration and subsequently to provisions such as medical inspection of all children and meals for underfed children. The ill-health of recruits in World War I played a part in hastening the introduction of the maternity and child welfare services. World War II engendered a sense of purpose that found expression in the Beveridge Report (HMSO 1942) and the necessity for collective action during the war made collective action to meet social needs after the war more acceptable.

Donnison's third strand is the *rising expectations* of ordinary people, aspirations often created by the social services themselves. Provision of new services tends to increase the demands made upon it. The provision of free medical care may lower our pain threshold. Need is often perceived only when a service that meets it is available, for example subsidized meals at a luncheon club for the elderly. Unwillingness to tolerate the housing conditions of the previous generations leads to families becoming 'homeless', knowing in the last resort the government must shelter them.

Donnison's fourth strand is that the *prices of services* which are supplied, for example education and medical care, are increasing in cost due to technological factors (i.e. the cost of renal dialysis), and rising labour costs (i.e. the higher pay for nurses after the Halsbury Report, HMSO 1974a). So, says Donnison, 'the development of social services does not hasten the day when people can provide for themselves through the normal mechanism of the market'.

The fifth strand is that the *recruitment and training* of growing numbers and varieties *of workers* play a part in extending and shaping the social services. He writes:

> the commitment of professional groups to the development of their work
> and status has repeatedly led them to demand more and better social

services . . . they have been disturbed by the knowledge that pupils cannot be taught unless they are first fed, that patients cannot be cured unless they are decently housed . . . for their primary responsibility is not to the taxpayer or the organization that employs them, but to their profession and the people whom they serve.

These professions expand, subdivide, multiply. Social workers now work with social work aides, home helps' work with maternity cases was once undertaken by the midwife and district nurses now work with bathing aides.

The Functions of the Social Services

Historians might disagree with these 'strands'. Radical historians prefer to explain the development of the social services in terms of *class antagonism*; the social services having developed to ensure the ruling classes kept their power. Social services have been described by some as the 'new opium of the people', and seen merely as means of social control. Other historians might explain the development of the social services as necessary for the stable development of the state. Views may be influenced not only by attitudes to welfare, but by views of the functions of the individual social services.

Here, Kahn (1973) offers us a useful classification of the functions of social services. He looks at social service functions in three groupings.

1. Firstly, *socialization and development*, where he includes social services which exist to 'protect, change or innovate with respect to many of the educational, child-rearing, value-imparting and social induction activities once assumed by the extended family, the neighbourhood and relatives'. He includes education, day care of children, family planning and even school meals in this grouping.

2. His second grouping is *social services for therapy*, help, rehabilitation and social protection, which would include family casework services, probation service and medical social work.

3. Lastly, he examines *access services*. He sees access not merely as giving information and advice but includes complaints machinery and services that facilitate participation (as do many community groups, such as tenants' associations and claimants' unions).

It may be that society is more ready to find the resources when it needs protection than when it merely wants to improve the knowledge of available services. The conflict within individuals who recognize their desire to spend money on their own individually chosen items, and also want to see improved social services is discussed in the next section of this chapter. It is hard, however, to disagree with Pinker when he writes:

> In the past the pattern of social justice was a product of the tyranny of rich minorities over a mass of poor people. In the future the persistence of injustice in our kind of society is more likely to arise from the indifference of a relatively prosperous majority to the welfare needs of a minority of poor people. . . . The real test of a civilized society is the degree of decency with which it treats its minorities irrespective of their lack of effective political power (Pinker 1974).

The Problem of Defining Need

Although we see the social services as having been developed to meet a wide range of human needs, the word '*need*' itself is hard to define. In ordinary conversation, we often say we 'need' when we simply mean 'want'. Bradshaw (1972) distinguished four definitions of need.

He first looks at *normative need*, which is what the professional would define as need in a given situation. He gives as an example the British Medical Association's nutritional standard used as a measure of the adequacy of diet. He reminds us that experts can disagree and that normative standards change over time because of developments in knowledge and changes in the values of society. Sometimes experts find it difficult to agree! If we take suspected child abuse as an example, we find social workers anxious to meet the child's needs by working to strengthen parental ties, while a health visitor might feel the child's needs would be best met away from the home environment. Increased understanding about possible contributory factors towards child abuse and the change in values and expectations of society in response to growing publicity, bring changes in definition of the needs of children. The need for a coordinated approach between health and social services is being promoted by the government and this involves the exchange of information between different agencies which might now take precedence over the previous stress on the need for confidentiality.

Bradshaw's second definition is *felt need* which is equated with want. This is a subjective definition. He sees this as an inadequate measure being limited by the knowledge and perceptions of the individual. People will not express a need for a service unless they know it exists: the disabled person unaware that he might obtain financial help from the local authority to adapt his home to make it more suitable, is unlikely to approach his local authority for such help. Bradshaw also mentions those who know there is a service but are reluctant to confess the loss of independence that asking for help implies: the low 'take up' of means-tested benefits like free schools meals and Family Income Supplement are examples of this. Bradshaw also reminds us that felt need might be inflated by those who ask for help without really needing it.

His third definition (similar to his second), is *expressed need* or *demand*. This is felt need turned into action as people demand a service. Whilst a service may not be requested unless a need is felt, it is common for felt need not to be expressed by demand. Expressed need is used in the health services, where hospital waiting lists are taken as a measure of unmet need, although as screening results show, it could be argued that such measures are not good definitions of 'real need'. The size of hospital waiting lists may depend more on the interpretation of the doctor concerned than the subjective feelings of the patient.

Lastly, Bradshaw identifies *comparative need*, found by studying the characteristics of those in receipt of a service and people with similar characteristics who are not in receipt of that same service. It is possible to argue that those not receiving the service are in need on a comparative basis. This definition is linked to the first, often depending on the views of professional people. One might compare the waiting list for council housing with one area and another and find the better endowed area still full of severe housing problems, as this definition of need cannot guarantee that provision is high enough to meet need. For individuals, Bradshaw's example is the attempt to complete a register of babies in need of special attention from the preventive services, on the basis of conditions such as forceps delivery or birth to older mothers.

Bradshaw's article then goes on to explain the significance of looking for need within all his four interrelated categories. Research workers, by producing evidence of these kinds of need, can help policy makers. He admits there are no easy solutions but argues decisions could be made on more clearly defined criteria than they often are if there was a more careful attempt to define need. This would be as true of planning a new service such as provisions for battered wives, as assessing need for services where supply is far short of demand, such as day nursery provision.

In a mixed economy like Britain, not all social needs are met by the social services. Housing 'need' is only relevant when the individual or family lacks the resources to satisfy their housing needs on the private market. The elderly lady who can employ a companion or pay for a hotel room does not need a home help or a bed in a local authority residential home.

Forder, discussing need, says that defining need is the crucial problem for the social services in that it defines the objects of the service. Need implies a goal, a measurable deficiency and a means of achieving the goal. He outlines five approaches to need ending with a discussion about national need which includes the economic and social framework in which social needs develop. The individual approach to meeting individual need may be no more than a palliative. He sees the development of the welfare state as 'the story of the gradual recognition of the importance for the nation of positive policies with regard to social and economic need, and widening of the concept of national need to include the welfare of all citizens and inhabitants of the national territory' (Forder 1974).

Meeting the needs of one group may conflict with the needs of another group, as illustrated by the opposition to the opening of a residential home for mentally handicapped adults in a middle-class suburb or a higher taxation to reduce inequalities in society. This kind of conflict is relevant to the discussion of public expenditure and social planning, which follows.

Public Expenditure and Social Planning

Whether, as an individual, one wants to increase or reduce spending on the social services relates to the attitudes to welfare discussed earlier in this chapter. Those seeing social service provision as an integral part of citizenship may seek to increase spending on the social services; those seeing the services as reducing the self reliance and independence of the population at large may well want to reduce it. But the economic circumstances of the moment are crucial in determining the amount of money that will be spent on social services. Inflation hits everyone, whether spending personal earnings or spending on behalf of the community: everyone gets less for money, although some suffer more as price increases differ on different items. As Isserlis reminds us:

> Although social policy is not always about money or money's worth, a lot of it is, and those who take part in the debate do well to remind themselves that the debate is about choice and that much of the choice is about who should spend how much of the community's total resources on what; how and at the expense of what else (see Klein 1974).

All that Britain produces and earns in a year is known as the Gross National Product (GNP). The percentage of the GNP that central and local government has been spending has risen rapidly during this century from 12.7 per cent in 1910, to 57 per cent in 1974. Within the overall increase in public expenditure there have been different growth rates. Between 1951 and 1973, expenditure on health grew fivefold, on social security payments sevenfold and on education, tenfold. The ways in which public funds are spent are clearly shown in Fig. 3.

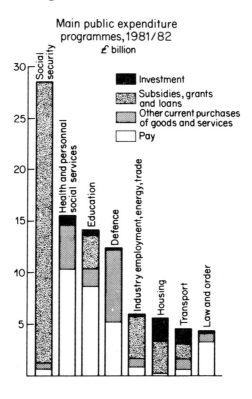

Fig. 3. Main public expenditure programmes 1981/2.
(Source: Economic Progress Report No. 135. July 1981. Published by the Treasury.)

The reasons why public expenditure increases vary, demographic factors being very important. Not only do longer life expectancy and technological advances in medicine keep the very handicapped alive longer, but also the number of elderly people, who make the most demands on the health, social service and social security provisions, is growing at a faster rate than the population in general. There were 6.6 million people over retirement age in 1951, and 9.4 million in 1979. Demand for housing is influenced by the rapid increase in the number of households. Longer life plays a part here too, as do increasing marriage and divorce rates, and the tendency of young people to set up independent households at an earlier age than a generation ago. The larger population is more willing than before to make use of the services offered, as the stigma associated with social service provision under the Poor Law leaves people's memories.

This rapid rise in demand is particularly marked in further and higher education which is a very expensive service. Health visitors may wonder at the contrast between this growth and the slow rise in provision for the under-fives. Population structure plays a part and the ability of students and the parents of potential students to argue for increases in higher education is stronger than that of mothers in deprived areas to argue for day care facilities for their children.

The cost of social services has risen, not only because of rising demands but because the public expect higher material standards in schools, hospitals and public housing. Obviously the workhouse had to be replaced by purpose-built homes for the elderly and the hospital building programme was long overdue when it began in 1962. The cost of the growing numbers working in public employment is increasing and public service pay has begun to match that of the private employee.

Between 1961 and 1973 central government employees grew by 14 per cent and local government staff by 53 per cent. These changes reflect new demands on local authorities (e.g. as a result of legislation such as the Chronically Sick and Disabled Act and new powers under the Rent Acts), as well as increased demand. The supply of a service at local level leads to demands as felt needs are recognized and become expressed needs, and there is a gap between the demands made on the social services and the resources available. As price is rarely involved, demands are not reduced by higher charges but by other methods of 'rationing'. The rationing can take place where the services are delivered, as when the overstretched general practitioners or health visitors give less time to a patient than they would like. It is seen in the increased employment of unqualified supportive staff, such as welfare assistants or social work aides in social service departments, also in lengthening waiting lists for minor surgery and/or public housing (Parker 1975).

It is easy to see the problems of those in control of allocating resources between different services, both at central and local government level. This applies also to the Treasury which makes the key decision about the percentage of the GNP personally kept for consumption or investment and the amount the government spends. When public expenditure is rising, there is bargaining between the spending ministries for their share of the national 'cake', just as there is bargaining to preserve their 'slices' when that cake is being reduced in size. Once the amount of central government grant to local government is known, plans for local services are then balanced with resources available at the local government level. The elected representatives, the councillors, advised by their professional officers, must take account not only of the needs they see around them and the views of fieldwork staff but also the limits they feel the ratepayers will tolerate and the views of local pressure groups, for example Gingerbread.

In a period of limited public expenditure, the need for re-appraisal of existing expenditure is even more acute. There are some who argue that cuts are 'good' for those responsible for running services, as they are made aware of the need to spend more effectively, which could produce a shift in spending away from institutional care and into community care.

We tend to find that spending on existing services continues, whilst newer needs, like those of the battered wife, or unpopular needs like those of the methylated spirit drinker, may be left to voluntary bodies or just ignored.

As ministers argue for their slice of cake (as do local authority chairmen of committees) certain pressures are exerted which influence the decisions being made, such as civil service advice and *pressure group* activities. Some pressure groups might be essential to the smooth running of a service and yet conflict: for example, the British Medical Association and the National Union of Public Employees. Public opinion is often judged through television and press reporting and individuals of outstanding ability who start pressure groups (such as the late Megan du Boisson who started the Disablement Income Group) can arouse public opinion which is useful when funds are being sought for particular groups in need. Professional groups who argue for their clients and not themselves have a particularly important role to play. Some would argue only economic growth can solve these problems, while others would prefer a growth of private provision for those willing and able to spend. Again some prefer charges as a means of reducing demand, while others argue that the inequalities of wealth and income that we see around us show that there is room for genuine redistribution of resources in the provision of social services.

It is difficult to plan for the future of the social services. There are those who would argue that a rational approach would ignore pressure groups instead of analysing all relevant factors to find the 'best solution' to a particular problem. Others see planning simply as seeking small changes: moving slowly from what exists towards what might be, accepting a balance between that goal, and what is feasible in terms of resources and the political constraints operating in a democratic society. Sometimes any attempt at planning disappears, and the government responds quickly to strong pressure and media attention, as in the case of money made available as the findings about Ely Hospital became known in 1969 (HMSO 1969).

Having read this section you may now be interested to read further about this important area, and to think out for yourself how you might like to rearrange the income and spending of the 'public expenditure pound'. Further discussion on the management problems of the social services is recorded by Brown (1973).

THE ADMINISTRATION OF THE SOCIAL SERVICES

This section aims to show something of the scope of the social services in Britain and the way they are organized.

Table 2 distinguishes three tiers of administration. At the top level there are the government departments, headed by politicians (members of the Cabinet), assisted by other politicians who are ministers of state. The Cabinet, with politicians advised by the civil service, decides the overall policy which determines what the different departments can and cannot do, or spend.

Civil servants administer one important service directly; that is, social security. The same amount of benefits must be paid out, and the same approach to claimants in need should be established throughout the country. Local government implements policies in a way that applies national legislation to fit local needs and priorities and this can lead to very wide variations in quality and quantity of provision between local authorities.

The government appoints the members of the ad hoc bodies (specially set up as opposed to elected) which administer the National Health Service and the universities.

Table 2. The organization of the social services

	Department of Health and Social Security	Home Office	Department of Education and Science	Department of Employment	Department of Environment
Central government	Health, welfare and Social Security. National Insurance Supplementary benefits, War Pensions, Industrial Disablement, Family Income Supplement, Mobility Allowance: network of local offices	Community Development, Urban Aid. Delinquent adults, prisons, courts, police, legal aid, police, probation service. Some juvenile delinquency. Anti-discrimination legislation–women, race relations. Community relations. Immigration/aliens	Policy in all sectors of education	Disablement resettlement officer, retraining, unemployment benefit/job finding, regional policy. Manpower Services Commission (youth opportunity schemes etc.)	Oversight of local government functions, finance. Land and housing policy, planning including appeals
Ad hoc bodies	*National Health Service* *Bodies* include RHAs and AHAs, family practitioner committees, community health councils.		University Grants Commission		

	Services	*Social Services Department*	*Local Education Authorities*	*Housing Departments*	*Planning Departments*
Local government	include hospital and specialist services; dental, pharmaceutical and G.P. Ambulances, health centres, domiciliary nursing and midwifery, health visitors, school health, maternity and child welfare, health education, vaccination	Residential, day and community care including homes, hostels, day centres, clubs, social work support, home helps, meals-on-wheels, occupational therapy, social work in hospitals. For elderly, deprived children, mentally disordered, under-fives physically handicapped	Schools, special schools, educational welfare, colleges of education, further and higher education, including polytechnics. Student grants, adult education, youth service. Where relevant to local area: help to community relations councils, applications for urban aid, help to community development projects	(now 400, before 1974, 1000) Council housing – building, allocation, management. Improvement grants, rent rebates and allowances, rent officers. Housing advice, mortgages.	Overall planning and applications

Local government is close to those for whom the services are designed, but central government exercises a great deal of control over its activities. Controlling local government expenditure is an important part of government's overall economic strategy. Local authorities can only provide services if Parliament allows them to. An Act of Parliament may make it a statutory responsibility for a local authority to do something (such as provide education for children from 5 to 16) or make it permissive for them to do something if they choose, such as providing swimming pools. Central government grants made up 51 per cent of local government expenditure in 1981–2 (out of a total budget of £28 200 million). Central government makes some specific grants towards particular services, such as the police force. The larger amount of grant is the Rate Support Grant.

Central government controls over local government expenditure have grown rapidly since the mid-1970s. By 1981 strict cash limits to capital spending were in operation, and it was illegal to spend more than specified sums. Rate Support Grant since 1981 has been based on central government's assumptions on what local authorities should spend. If more is spent, central government grants are reduced, forcing local authorities to raise more by higher rates. Further controls on rate rises were under discussion by the end of 1981.

The government might send circulars advising local authorities on particular policies, such as one asking them to cooperate with health authorities in the setting up of area review committees for cases of suspected child abuse. Overall, the economic situation and the policies of the government in power are particularly important factors explaining the balance between central control and local authority freedom at any one point in time.

The maintenance of full employment is an important part of government policy and relevant aspects of the work of the Department of Employment include retraining schemes, improving the image of the job-finding services, and offering specialist advice to the disabled through the disablement resettlement officer. The Home Office has a wide range of functions and those concerned with penal policy and with community relations are of most interest to health visitors.

Social Security and the Problem of Poverty
The social security system is designed to maintain income when it is

interrupted (e.g. by sickness) or stops (e.g. through death of the breadwinner or retirement). There are two major kinds of benefit. The National Insurance benefits are decided upon in terms of a person's contribution record. Benefits include maternity grant, sickness and unemployment benefit, as well as retirement benefit and death grant.

For those who have not contributed, who have been unemployed for over a year or who cannot manage on the National Insurance benefits, there is the Supplementary Benefits Scheme which was known until 1966 as National Assistance. A means test is administered, either at the social security office or in the claimant's home, to establish income, savings and needs before deciding on eligibility and the amount to be paid. Apart from regular weekly payments, special allowances may be paid to cover additional heating costs or special diets in particular situations. Grants may be made to meet exceptional needs, such as the replacement of clothes.

From 1948 until 1976, the universal Family Allowance was payable for the second and subsequent children only. From April 1976 the Family Allowance became payable for the first child of the single parent and this was the first step in changing to a scheme which would benefit all children (child benefit).

There are other social security benefits. The low wage earner working at least 30 hours a week may be able to claim Family Income Supplement. The Attendance Allowance and Mobility Allowance are of particular interest to the disabled and to those looking after disabled adults and children.

Social security staff are civil servants who do not choose to operate the social security system, but choose a career in the civil service and are then told where the vacancies are. They have a difficult job. Claimants are usually apprehensive and sometimes aggressive. The schemes are complex to administer and very difficult to explain to the claimants who are often vulnerable, deprived and desperate.

When health visitors find their clients have financial difficulties it is important to advise them to contact the local social security office to see if they can be helped. A useful booklet called *Which Benefit?*, known as FB2, is available free from social security offices for members of the helping professions in contact with the public. It is revised regularly.

There is a large range of other means-tested benefits. Outside the scope of the social security system itself, there is relief from paying prescription charges or a family may be entitled to free school meals or a uniform grant. Council tenants may be entitled to rent rebates, private tenants to rent allowances and both to rate rebates.

An individual's basic attitude to welfare will determine overall attitudes to social security. Some are most concerned with possible

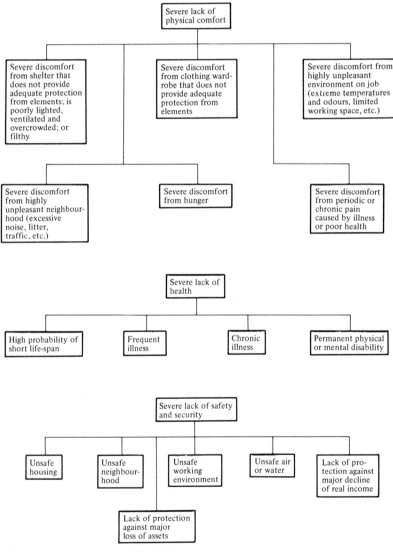

Fig. 4. Sub-dimensions of poverty.

abuse and would prefer to see more selective, means-tested, benefits introduced (HMSO 1973). Others are more worried about the lack of use of benefits due to ignorance and the fear of stigmatization. The low level of social security benefits means living at a level which

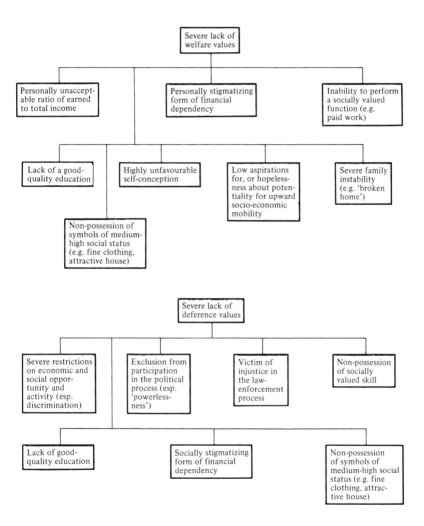

Fig. 4. (*continued*). Source: Baratz, M.S. and Grigsby, W.G. (1972).

is hardly a comfortable life-style. Large numbers of retirement pensioners claim Supplementary Benefit in addition to the retirement pension and as unemployment rises, more and more people are relying on social security provision. Inflation makes it harder than ever to manage, although at the time of writing benefits are reviewed annually.

In the years following the introduction of the social security scheme in the late 1940s and early 1950s it was thought poverty would disappear. However, research from the mid-1950s onwards has shown this is not so. Low wages continue to play a continuing role in poverty, especially where young children or a shortage of jobs prevents the wife from earning. The growing numbers of one-parent families contribute to the numbers living at the poverty level, as do the fact that our very definition of poverty is changing.

Poverty itself is too complex a concept to deal with briefly but its relative nature compared to the average standard of living, and its cumulative effects, will be obvious to any practising health visitors. The Social Science Research Council (1968) summarized the main categories and causes of poverty, as follows.

1. *Crisis poverty*. Hardships following directly from bereavement, injury or unemployment.
2. *Long-term dependency*. Where people never recover from such a crisis, or perhaps are born disabled.
3. *Life cycle poverty* affects people during childhood, in parenthood when their own children are young stopping the wife working, and then during old age.
4. *Depressed area poverty*. There are regions like the North East which are left behind as old industries decline and new industries are slow to take their place.
5. *Down-town poverty*. Describes the pattern which appears in many cities, with investment tending to concentrate on the suburbs and commercial centres, leaving whole parts of the central city with decaying housing, poor schools and so on.
6. This category suggests a combination of financial hardship, squalid environment, family structure and personal relationships producing a life-style making it hard for the families to escape from poverty.

A further complication for the low wage earner is the *poverty trap*. Because of the growth of means-tested benefits, when a low-paid worker with dependants receives a rise in wages it can be an actual loss in real terms. A small rise of £4 or £5 can be lost as income tax becomes payable, National Insurance contribution rises and the family may lose free school meals, part of their Family Income Supplement, part of a rent rebate and so on.

It is important not to see poverty only as low income. It can be more realistically thought about along several different dimensions. This wider way of looking at poverty is well illustrated in Fig. 4, which was drawn up by two American sociologists (Baratz & Grigsby 1972).

HOUSING

In many parts of the country, housing is likely to be the biggest problem facing those whom health visitors help and advise. Not only is family housing in short supply, but also are community facilities for the mentally ill, sheltered housing for the elderly and purpose-built accommodation for the disabled. Since the war the number of dwellings owned by their occupiers has risen to over half the total. Local authority housing now accounts for about one-third of the total number of dwellings and the private landlord's role is shrinking fast. A growing number of people who would like to buy their own home now find this difficult as house prices have risen rapidly and so have mortgage interest rates. Competition for the shrinking number of privately rented flats is fierce, with rents high and conditions often poor.

This leaves the local authority housing departments to fill the gap between supply and demand. They have no responsibility for those without children, except the elderly and handicapped. The extent to which local authorities build council housing is partly related to local policy (Alfred & Boaden 1973). Local authorities may add to their stock of housing by the destruction of existing buildings and the redevelopment of an area in the larger cities.

Local authority housing departments keep waiting lists of those in housing need who have been resident within that area for a certain length of time, but rehousing from the list is slow, particularly in large cities. This is partly because priority goes to those whose housing is required for redevelopment and partly because of the help that is given to homeless families. Policy and practices vary greatly from one local authority to another and certainly those accepted as homeless families and accommodated, are only a small proportion of those in acute housing need. Of the 48 750 children received into care in 1978, 13 per cent were admitted due to homelessness or unsatisfactory home conditions.

Homelessness is a reflection of the cost and the shortage of housing. It is not a problem facing people uniformly over the country: nearly half the officially recognized homeless families are newcomers to an area; others have been evicted (although the numbers of evictions are reduced as more tenants are now covered by legislation granting security of tenure).

Another reason for homelessness is family disputes. This might mean parents who are unable to tolerate married children living with them, or marital disputes. It would be essential for a health visitor to find out how the local authority housing department operates and how the badly housed and homeless are helped. Unfortunately, housing has been the service most affected by public expenditure cuts, whilst at the same time, the economic recession has reduced the amount of private house building.

EDUCATION PROVISION

Local authorities have a responsibility to provide school places for children aged from 5 to 16 within their boundaries. Since the 1944 Education Act, the emphasis in secondary education has slowly moved away from selection at 11, which resulted in either success and the grammar school, or failure and the secondary modern school. Because local government can interpret central government policy to suit local needs and wishes, this trend has not been smooth. Many parents have been indifferent; some have organized themselves into pressure groups to fight for comprehensive education. The 1964 Labour Government sent local authorities a circular asking them to produce plans for comprehensive schools and whilst many councils did produce plans, Conservative councils that had not done so welcomed the withdrawal of that circular by the newly elected Conservative Government in 1970. In 1975 the Labour Government decided to draw up legislation for comprehensive schools; the 1979 Conservative Government subsequently repealed that Act.

Some argue that comprehensive schools reduce choice, others that for the 80 per cent who were labelled 'failures' at 11, there never was a choice! Many of the problems thought to arise from comprehensive schools reflect the problems of a society changing its values—becoming less authoritarian for example. In the deprived areas of the inner city the school can have little influence on correcting the inequalities from which so many children suffer (Field 1973; see also Chapter 5).

One effect of the ending of the eleven-plus examination has been to reduce the pressures on primary schools, as it was no longer necessary to gear the curriculum to the demands of an examination at 11. It removed stress from young children and widened the opportunities available to all young people as they progressed through their secondary schooling.

Provision for children under five is divided between nursery schools and nursery classes provided or supervised by the social services department. The major sources of provision at present are not the day nurseries but playgroups or child minders and quality and quantity vary. Local authorities make special provision for children with special needs, e.g. the educationally subnormal, maladjusted and physically handicapped. Legislation implementing proposals for a more integrated approach to the education of children with special needs was being discussed in 1981, following publication of the Warnock Report in 1978.

THE HEALTH AND WELFARE SERVICES

The National Health Service and the personal social services are two closely related services, separate examination being necessary as they are separately staffed, financed and organized, although it is difficult to define the line which separates a health from a welfare problem. Health visitors are the occupational group most closely involved in bridging the health and welfare gap and those entering the service now might well, within their working lives, see further reorganization to integrate the services more closely.

The National Health Service

Health provision in Britain before 1948 was complex. Hospitals were provided by local authorities or voluntary bodies. There were enormous variations in quantity and quality of hospital provision, with voluntary hospitals the most likely to treat the private patient and the individual with insurance cover. For general practitioner services, some workers were insured but in most schemes wives and children were not covered at all. Local authorities were responsible for 'public health' services such as maternity and child health services.

When the Beveridge Report was published in 1942 (HMSO 1942), it recommended the setting up of a comprehensive health service. Just as the new social security scheme would conquer the giant of 'Want', so a health service was needed to conquer the giant of 'Disease'. Beveridge envisaged that the health service would cost less money as the health of the nation improved: but for reasons we shall discuss later, this was not to be.

The National Health Service Act was passed in 1946 and the service went into operation in 1948. It aimed to establish a national comprehensive health service, securing improvements in the physical and mental health of the population and concerned with prevention, diagnosis and treatment. It was to be financed out of general taxation—a crucially important decision. It was this that enabled the British medical services to become truly comprehensive, treating people on the basis of need, not ability to pay or membership of insurance schemes.

The pattern of the National Health Service organization between 1948 and 1974 is shown in Fig. 5. There were changes that followed

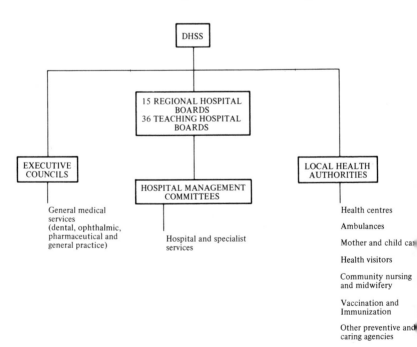

Fig. 5. The NHS structure before reorganization (Office of Health Economics 1975).

the setting up of the Social Services Department in 1971 in that local health authorities lost responsibilities in relation to mental health and children under five as well as the home help service.

The 1948 organization was the result of compromise, partly related to the medical care services that preceded the National Health Service and partly because of the need to ensure the cooperation of doctors who were then, as now, the most powerful of all professional groups. The story of the creation of the NHS is a fascinating one, well told in a short book by Wilcocks (1967).

The National Health Service was like a three-legged stool, and we shall look quickly now at the functions of those three 'legs' of the tripartite system.

Services administered by the executive councils General practitioners' services were free to patients and patients could be seen at either home or surgery, once having registered. The general practitioner had an independent contractor status with the executive council, an 'ad hoc' body on which the professions had 50 per cent representation. The pay and fees of all the professions contracted to the executive council (they also administered the ophthalmic, pharmaceutical and dental services) came directly from the Ministry of Health (later the Department of Health and Social Security). Because of their horror of a salaried service the general practitioners were paid out of a pool which was related to size of list which did not encourage good standards of practice. After 1966 the payment system changed with a larger element of standardized payment, seniority payments linked to postgraduate courses and 70 per cent reimbursement on money spent on improving practices including employment of staff such as receptionists and practice nurses. This raised the standards of most practices gradually, as did the gradual move towards group practice. Yet there was in some practices the fresh barrier to patient–doctor contact represented by the receptionist.

The hospitals The hospital services were then run for the Ministry by 'ad hoc' bodies, the regional hospital boards, appointed by the Minister, grouped into 14 regions and managed either separately, but usually in groups, by hospital management committees. The members of these committees were also appointed, but consultation with local authorities meant some local councillors were members. Teaching hospitals were separately managed under their own boards of governors.

Local health authorities The local health authorities had a wide range of functions, as listed in Fig. 5. They were given additional responsibility after 1959 for the community care of the mentally ill. As in all local authority services, there were variations in quantity and quality of service. Each local health authority was headed by a medical officer of health who was a doctor with additional qualifications in public health. Health visitors were local health authority employees until reorganization. Before going on to look at some of the criticism made of the tripartite system, it is useful to look at five main areas of change between 1948 and 1974 that affected medical care.

1. Demography The population is growing—from 48 million in 1954 to 56 million in 1976. The percentage of those aged over 75 in the population rose from 1.3 million in 1941 to 2.8 million in 1974. The elderly make the heaviest demands on the health services and these heavier demands are a significant factor in explaining the rising costs of the National Health Service.

2. Technological change Advances in technology have played a large part in keeping people alive longer. The drug revolution in the sphere of mental illness is equally important. With the drastic reduction in deaths from infectious diseases due to prevention and the development of modern drugs, people live longer—long enough to contract the disabling diseases to which the elderly are most prone. Those who are born or become disabled, victims of accidents and the mentally subnormal are other groups now living longer due to drugs and other developments. Techniques such as dialysis and open heart surgery which keep alive those who might otherwise die are expensive. The use of expensive diagnostic equipment is growing (and is not without its critics, Teeling-Smith 1976).

3. Changing ideas about health The definition of health is one that varies, subjectively, from one person to another and from one doctor to another and our pain threshold seems lower than that of the previous generation. There is a cost to the community when demands are made on the National Health Service as there is economic significance in the days lost from work due to sickness. Demands for health care may suddenly rise because a service becomes available (e.g. renal dialysis) or because a particular treatment receives a lot of publicity in the press (e.g. hormone replacement therapy).

There is also the trend which has seen social problems being turned into medical episodes with help sought from a doctor. Housing or marital problems may well be met with prescriptions for tranquillizers when the problem is not necessarily a medical one and doctors may see such consultations as a waste of time but fail to refer them to other agencies. The medicalization of social problems is discussed in a provocative and stimulating way by Illich (1975).

4. Changing workload Increasing numbers of elderly people, those who contract disabling diseases and those who survive accidents change the role of those involved in medical care. From becoming people who cure and treat, they become people who care and alleviate. Although this is just as important a role for the patient, it may appear less satisfying to some of the caring personnel, for example the status of the consultant surgeon compared unfavourably with that of the consultant geriatrician.

5. Growing awareness of inequalities within the National Health Service There are wide differences in the spending of different regions and these inequalities were at the time of writing being investigated by a departmental working party, aiming progressively to reduce the disparities between the different parts of the country in terms of opportunity for access to health care of people at equal risk, taking into account measures of health need and social and environmental factors. The effect of the recommendations of the working party will be felt slowly, but they are a beginning in the direction of correcting these regional inequalities.

Inequalities can also be seen in terms of social class. The infant mortality rates are higher in social classes IV and V than in the higher social classes, I and II (Townsend 1974). The regions receiving the lower amounts of money are those with higher proportions of people from the lower socioeconomic groups.

A third way of looking at inequalities is to examine the differential treatment of those in the acute hospital and those in the chronic wards. The comparison between the standards of staff and housekeeping in wards for acute patients and those for the mentally subnormal is marked. The disadvantageous situation found in geriatric and other long-stay facilities is commented on frequently in the annual reports of the multidisciplinary Hospital Advisory Service (HMSO, Annual Report).

These background problems affecting the demands for and

supply of medical care in the years after the foundation of the National Health Service form a background to the criticism made of the tripartite system. In this period the percentage of the gross national product spent on the Service varied, rising from 3.87 per cent in 1951 to 4.7 per cent in 1979, when the cost of the Service rose to over £7284 million. The Service employs about one million staff and as pay, as well as working conditions in terms of hours and holidays, improve, the supply side is going to continue to cost more, whatever happens to the demand side of the equation.

Criticism of the tripartite system The divided administrative and financial responsibility of the three parts of the National Health Service was the root of most of the criticism. This led to gaps and overlap in terms of services available, discontinuity of care for patients and inflexible use of staff. Coordination on behalf of the patient was difficult. The service was dominated by the hospital services, as is shown in Fig. 6—although it is important to remember that the hospital service, by expanding throughout, which involved heavier workloads for staff, especially in surgical wards, helped to keep costs lower than they would otherwise have been. The consumer had no say in the way the service was run, apart from the Patients' Association, a small voice trying to speak for all patients.

Efforts to overcome some of these problems were, however, being made. Joint appointments of social workers, whose pay was shared between the NHS and the local health authority (later social services departments) helped to integrate social work care, especially for the mentally ill, in some areas. The attachment of district nurses and health visitors to general practitioners' teams is another example of action taken before reorganization to coordinate care at the patient's level. The growth of health centres, from about 20 in 1964 to about 600 in 1976, was also important in integrating services, but these efforts were spasmodic and unevenly spread around the country, and the arguments for reorganization were widely accepted by politicians and the public as well as National Health Service employees (Office of Health Economics 1975).

The 1964 to 1970 Labour Government produced two Green Papers—publications aimed to stimulate discussion—about National Health Service reorganization with proposals for reorganization of the health service at the same time as reorganizing local government and creating the social service departments. A change of government in 1970 meant delays in the formulation of new policies.

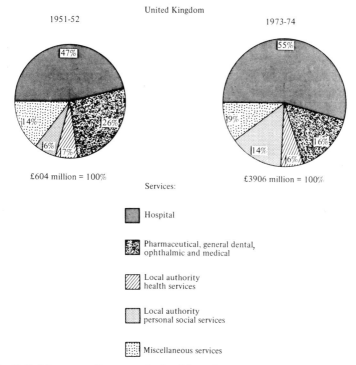

Fig. 6. Public expenditure on the health and social services. Source: HMSO (1975)

The latest NHS reorganization (1982) is discussed at the end of this section.

The Reorganized National Health Service

The pattern of the reorganized NHS is shown in Fig. 7. The reorganization is based on ideas put forward in a Consultative Document published in 1971 followed by a White Paper of 1972 and an Act of 1973. Some services were left outside the unified service, including the occupational health service which is under the auspices of the Department of Employment, and the environmental health services under the local authorities.

The aims were to ensure integrated planning of all health services within unified geographical areas and closer coordination of health service and social service planning. In so doing, it was hoped to

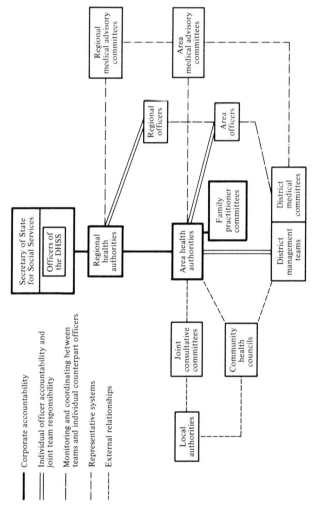

Fig. 7.   The reorganized National Health Service, 1974–82 (HMSO 1972).

ensure a reallocation of resources from hospital-based to community-based medical care. This would provide for the growing numbers of elderly people in the community and be in line with the philosophy of community care that groups such as the mentally ill, the disabled and the mentally subnormal should live in the community wherever possible. This aim might well be the most difficult to achieve, as over 66 per cent of the total costs of the health service in the mid-1970s was going to hospital services, while many of the resources needed for community care facilities came out of the budget of social service departments.

The National Health Service then contained three major tiers. It was hoped that reorganization would achieve maximum delegation downwards and maximum accountability upwards. There were 14 regional health authorities providing the services shown in Fig. 8 and having overall responsibility for allocating the resources made available to them by the DHSS. The 15 members of the regional health authority were appointed by the Secretary of State and these lay policy makers were supported by a team of regional officers.

There were 90 area health authorities whose boundaries corresponded to the new units of local government which were formed in 1974. Their boundaries corresponded to metropolitan districts, to non-metropolitan counties and to groups of London boroughs. Area health authorities usually had 15 members, 4 appointed on the recommendations of the local authority and the rest chosen by the regional health authorities. The chairman, who received a payment, was chosen by the Secretary of State. In areas with teaching hospitals there were two additional members. Figure 9 shows the make-up of the area management team and the responsibilities of its members.

A major responsibility of the area health authority was to assess needs, plan, organize and administer the medical services within its boundaries. Particularly important was the responsibility to ensure that their own services and the social services of the local authorities were organized in a way that was complementary, avoiding some of the gaps and overlaps of the previous system. Apart from the fact that some of the AHA members were local authority councillors, joint consultative committees were set up. These ensured that discussion and therefore coordination of policies would take place. In non-metropolitan counties, relevant services such as housing and environmental health were administered on a lower administrative tier than social services, so different patterns of joint consultative committees were being organized and health visitors needed to find

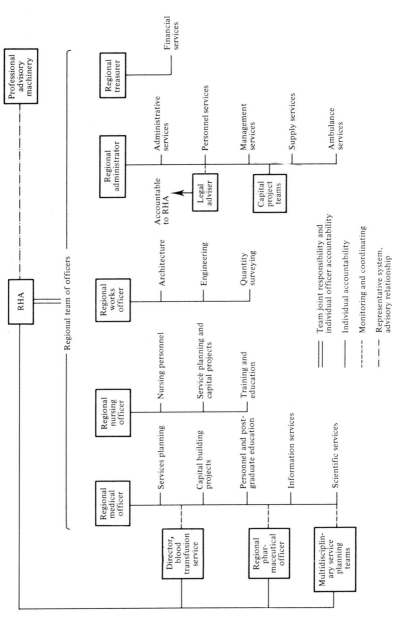

Fig. 8.   The regional health authority (Office of Health Economics 1975).

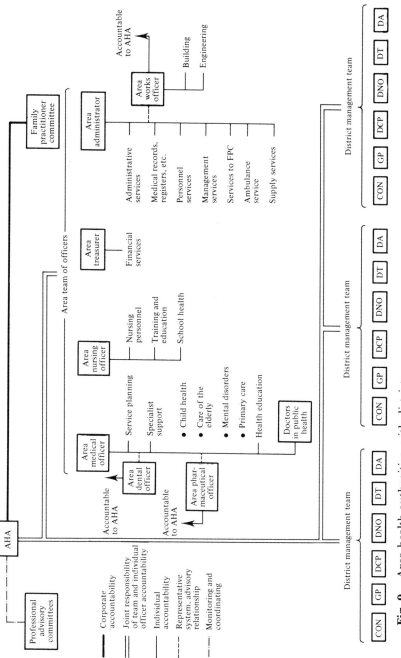

Fig. 9. Area health authorities, with districts.

out the pattern in their own areas. This was a vital committee to enable health and social services to work closer together.

The area health authorities employed most of the National Health Service staff, although many actually worked at district level, and they arranged the finance and staff for the family practitioner committees. These committees were similar in functions and composition to the former executive councils, responsible for the independent contractors—general practitioners, pharmacists, dentists and ophthalmic personnel. The family practitioner committee had 30 members, half appointed by local representative committees of the professions (8 doctors, 3 dentists, 2 pharmacists, an ophthalmic medical practitioner and a dispensing optician). The 15 lay members were divided between 11 area health authority appointments and 4 local authority appointments. Each family practitioner committee had many subcommittees, some concerned with ensuring that the professional groups did not break conditions of service.

The area medical officer played a key role in the provision of medical care in the district and in the building up of an effective health education service.

Small area health authorities covered only one district but others covered up to six districts. Figure 10 shows the shape of the district services. There were no lay people at the district level and the district management team was responsible for health care planning and coordination. The district management team consisted of four officers who ran their own services within the district, plus two medical practitioners elected by the district medical committee—one a GP, the other a consultant. Officers of the district management team were not meant to be subordinate to the area officers, but provide them with information and advice. However, should the district management team be unable to make a collective decision on any issue, it was passed to the area health authority to be resolved.

The average district had a population of 250 000 and the main health care groups within that average district were approximately as follows.

60 000 children of whom 500 were physically handicapped and 200 severely mentally handicapped.

35 000 people aged over 65; 4500 of them severely or appreciably physically handicapped. About 800 in hospital at any one time and a similar number in old people's homes. A further 1000 would require domiciliary services.

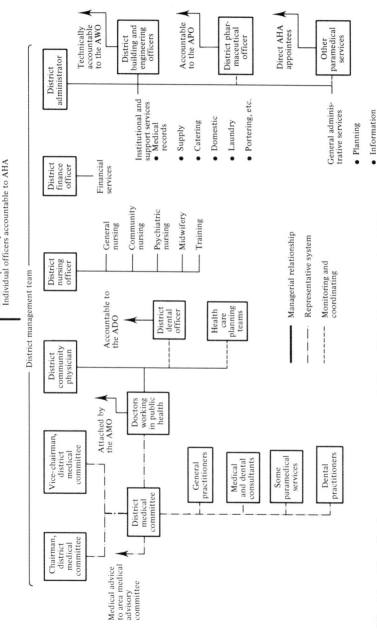

Fig. 10. The district management team (Office of Health Economics 1975).

2000 severely or appreciably physically handicapped people of working age living in the community.

About 700 people officially classified as severely mentally handicapped of whom over half would be living outside hospitals. About 300 were likely to be hospital in-patients.

Around 2500 people thought of as being mentally ill and in contact with hospitals. Of these nearly 600 would be in-patients at any one time.

About 19 000 people would need acute medical or surgical care each year as hospital in-patients, about 550 of them being in hospital at any one time (HMSO 1972).

Although districts were the most important level for the consumer, they were the level of the new National Health Service where the concept of boundaries coterminous with local authority boundaries broke down. When the boundaries were discussed at local level, hospital catchment areas rather than social service links sometimes took priority. This means that in London, for example, district boundaries could cut through London boroughs.

District officers manage and coordinate services within their localities and help to formulate plans for the future. Members of the district management team participate in the planning sequence, identifying needs and then asking for the resources to meet them. The claims from district level go to area and then regional level involving continuous consultation rather than imposition of the views of the higher tiers. Implementation of plans ultimately depends on the resources allocated nationally to the National Health Service by the Department of Health and Social Security.

Two important groupings at district level were the health care planning teams and the community health council. Several health care planning teams were set up in each district. They focus on particular patient groups, such as the mentally ill or the young chronic sick, and by drawing in a wide range of professionals involved in the care of the group, integrate provisions for them. Where they work effectively, the health care planning team provides an important method of ensuring that community health needs are brought to the attention of the district management team.

The community health councils were a way of involving the consumer in the health service and they vary in size, with a maximum of 30 members. In 1974 the original proposals for membership and functions of the community health councils were extended. Five-sixths of the membership were appointed by local authorities and voluntary bodies and had power to obtain information about the health services in their district and to enter and inspect hospitals and other health premises. They were to be consulted before decisions were taken on any substantial development or variation in services. There was no formal link with the district management team, but the area health authority had to meet the council at least once a year and each community health council presented an annual report and its meetings were open to the press and public. Its value to the community it served depended on the ability and commitment of its members.

The community health council had a paid secretary and, wherever possible, its own premises. The council tried to find premises in shopping parades so that the public could be encouraged to call in and express views or ask advice about any aspect of the health services, while others held evening advice sessions advertised in the local press. When proposals for closing hospitals were made the council had to be consulted and if the proposal was accepted no further permission was needed but if the council objected the Department of Health and Social Security became involved.

There was a National Association of Community Health Council with a budget provided by central government and a paid director. The National Association advises and assists as it works towards consumer participation within the Service. Now that consumers had to be consulted about changes in the services at local level, it was to be hoped that the National Health Service would become more responsive to patients' views than hitherto.

One other innovation introduced in connection with, but before, reorganization was a complaints procedure, through the health services commissioner. These innovations together with the community health councils were aimed at making the Service more sensitive to consumer demands.

Before turning to criticism of that reorganized National Health Service, we might remember the conclusions of the White Paper on which it was based: 'In the final analysis health care depends on the effective delivery at the right time and the right place of the skills and devotion of those providing the services required' (HMSO 1972). Brown's discussion *The Changing National Health Service* (1973) also gives useful background here.

Criticism of the reorganized National Health Service A major criticism of the NHS to emerge was that it had become too bureaucratic—and too inflexible to be responsive to changing demands (Draper & Smart 1973). Certainly those working in the Service felt that simple requests for resources took longer to be accepted or rejected than before. Increasing numbers of meetings, whilst valuable in terms of increasing cooperation between different parts of the newly integrated National Health Service, consumed a disproportionate amount of time. A study of the Humberside Region concluded that the reorganization was expensive, inefficient and damaging to staff morale. It had cost £25 000 in that region alone, with the employment of over 25 per cent additional administrative staff (Institute of Health Studies 1975).

Major criticism continues to surround the separation of the health and welfare services. The joint consultative committees lack means of enforcing their collective views. The problem remains, as under the tripartite system, that ways of reducing the demands on the health service budget shift the cost onto the local authority. For example, it is a well-documented fact that many of those in psychiatric hospitals could be discharged if sheltered accommodation and hostel accommodation were available. Such new facilities are unlikely to develop rapidly in a period of restraint in local government expenditure. In 1976 it was announced that health service money would become available to local authorities to help build up their community mental health, and other services.

The 1972 White Paper argued that health services depended on the humane provision and planning of the personal social services. It talked about unifying health and social services, but said the practical difficulties ruled this out as a realistic conclusion, requiring instead concentration on ensuring that the two authorities with their separate statutory responsibilities worked together in partnership for the health and social care of the population (Brown 1973).

It may be argued that the continued dominance of the medical profession in the National Health Service is one factor making this partnership difficult. The need for teamwork is stressed throughout this book, but the medical profession still retains a key role. The role of the consultant may perpetuate the dominance of hospital over community medicine. The teaching hospitals influence the kind of doctors we train and the education they receive. The family practitioner committee perpetuates the independent status of the general practitioner although the growth of health centres is an important countervailing pressure.

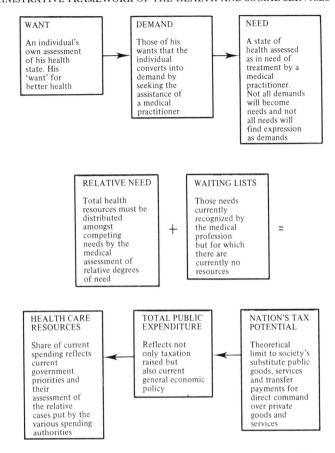

Fig. 11. The accommodation of wants to supply (Cooper 1975).

The issue of medical dominance in the decision-making machinery of the National Health Service and in relation to the way it really works is linked to further areas of criticism of the National Health Service itself. Cooper (1975) argues that doctors' clinical freedom is such that it is they who determine allocation of resources and they act as a rationing device in a situation where demand for medical care is outstripped by the supply (Fig. 11). The key rationing role of the medical practitioner is seen in translating 'wants' into those 'needs' that the health services should meet. Cooper stresses too the way in which supply is constrained by our own willingness to pay taxes for the health services rather than to keep our money to buy other kinds of goods.

Another problem raised by Doctors Cochrane and Doll concerns our failure to evaluate health services. Cochrane (1972) argues for 'a marked reduction in the use of ineffective remedies and of effective remedies used inefficiently', while Doll (1974) says that we need to find a means whereby the benefits of this service can be measured in the same units as are used to estimate its costs. In other words, we need to express in the same units the value of preventing mental deficiency in a child, of saving the life of a 70-year-old man and of relieving a chronic duodenal ulcer. This is a point made in the context of the argument for measuring progress towards the goal of providing equal opportunity for equal treatment regardless of financial means, age, sex or employment.

If we could look at existing health needs in Britain today and then begin to build up our health services afresh, we should not have the kind of service that we have now. Our services, however, are based not only on the 1948 legislation but on what existed previously, although operating in different demographic, economic and other circumstances. Vested interests fight hard, but even so our medical care system compares favourably with those of other countries, as the Royal Commission on the National Health Service (1979) confirmed.

The New National Health Service: 1982 Reorganization

The 1974 reorganization of the NHS, however traumatic for staff at the time, was planned and implemented in a period of optimism within the health service. But since the mid-1970s the NHS has been faced with the problem of a reduction in the rate of planned expenditure. The funds for the NHS were not actually cut, but due to inflation and rising demands, there was effectively a real reduction in funds. At the same time, social services provision, which is often complementary to health service provision, was even more severely hit by public expenditure cuts. The 1982 reorganization therefore took place in a period of acute anxiety about the quality and quantity of health care—an anxiety which practising health visitors and all nurses will be well aware of.

Within months of being elected in 1979, the new Conservative Government published a Consultative Paper on the Structure and Management of the NHS in England and Wales, (Patients First). It summarized the major criticisms of the 1974 structure

too many tiers
failure to take quick decisions
too many administrators
money wasted.

The Government therefore proposed a further reorganization of the NHS, which came into effect by 1982. Area health authorities disappeared, and district health authorities, (DHAs) replaced them. In single-district AHAs the changes are less drastic than in multi-district AHAs. It is hoped that the new structure will strengthen the management arrangements at the local level, with greater delegation of responsibility to those in the hospital and community services; simplify the professional advisory machinery and simplify the planning system. The DHAs are responsible for the planning, development and management of health services, within national and regional strategic guidelines. Most—but certainly not all—are co-terminous with the boundaries of the local authority, to help relations with other relevant services—and, indeed, joint consultative committees linking the NHS and local authorities will remain.

The chairman of the DHA is appointed by the Secretary of State. The regional health authority appoints the other members, who will include one consultant, one GP, one nurse, midwife or health visitor, a medical school nominee, a trade union nominee, 4 members appointed by the local authorities, and additional generalist members will be appointed to make the total 16. Family practitioner committees remain as they are, and may well cover more than one DHA. Community health councils also remain, although their role will ultimately be reviewed.

The management structure is similar to that outlined for the district management teams earlier in this chapter, although the Government is concerned that officers will be accountable *individually* for the performance of their own functions as well as being members of a team. Indeed, the district administrator has responsibility for seeing that DHA policies are implemented.

Services are to be organized into 'units of management', e.g. a single large hospital, community services, maternity services, several small hospitals. Each has an administrator and a director of nursing services, accountable to the district administrator and the district nursing officer. The Government envisages that DHAs will exercise financial responsibility, giving maximum local delegation consistent with overall control via cash limits. It was hoped to reduce management costs by 10 per cent by 1984. Regional health authorities retain important functions, including the coordination of strategic plans, resource allocation, ensuring expenditure is kept within cash limits and manpower planning. This latter is a major task: in 1979 the

NHS employed over 770 000 staff, with nursing staff the largest group at 358 000.

These proposals being implemented in 1982 indicate that the ways in which the guidelines outlined above are interpreted will vary. Community staff are concerned that the units of management based on hospitals are stronger within the DHA than the community services.

The NHS in the eighties is facing new problems, yet as the Secretary of State said in his foreword to *Care in Action*, (see Further Reading section for details): 'The Government's top priority must be to get the economy right; for that reason it cannot be assumed that money will always be available to be spent on health care'. Indeed, this document looks to an expansion of private medical care and voluntary activity as well as increased efficiency and financial controls. Apart from the personal, unsettling effect of NHS reorganization, nursing staff will be concerned to effect these changes with the minimum impact on patient care. Patients are more aware of their rights and more anxious to participate in the health services than ever before. Although the Government's 1979 Consultative Paper was entitled 'Patients First', whether that becomes a reality will depend, as ever, on the sensitive implementation of the reorganization by NHS staff, as well as on adequate finance for the NHS throughout the 1980s.

THE PERSONAL SOCIAL SERVICES

The social services that developed after World War II were geared to supplying a service to defined groups in the population identified as needing such help. These groups were as follows.

1. *The elderly, physically handicapped and homeless*, for whom responsibility was given to welfare departments under Part III of the National Assistance Act, 1948. Welfare departments were responsible to the Ministry of Health at central government level (later to the DHSS when it was formed in 1966).

2. *Children who were deprived* of a normal home life (for reasons including death or desertion of parents, or parents being unfit, or the child being in need of care, protection or control) were made the responsibility of another new local authority department, the children's department under the 1948 Children Act. This department, like the welfare department, had its own chief officer and its own

committee. It was then, however, responsible to the Home Office at central government level.

3. *The mentally disordered* were the responsibility of local health authorities in terms of running junior training centres (before their transfer to the education service) for subnormal children, and adult training centres for subnormal adults. Some aspects of local health authority work were relevant to other groups in need, for example the local health authority organized the home help service which served the elderly as well as new mothers.

Overall, these services developed in their own way but they were all affected by certain trends. The most important of these trends was the increasing emphasis on community, as opposed to institutional care, during the post-war years. Jones (1975a) reminds us that institutional care has a long history. She writes:

> In the second half of the eighteenth century, the need for refuges from an increasingly hard and competitive world was accentuated, and they increased both in number and in variety. Social problems proliferated and our system grew, because there seemed no alternative to it . . . Before the century ended, attempts were being made to break down or by-pass the monolithic structures—orphanages, asylums, prisons, workhouses—which had been created. In our own day, this policy has been sharpened and given shape by the community care movement and the extension of social work training.

Although the trend since the 1950s has been towards community care, this does not mean the end of institutions which heal, shelter, confine, teach or protect different groups in society (Jones 1975a) *Community care* implies groups or individuals receiving care in the community rather than in an institution. For some groups, such as the elderly, community care means domiciliary services in their existing home, or a new home such as a sheltered flatlet, rather than a bed in a local authority residential home. For other groups, taking a bed in a local authority residential home means community care—as hostels are based within the community, unlike most of the beds for the mentally ill and subnormal.

The movement towards community care has occurred for two major reasons. Firstly, it is cheaper to keep people out of residential care, for example fostering a child is cheaper than offering a place in a residential children's home. Those who enter institutions are increasingly dependent, or difficult (e.g. children in care) and the denigration of residential institutions does not help staff morale as they care for their residents.

The second reason for increased emphasis on community care is the growing criticism of institutions. Jones (1975a) says, however, that the movement towards community care has been accompanied by literature concerned with what is wrong with institutions rather than with how they can be efficiently organized. Townsend (1964), in his study of residential homes for the elderly, summarized the criticisms of institutions:

> in the institution people live communally with a minimum of privacy and yet their relationships with each other are slender. Many subsist in a kind of defensive shell of isolation. Their social experiences are limited, they lack creative occupation and cannot exercise much self-determination and they are deprived of intimate family relationships. The individual has too little opportunity to develop the talents he possesses and they atrophy through disuse. In some of the smaller and more humanely administered institutions these various characteristics seem to be less frequently found but they are still present.

Similar conclusions have been reached after studies of mental hospitals, children's homes and prisons (Morris 1969; King et al. 1971). Townsend also notes that many old people living at home also experience serious deprivations.

There are sociological and economic arguments favouring care in the community. People rarely choose to move away from a familiar neighbourhood and the groups needing help are most likely to prefer support at home or accommodation or care locally.

The trend towards community care is not uniform throughout Great Britain, but depends on the policy and resources of each local authority, as well as local opinion. This trend, together with demographic changes, has dominated the history of the social services since World War II. Demographic changes include the increasing number of elderly people and those handicapped groups that live longer due to advances in medical technology. Changes in family structure also affect the demand for social service intervention, for example the increasing number of single-parent families (see Chapter 5).

The details of the way in which the three local authority departments concerned with social service provision developed since World War II have been well documented (see the Further Reading list), and are not discussed here. We shall look, however, at the Report that led to the replacement of these departments by the local authority social service departments, which came into being in 1971.

The Seebohm Report
The Committee on Local Authority and Allied Personal Social Services was set up under the chairmanship of Lord Seebohm in 1965. Its brief was to 'review the organization and responsibilities of the local authority personal social services in England and Wales and to consider what changes are desirable to secure an effective family service' (HMSO 1968).

It is perhaps helpful to define the term *personal social services*. Parker (1970), a member of the Committee, subsequently wrote, 'The personal social services are usually considered to be those lying outside the general fields of health and education, which are adjusted in some special way to the particular social needs of individuals, families or groups and which require personal contact between provider and recipient. The skill involved is often labelled *social work*'. He goes on to say that this is interpreted to include such things as provision of straightforward information or domestic help as well as residential care of the old, or work in the community supporting groups such as the mentally disordered and their families. The health visitor reading this definition may wonder why health visiting is not included as a *personal social service*, and the absence of a health visitor from the Committee may be a relevant factor!

The Committee looked at the whole range of social service provision, not only the work of the welfare department, children's department and the local health authority. It looked at the needs of, and provision for, children, the elderly, physically handicapped, mentally ill and mentally subnormal (both in terms of statutory and voluntary provision). Occupational groups such as medical social workers, educational welfare officers and probation officers as well as the staff of child guidance clinics were discussed.

Findings and recommendations The Committee members were concerned at the lack of resources for social care. They found inadequacy in terms of many provisions, such as shortage of places in training centres for the mentally subnormal, and also in terms of the range of care offered. They found inequalities of service, poor coordination between services and poor cooperation between staff of the various services examined. The Committee felt the services were not adaptable and were slow to meet the needs of families and individuals as new needs became apparent. The Committee was concerned with problems of access for those seeking help. With so many different departments operating, those seeking help were often turned away by one department and sent to another. This led both to duplication of facilities and gaps.

Seventeen years after the Report one could still make the same criticisms of the social service provisions. The problems of cooperation and coordination have been brought out in every report examining cases of child abuse (HMSO 1974b). Slow adaptation to needs is still apparent in the situation of battered wives. Yet the recommendations that came from the Report were implemented, the first being the recommendation that the junior training centres for the mentally subnormal child seen as unfit for education should become part of the Special Schools Service. This has been of great value in terms of the training of staff and the resources made available for these children, now attending schools for the severely subnormal.

The most important recommendation was that a new local authority department was needed which would be geared to the needs of the whole population served. It would form a large, powerful department, headed by someone with status and backed up by a committee of councillors able to argue on equal terms with other important local authority committees, such as housing or education. There would be better career prospects for staff and the need for more training of social workers was stressed in the Report. There was stress too on accessibility: the social service department was to operate from area offices, several to each local government area, which would make the service more sensitive to local needs. In the event, the shortage of resources has proved more important than the location of the area office. It was hoped that with the service more localized, the barrier between giver and receiver could be broken down. With the stress on training for social workers came the idea of the *generic* social worker: one able to cope with the wide range of problems that would present itself to the local office.

The Social Services Act was passed in 1970, with the new departments operational from April 1971. One of the problems of the previous arrangements was that whilst welfare departments and local health authorities were responsible to the DHSS, the children's departments were the responsibility of the Home Office. Under the Act, the Department of Health and Social Security became the directing central government department.

Criticism of the Seebohm Report and its implications for social workers One criticism of the Seebohm Report was that, like the Report of the Committee on Nursing, it undertook no research. In particular, the lack of consumer research was regretted. When formed, the social services departments provided a large number of senior posts, which meant that qualified and experienced social workers were promoted to management level leaving the inexperienced and often unqualified staff at the field level. Some local authorities are trying to solve this dilemma by the creation of senior practitioner posts.

The problems not resolved by the proposals in the Seebohm Report remain unresolved, such as the question of what kind of family relationship the State should support. One social service department is experimenting with relatively high financial payments to relatives who stop work to care for dependent relatives. With safeguards to prevent abuse, this is a recognition of what families save the State when they care for those who would otherwise be in hospital or residential care.

Another problem relates to the nature of social work. Some social workers feel that much of their work arises simply because of poverty and bad housing and they find it difficult to help those whose problems the State could solve by redistribution of income and changes in priorities, perhaps at the cost of neglecting those with the more intangible problems that need social work skills. This can lead to conflict between social workers and their employing local authority. Social workers may resent being used to help people to adjust to situations they see as created by the society in which we live. Others see social workers as not willing to work for social change. Sinfield (1969) and Lees (1972) both put this view clearly.

Rising expectations of the community, shortage of trained staff, and economic policies make it harder than ever for social services departments to function at the level society expects. Social workers perhaps also suffer from the fact that when other professionals find a problem insoluble, they tend to ask the social services to cope. The mentally disturbed adult discharged from the mental hospital on the grounds that nothing more can be done for him is left to the local social worker. Medical developments have led us to avoid issues like death and pain. In a similar way, perhaps we now expect social workers to prevent the unhappiness and failures of relationships that cannot in fact be resolved.

The limitations of the role of the social worker were discussed in an editorial in the press following the death of Steven Meurs, who died from starvation at the age of 15 months, noting the way the system failed for him:

the sheer multiplicity of official callers at his door shows that the apparatus was deployed and defeated. But it is a big step from there to the contention that new procedures must be instituted, new ministries set up, more social workers hired, more case conferences called, until human sinfulness has been abolished. Taken to the end it would prove a remarkably expensive thesis . . . but it has worse faults than that. It threatens certain kinds of freedom, since the attempt at forestalling domestic wrong-doing could only be pushed wider than at present by a more marked infringement of privacy; and it attacks the corollary of freedom, which is responsibility (Editorial 1976).

We now turn from the problems left for us after the Seebohm Report and the subsequent legislation to look at the actual work and achievements of the social services departments.

The Social Services Departments

The Local Authority Social Services Act required local authorities to set up a social services committee and to appoint a director of social services who should be a qualified social worker with managerial experience. This Act was passed by the Government as part of a comprehensive series of reforms which included reorganization of the health services and of local government, but as the Labour Government was defeated before its other plans were legislated for, the social services departments preceded the other changes. This meant that as the departments were staffed, all areas outside London knew that when local government was reorganized there would be further changes in administrative boundaries and committee members, with possible changes of policy.

Following the local reorganization that came into effect in April 1974, social services departments became the responsibility of the London boroughs, non-metropolitan counties and metropolitan districts. The departments were created at the same time as they were given additional responsibilities through two important Acts, The Children and Young Persons Act, 1969 and the Chronically Sick and Disabled Act, 1970, and through a circular bringing in parts of an earlier Act relating to welfare services for the elderly.

The new demands on and responsibilities of the departments combined with the desire of the councillors and officials involved to assess and meet needs in their own areas. The result was a rapid rise in the spending of the departments. After looking at general changes in the role of the new social services departments, we now look at some of the major groups the department serves.

Services for children The social services departments concentrate on helping the most vulnerable children, and of course families, in our society: children in need of care, protection and/or control, to use the words of the relevant legislation. In some areas social services departments may ask (and pay) specialized voluntary agencies such as the family service units to work with these families.

In looking at social work with children and families, it is important to remember it is but one part of a range of policies relevant to families in general. Wynn (1970) argues for a comprehensive family policy which she sees as including arrangements for the employment of mothers, including its effect on education authorities and on social security; the adaptation of working hours to school hours; counting sickness of children as a reason for absence of work and the adaptation of social security contributions to encourage part-time work. Fiscal policies affecting child tax allowances are equally relevant. She goes on to argue that:

> Poverty and hardship have been the lot of most of mankind throughout history. The good society can still only be achieved by further economic growth. . . . Our future is in our children and, therefore, in our families with dependent children. The redistribution of wealth is today a feature of all advanced societies. Wealth may, however, be redistributed to promote economic growth by improving the upbringing and environment and education of the coming generations, or wealth may be redistributed in ways that retard economic growth by diverting the flow of wealth away from families with dependent children. . . . The good of the citizen must always be the first objective of public policy, but there is a contradiction at some points between the good of the citizen today and the citizen of tomorrow.

Health visitors may well have more interest than other professional groups in the good of the citizen tomorrow, but the tax implications of the proposals Wynn is arguing for may well bring out the very contradiction within ourselves that she warns about.

The work of the social services departments in relation to children is governed by four major pieces of legislation. The Children Act, 1948 was the basis for the former children's department, and was absorbed by the social services department in 1971. It stemmed from the Curtis Report, set up through concern at the fragmentation of services for children in need, as well as the low standards of child care (HMSO 1946). Under the 1948 Act, the children's departments were responsible to the Home Office. Set up at local government level, the departments had a duty to receive into care a child who had no parent or guardian, or who was abandoned. There was also a duty to intervene in any situation where it was in the welfare of the child so to do, for example in the case of a parent who was physically or mentally incapacitated or who was leading a life which made him or her unfit to care for a child.

Receiving children into care, and then arranging for them to live in a residential home, to be fostered or, more rarely, to be adopted, was seen increasingly as an unsatisfactory way of helping—in that such intervention was often too late. In the 1963 Children and Young Persons Act the local authority was allowed and encouraged to undertake preventive work to keep children out of care. They had the duty to give advice, guidance and assistance to promote the welfare of children and so reduce the need for them to be received into care. This might mean the setting up of advice centres, or giving practical assistance, including financial assistance. An electricity bill might possibly be paid or a relative's fares might be paid to enable care for the child during a parent's absence in hospital. The interpretation of this Act, and the money allocated to pay for such services, varies widely from one local authority area to another.

The legislation dealing with children whose behaviour brought them into conflict with the law is the 1969 Children and Young Persons Act. The philosophy of this Act was concerned to prevent deprived and delinquent children from becoming deprived, inadequate, unstable or criminal citizens. It was thought this could be achieved by social work support and by offering a wide range of provisions, residential and community-based, to meet the needs of any child appearing before the court. The criteria for court proceedings were to be a kind of double test. The child might be neglected or ill-treated, or exposed to moral danger or beyond the control of his parents or guardian. Alternatively he may have been guilty of an offence—and in addition the child must be 'in need of care or control which he is unlikely to receive unless the court makes an order under this section in respect of him', to quote the Act itself.

The integration of such provision, formerly known by various names (approved schools, residential homes, remand homes) now all known as *community homes* run by local authority social services departments, has come about. However, low priority for the children's services means there are shortages of suitable accommodation, especially secure accommodation. There was discussion about the philosophy of this Act, which was passed well before there were sufficient social workers or the range of facilities envisaged. The Act itself, and the context in which it operates, is well explained by Berlins and Wamsell (1974).

The most recent Children Act, that of 1975, is also controversial. It makes it a duty for local authorities to establish an adoption service. It enables the mother to give consent six weeks after a child's birth, so decreasing the anxiety of the adopters. The Act allows foster parents who have looked after the child for five years to apply for adoption and introduces the concept of legal guardianship whereby foster parents can have a stronger link with the child they care for after a year if the parent or local authority agrees, and after three years such permission is not needed. Since the concern felt at the death of Maria Colwell, who could not speak for herself when her mother applied to the courts to have the child removed from her foster home, the Act provides that a court may appoint a 'guardian ad litem' to safeguard the interest of the child, if it is felt that the parent does not represent the child. The Act provides that private foster children should be visited as often as local authority foster children and gives as a basis for reaching decisions on children in care, the need to safeguard and promote the welfare of the child throughout his childhood, and to ascertain the wishes and feelings of the child regarding such decisions.

This Act is controversial because it expressed the question of the rights of parents as against the right of the child. For example, Rowe (1975) wrote:

> Although at present surrounded by confusion, controversy and delay, I believe that the Children's Bill will go down in history as another milestone in the long progress towards recognizing children as persons and not the possessions of adults. To describe the Bill as anti-parent is to distort both its spirit and its provisions. But it stands to reason that an increase in children's legal rights must inevitably involve curbing adult rights whenever these are in conflict with the essential welfare of the child. And since children cannot speak for themselves, protecting their rights must involve giving greater powers to courts and social agencies.

Holman (1975) saw the Act as constituting a serious threat to the rights of natural parents and argued:

> So pronounced are the new custody powers that it might actually be counter-productive. Fear of losing access to their children might provoke some parents to remove their children before the time period is reached just to forestall the possibility of an order. Thus some fosterings might be broken that would otherwise have remained intact. Further, the British Association of Social Workers has expressed the view that some parents will now not approach social services departments at all for fear that they

will permanently lose their children. In the case of parents under great temporary stress, this will mean that children will be subject to ill treatment at home which could otherwise have been avoided by short-term fostering.

It is difficult even some years after the Act to assess this issue, but observation and experience in the field will help health visitors make up their own minds. Despite efforts by the social services departments to prevent children being received into care, the numbers continue to rise. In 1978 in England and Wales, 100 700 children were in care, compared with 87 000 in 1971. There is a tendency for children to stay longer in care, although most are in care for short-term reasons, e.g. short-term illness of parent.

Of the children in care in 1978, over 34 000 were in foster homes, 18 000 were in the charge of a relative, guardian or friend and the rest were in a wide range of institutions provided by voluntary organizations as well as local authorities. The shortage of the right accommodation in the right place at the right time is likely to continue, as is the shortage of social workers. It would be a mistake to assume that because a child is officially in care someone is actually doing any caring.

It is also depressing to consider that of those children received into care, some are there for preventable reasons, e.g. the 4700 in care because of the homelessness of their parents. Apart from the distress to the families, it hardly makes economic sense to receive into care, at considerable cost, a child whose parents could be re-housed at a much smaller cost!

Apart from the responsibilities outlined above, the social services departments are concerned with other facilities for children. They register *child minders* and some areas take this responsibility seriously, offering training courses, toy libraries and the like to registered minders. They are responsible for the *day nurseries* (as opposed to the local education authority nursery schools), and health visitors are more aware than most of the population of the inadequacies of our day care provisions for the under-fives.

One of the most vulnerable groups of all are the children in *one-parent families* whose needs have been well documented but badly provided for (HMSO 1974c).

From the point of view of public opinion as expressed through the media, the major problem of the social services departments in relation to children is one that cannot be solved by legislation or money: the problem of *child abuse*. Increasingly well documented, child abuse involves health, education and social services workers. The policy initiative taken by the DHSS urged social services departments and health authorities to set up area review committees as policy-making bodies for the management of cases of child abuse. They should meet three or four times a year. Health visitors are more likely to be involved in the case conferences recommended by the Memorandum, which would bring together those with a statutory responsibility for the child (a consultant perhaps), and those people directly concerned, e.g. the health visitor, social worker and general practitioner. Central records are recommended and the need for staff training stressed. The Memorandum argues for more preventive work (DHSS 1974) but the existing studies show how complex are the causal factors in child abuse and thus how difficult effective preventive programmes are to devise. Much valuable work in child abuse is undertaken by a voluntary agency, the National Society for the Prevention of Cruelty to Children, whose research workers and officers play a key role in this issue.

Provision for the elderly and handicapped   These groups have in common not merely the likelihood of poverty and dependence on others, but they suffer from the kind of stigma that a society valuing speed and earning powers tends to lay on its slower and more dependent members. Modern medicine ensures these groups are growing larger and living longer. Yet attitudes are slow to change! It is easy to say how many people in Britain are 'old', taking as 'old' the retirement ages of 60 for women and 65 for men. In 1979, 17.4 per cent of the population, well over 9 million individuals, were 'old'. It is more difficult to measure the numbers of physically handicapped people, because of the problems of definition. In her national survey of the handicapped in Great Britain, Harris (1971) used as her definition of impairment, 'lacking part or all of a limb' or 'having a defective limb' or 'having a defective organ or mechanism of the body which stops or limits getting about, working or self-care'. She estimated that there were about 3 million people in Britain impaired according to this definition. Many elderly people are of course impaired and perhaps the proportion over the age of 75, likely to be more dependent, are more important than the overall numbers over retirement age.

Local authorities have had a duty to provide *residential accommodation* for the elderly and handicapped since 1948, but community provision has been slower to develop. Voluntary organizations and individual volunteers have been filling many of the gaps in provision for the elderly and handicapped. Many of the needs of these groups are met by suppliers of services outside the social services departments. Geriatric services meet some of the health needs of the elderly, the general practitioner is important and the proportion of elderly patients in ordinary hospital beds continues to grow. There is evidence that the health needs of the elderly are inadequately met (Barker 1974) and the use of geriatric beds for the younger chronic sick, although against the letter and spirit of the 1970 Chronically Sick and Disabled Act, continues.

We know that the financial resources of the elderly are low and despite the growing and complex range of social security benefits for the handicapped under retirement age, they too are a group that tend to suffer financial hardship.

The most acute shortage within the housing market is for purpose-built dwellings for the elderly and the handicapped. It is therefore impossible to expect the social services departments to be able to make up for the many deficiencies in the range of provision for the elderly or handicapped. Since 1948 when the Poor Law was repealed, local authorities have had a duty to provide residential accommodation for these groups. After the war it was often provided in old workhouses, but gradually new, or newly adapted, accommodation has been provided. Buried in the 1968 Public Health and Services Act was a Section 45 which gave local authorities permission to promote the welfare of old people. That Section came into force in 1971 with the formation of the social services departments. The departments could pay voluntary agencies to promote the welfare of the elderly or could promote it themselves.

Welfare covers services such as meals-on-wheels, recreational facilities at home or outside the home, as well as visiting and social work support services. It also covers provision of practical assistance in the home, which means adapting a home to make it more suitable, or issues aids such as a bath seat. (Services vary from one local authority area to another.) The voluntary component of the work for the elderly is well developed, but as most volunteers tend to be middle class, working-class areas, like inner London tend to be left with large numbers of elderly people in need and a limited number of the traditional type of volunteer. The growth of *community work* and community-based groups such as tenant's associations is but one way in which this imbalance may be partly corrected.

The community needs of the handicapped were slow to develop

and uneven within the different kinds of handicap. The services for the blind developed first. Those for the other, general, group of handicapped people later. The deaf remain a rather isolated and ill-served group. Only since the passing of the 1970 Chronically Sick and Disabled Act have provisions developed in a way that seeks to try to integrate the handicapped into society. The Act was introduced into the House of Commons as a Private Member's Bill by Alf Morris, who was advised about the Bill by a committee of disabled people. His Bill was, therefore, governed by the needs and wishes of those who were *consumers* of the provisions being debated, something rare in the history of British legislation. The legislation was ambitious and imaginative and if progress has been slow and uneven, it is an important landmark on the way to creating a society which treats its handicapped members as equals.

The first major provision of the Act was that each local authority must inform itself of the numbers and needs of the disabled in its area. Some did this by delivering leaflets, others by house-to-house survey. Once found, the handicapped person is registered with the local authority, and can be provided with a wide range of services including the following.

1. Radio, TV, or similar recreational facilities at home.
2. Recreational and education facilities outside the home.
3. Help with travel.
4. Help with adapting the house to make it safer, more comfortable or more convenient.
5. Meals in the home or elsewhere.
6. Help with holidays.
7. A telephone.

There was great stress in the Act on *access*; special accommodation for the disabled was to be provided and new buildings were to be designed so that disabled people could use them. Public toilets were to be made available to disabled persons, both local authority toilets and those in hotels, theatres and the like. Parking facilities were improved both for the disabled themselves, and those driving a disabled passenger.

Figure 12 illustrates the general growth in community health and welfare provision for the elderly and handicapped. In particular, when we look at the rapid increase in the number of handicapped people registered, it shows the tangible effects of the Chronically Sick and Disabled Act.

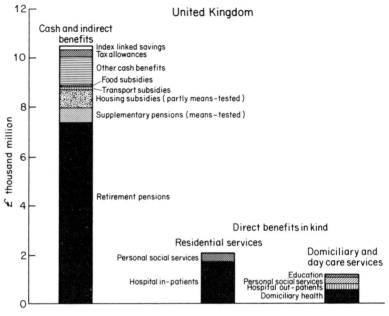

Fig. 12. Principal public sector social expenditure on the elderly, 1978. Source: Social Trends 11, 1981 edition (HMSO).

We have, as a society, now raised the expectations of these two groups and in recognizing that provision has not kept pace with these expectations, it is important to acknowledge the progress that has been made, but is slowing down. As a recent government publication on priorities shows (HMSO 1976), spending on domiciliary services for the elderly has been rising at a rate of 15 to 20 per cent in the last few years. Whilst those of us at work may feel we are making sacrifices in the fight against inflation, the real burden is in fact falling on the most vulnerable groups—like the elderly and handicapped.

The mentally disordered The turning point for the provisions for the *mentally disordered* was the 1959 Mental Health Act which put into effect most of the recommendations of the Royal Commission which reported in 1957 (HMSO 1957). The Act introduced new terminology and used the term 'mentally disordered' to cover *mental illness, arrested* or *incomplete development of mind* and *psychopathic disorder*. The Act was concerned to move more rapidly from compulsory to voluntary admission to psychiatric hospitals, also to reduce the stigma attached to mental disorder and to promote community care facilities. The background to legislation was the revolution in the treatment of mental illness brought about by the drugs developed after World War II. From playing a custodial role only, the mental hospital was beginning to play a 'curing' role, the closed door being replaced by the open or perhaps revolving door.

The 1962 Hospital Plan envisaged a reduction of the number of beds allocated to mental illness and the development of psychiatric wards in district general hospitals. Although about half our hospital beds are occupied by those suffering from some kind of mental disorder, the service is underfinanced: about £14 of every £100 spent on the NHS is spent on the mentally disordered.

Apathy in the field of the mental subnormality hospitals has shown itself in many reports, started by the one on Ely Hospital in Wales (HMSO 1969). Concern for the poor quality of hospital provision for the mentally disordered has not been matched by a concern to build up community care facilities.

Recent estimates of the need for hostel provision, adult training centres and for social workers have been made and in the foreword to a White Paper, Barbara Castle, then Secretary of State for Health and Social Services wrote, 'Very little material progress in the shape of new physical development is to be expected in the next few years. Moreover the time scale for further significant progress must depend on the general economic situation and has therefore at present to be left open' (HMSO 1975a).

The White Paper also adds 'The Government is well aware that the pattern of services described in the preceding chapters is a far cry from that which exists today. While there are many general hospital units already in being, probably only about a third are of adequate size or offer standards of facilities for both day and in-patients capable of providing the focus of a full district service' (HMSO 1975a). It goes on to show that specific statutory duties often take priority over long-term preventive work and recognizes the effects of recent reorganization on health and social services. The kind of services envisaged are as in 1959: hostel provision, day hospitals, sheltered employment, social work support, day centres and so on.

The history and problems of the services for the mentally ill and mentally handicapped are well documented by Jones (1972 & 1975b) and make interesting background reading for students who wish to make further study of this area.

The future of the social services departments We have already discussed the effect on the morale of staff who felt specialist knowledge was being devalued by the growth of generic social work. There is now a return to recognition of the need for specialized social work, particularly in relation to the mentally ill. Th_ 'rend towards community care as shown in legislation and government policy statements has put an enormous burden on the field staff of the new departments. Spending on the social services rose rapidly after the creation of the new department, but they now face a period of virtual standstill.

Social workers feel very vulnerable when publicity over cases of child abuse tends to blame them for the lack of cooperation and coordination between health and social service personnel at consumer level. They are conscious of the pressures arising from growing demands being made upon them following the raising of expectations that the creation of the social service department itself created. There are pressures for increased capital expenditure on hostel accommodation to meet new needs such as those of the battered wife, and yet much of their workload could be reduced, if perhaps, instead of concentrating on unmet needs, resources were concentrated on reducing some of the preventable problems arising from poverty and bad housing with which the social worker is forced to deal.

SOCIAL POLICY: THE NEED FOR COORDINATION

This chapter has tried to show something of the complexity of provision made in this country to meet social needs. One major problem is that of coordination. Coordination at field level can only come with understanding of, and respect for, the role of other professional groups within the caring professions. A hierarchical organization which demands that messages go up one organizational pyramid and down the next in order that two fieldworkers know what each is doing leads to delay. Forging personal relationships between other fieldworkers can only aid the way services are delivered. For the consumer, it is this delivery that matters, not the activities of the relevant cabinet minister or civil servants.

Coordination at the level of provision of services is therefore vital. But so is coordination of provision and there is hope that there will be less fragmented social policies in the future than in the past. This hope appeared in a document (HMSO 1975*b*) prepared by the Central Policy Review Staff, a group that advises the Prime Minister. The document was concerned with the way in which public expenditure has been growing faster than production, and expenditure on social programmes growing faster than the rest of public expenditure.

They argued:

> It has led to unrealistic expectations about the scope for improvements and extensions. It has also reduced the incentive to increase the efficiency of existing policies and programmes. . . . If the structure on social expenditure is not to become increasingly arbitrary some better basis is needed for defining priorities. . . . Ministers also need to ensure that their priorities are adequately reflected in policies which are actually being carried out; and that in practice these policies are having the effects intended

They said their review aims were:

    (a) improved coordination between services as they affect the individual;
    (b) better analysis of, and policy prescriptions for, complex problems— especially when they are the concern of more than one department;
    (c) the development over time of collective views on priorities as between different problems and groups.

They recommended that ministers should meet regularly to discuss social policy strategies; that there should be an improvement in the gathering of information about social policies and social problems and that there should be studies of specific topics, for example: the implications for demand of the decline in the birth rate; the possible declining capacity and willingness of the family and local community to care for their own social casualties; the implications of this for community care and the scope for reversing the trend. They suggested other topics for study, such as social aspects of housing and disadvantaged youth.

Hope for better coordination comes not only from this document concerned to look at social problems across departmental boundaries. It comes too from agreement to finance some local authority projects (which will relieve the health services), from National Health Service money, if put forward by the joint consultative committees which bring the area health authorities and the local authorities together. It comes too from the plan to widen the scope of the Hospital Advisory Service to become the Health Advisory Service and to liaise with the Social Work Service within the Department of Health and Social Security. It will examine local authority as well as

National Health Service provisions for the elderly and mentally disordered and a new team will be set up to look at provision for children in long-term hospital care.

In the last analysis, coordination of provision and wider government monitoring of services, while of central importance to the health visitor, is not the concern of most clients. They judge the social services by the attitude and action of the personnel delivering that service to them. In this way, health visitors are as important a factor in the delivery of effective social policies as the cabinet minister or the civil servant.

SUMMARY

This chapter has attempted to explain to student health visitors how the health and other social services are organized and function, and some of the problems being faced. The latest NHS reorganization has been described. There is a very close link between economic and social policies, and the chapter has been revised when there is much uncertainty in both spheres. The continued public expenditure cuts, the exceptionally high rate of unemployment (especially among the young), and the way in which the acute problems of the inner cities erupted into public consciousness in the summer of 1981 are issues we must all think about—as student health visitors and as citizens.

QUESTIONS FOR ESSAY OR DISCUSSION

1. 'The encouragement of smaller families is the best way to reduce the incidence of family poverty in Britain today.' Discuss.
2. 'The housing problem is easier to describe than solve.' Discuss with examples from your experience as a health visitor.
3. Discuss the relative merits of the universalist and selectivist approach to the social security system.
4. Briefly outline the major problems that faced the National Health Service before the 1974 reorganization. To what extent did reorganization solve these problems?
5. What factors explain the constantly rising level of demand made upon the National Health Service?
6. Analyse the concept of *community care* and discuss the adequacy of community provision for: *either* the elderly; *or* the mentally disordered; *or* the physically handicapped.
7. To what extent are the social services the inevitable response to the social problems of urban industrial societies?

8. 'It is the British habit to legislate first and investigate afterwards.' Discuss with relation to the development of the child care services.
9. 'The comprehensive school creates more problems than it solves.' Discuss this statement.
10. How would you define social need? Discuss the concept with reference to one area of social policy where you, as a health visitor, see unmet needs.
11. To what extent is increased economic growth a feasible solution to the problems of poverty in Britain today?
12. Outline the major problems facing the social services departments in a period of rapid inflation. How do these affect the work of the health visitor?
13. 'Social policy should aim to eliminate poverty not pursue equality.' Discuss.
14. 'Public expenditure cuts in the health and social services enable service providers to concentrate on real "needs".' Discuss.

REFERENCES

Alfred, R.R. & Boaden, N.T. (1973) Sources of diversity in English local government decisions. In: *Social Administration*, ed. W.D. Burrell. Harmondsworth: Penguin.

Baratz, M.S. & Grigsby, W.C. (1972) *Journal of Social Policy*, Vol. 1, Part II.

Barker, J. (1974) *Hospital and Community Care for the Elderly*. London: Age Concern.

Berlins, M. & Wamsell, G. (1974) *Caught in the Act: Children, Society and the Law*. London: Pelican.

Bradshaw, J. (1972) The concept of needs. *New Society*, *19*, 494, 640 (30 March).

Brown, R.G.S. (1973) *The Changing National Health Service*. London: Routledge & Kegan Paul.

Cochrane, A.L. (1972) *Effectiveness and Efficiency: Random Reflections on the NHS*. London: Nuffield Hospital Provincial Trust.

Cooper, M. (1975) *Rationing Health Care*. London: Croom Helm. DHSS (1974) *Non-Accidental Injury to Children. A Memorandum (22 April)*. London.

Doll, R. (1974) *To Measure NHS Progress*. Fabian Occasional Paper, 8. London: Fabian Society.

Donnison, D. *et al*. (1975) *Social Policy Revisited*. London: Allen & Unwin.

Draper, P. & Smart, T. (1973) *The Future of Our Health Care*. NHS Reorganization Project. London: Guy's Hospital.

Editorial (1976) The state and sin. *Sunday Times*, 18 January.

Field, F. (1973) *Unequal Britain*. London: Hutchinson.

Forder, A. (1974) *Concepts in Social Administration*, pp. 35–9. London: Routledge & Kegan Paul.

Harris, A. (1971) *Handicapped and Impaired in Great Britain*, Part I. London: HMSO.

HMSO. *Annual Report of the Hospital Advisory Service to the Secretary of State for Social Services*. London. (Published annually since 1970.)

HMSO (1974) *Beveridge Report. Social Insurance and Allied Services*. Cmnd. 6404. London.

HMSO (1946) *Curtis Report. Report of the Committee on Care of Children*. London.

HMSO (1957) *Royal Commission on the Law Relating to Mental Illness and Mental Deficiency*. Cmnd. 169. London.

HMSO (1968) *Seebohm Report. Report of the Committee on Local Authority and Allied Personal Social Services*. Cmnd. 3703. London.

HMSO (1969) *Report of the Committee of Enquiry into Allegations of Ill Treatment of Patients and other Irregularities at the Ely Hospital Cardiff*. Cmnd. 3975. London.

HMSO (1972) *National Health Service Reorganization, England*. Cmnd. 5055. London.

HMSO (1973) *Fisher Report. Report of the Committee on Abuse of Social Security Benefits*. Cmnd. 5223. London.

HMSO (1974a) *Halsbury Report. Report of the Committee of Enquiry into the Pay and Related Conditions of Service of Nurses and Midwives*. London.

HMSO (1974b) *Report of the Committee of Enquiry into the Care and Supervision Provided in Relation to Maria Colwell*. London.

HMSO (1974c) *Finer Report. Report of the Committee on One-Parent Families*. London.

HMSO (1975a) *Better Services for the Mentally Ill*. Cmnd. 6233. London.

HMSO (1975b) *A Joint Framework for Social Policy. A Report by the Central Policy Review Staff*. London.

HMSO (1976) *Priorities for Health and Social Services in England*. London.

Holman, R. (1975) Why custodianship is such a paradox. *Community Care* (7 May).

Illich, I. (1975) *Medical Nemesis*. London: Calder and Boyars.

Institute of Health Studies (1975) *New Wine: Old Wine?* Humberside Reorganization Project. Hull: University of Hull.

Jones, K. (1972) *A History of the Mental Health Services*. London: Routledge & Kegan Paul.

Jones, K. (1975a) The development of institutional care. In: *Social Welfare in Modern Britain*, ed. E. Butterworth & R. Holman. London: Fontana.

Jones, K. (1975b) *Opening the Door: A Study of New Policies for the Mentally Handicapped*. London: Routledge & Kegan Paul.

Kahn, A.J. (1973) *Social Policy and the Social Services*. New York: Random House.

King, R.D., Raynes, N.V. & Tizard, J. (1971) *Patterns of Residential Care: Sociological Studies in Institutions for Handicapped Children*. London: Routledge & Kegan Paul.

Klein, R. (1974) *Social Policy and Public Expenditure*, Foreword by A.R. Isserliss. London: London Centre for Studies in Social Policy.

Lees, R. (1972) *Politics and Social Work*. London: Routledge & Kegan Paul.

Marshall, T.H. (1970) *Social Policy*, p. 9. London: Hutchinson.

Morris, P. (1969) *Put Away: A Sociological Study of Institutions for the Mentally Retarded*. London: Routledge & Kegan Paul.

Office of Health Economics (1975) *The NHS Reorganization*. London.

Parker, R. (1970) The future of the present social services. In: *The Future of the Social Services*, ed. B. Crick & W.A. Robson. Harmondsworth: Penguin.

Parker, R.A. (1975) Social administration and scarcity. In: *Social Welfare in Modern Britain*, ed. E. Butterworth & R. Holman. London: Fontana.

Pinker R. (1974) Social policy and social justice. *Journal of Social Policy*, *3*, 1, pp. 1–19.

Rowe, J. (1975) A charter for children. *Community Care*, 84 (5 November).

Social Science Research Council (1968) *Research on Poverty*. London: Heinemann.

Sinfield, A. (1969) *Which Way for Social Work?* Fabian Tract 393. London: Fabian Society.

Teeling-Smith, G. (1976) Cost-benefit paralysis. *Nursing Times*, *72*, 3 (22 January).

Titmuss, R.M. (1974) *Social Policy, An Introduction*, pp. 23–32. London: Allen & Unwin.

Townsend, P. (1964) *The Last Refuge*, pp. 171–2, 226. London: Routledge & Kegan Paul.

Townsend, P. (1974) Inequality and the health service. *Lancet, i*, 7868 (15 May).

Wilcocks, A.J. (1967) *The Creation of the National Health Service*. London: Routledge & Kegan Paul.

Wynn, M. (1970) *Family Policy*, pp. 261 & 273. London: Michael Joseph. (Also available in Pelican.)

FURTHER READING

Abel-Smith, B. (1976) *Value for Money in the Health Services*. London: Heinemann.

Brearley, P. *et al.* (1978) *The Social Context of Health Care*. London: Martin Robertson/Oxford: Basil Blackwell.

Brown, M. (1975) *Introduction to Social Administration*. London: Hutchinson.

Brown, R.G.S. (1975) *The Management of Welfare*. London: Fontana.

Davies, B.M. (1980) *Community Health, Preventive Medicine and Social Services*. London: Baillière Tindall.

Department of Education and Science (1978) *Special Education Needs. Report of the Committee of Enquiry into the Education of Handicapped Children and Young People (Warnock Report)*. Cmnd. 7212. London: HMSO

DHSS (1976) *Priorities for Health and Personal Social Services in England: A Consultative Document*. London: HMSO

DHSS (1976) *Sharing Resources for Health in England: A Report of the Resources Allocation Working Party*. London: HMSO.

DHSS (1977) *Priorities in the Health and Social Services: The Way Forward*. London: HMSO.

DHSS (1978) *A Happier Old Age: A Discussion Document on Elderly People in our Society*. London: HMSO.

DHSS (1978) *Review of the Mental Health Act*. Cmnd. 7320. London: HMSO.

DHSS (1979) *Patients First: A Consultative Paper on the Structure and Management of the NHS in England and Wales*. London: HMSO.

DHSS (1980) *Health Service Development: Structure and Management*. HC (80)8 LAC (80)3. London: HMSO.

DHSS (1980) *Inequalities in Health: Report of a Research Working Group*. London: HMSO.

DHSS (1981) *Care in Action: A Handbook of Policies and Priorities for the Health and Personal Social Services in England*. London: HMSO.

DHSS (1981) *The Primary Health Care Team*. London: HMSO.

Gaffin, J. (ed.) (1981) *The Nurse and the Welfare State*. London: HM&M Publishers.

Holman, R. (1978) *Poverty: Explanations of Social Deprivation*. London: Martin Robertson.

Lahiff, M. (1981) *Hard to Help Families*. London: HM&M Publishers.

Layard, R. *et al*. (1978) *The Causes of Poverty*. Background Paper No. 5. Royal Commission on the Distribution of Income and Wealth. London: HMSO.

Lonsdale, S. *et al*. (1980) *Teamwork in the Personal Social Services and Health Care*. London: Croom Helm.

Moroney, R.M. (1976) *The Family and the State*. London: Longman.

Royal Commission on the NHS (Merrison Report) (1979) Cmnd. 7615. London: HMSO.

Watkin, B. (1978) *The National Health Services: The First Phase 1948–1974 and After*. London: Allen & Unwin.

7. The Social Aspects of Health and Disease

SECTION I UNDERSTANDING THE SOCIAL ASPECTS OF HEALTH AND DISEASE

Grace M. Owen

Students entering the health visitor's course come with a considerable level of skills, knowledge and attitudes to sickness and health acquired during nursing experience. Most of this experience, however, has been gained in caring for people during short episodes of acute illness in the clinical setting, or during longer periods of chronic sickness, and inevitably the emphasis has been on understanding the clinical aspects of the disease and care leading to cure.

The section of the health visitor's syllabus dealing with the social aspects of health and disease is planned to complement and round off this perspective, by introducing a more comprehensive approach to the changing patterns of health and disease in society. Students are introduced to the relative concepts of health and sickness and learn to examine some of the causes that determine the patterns of disease; also the population distribution, the organization of care and determination of priorities within the health services.

Some discussion on priorities and the administration of the health services has been included in Chapter 6. This chapter, therefore, will concentrate mainly on the patterns of health and disease and the methods of measuring and assessing them, in order to determine need and provide a service both nationally and locally.

ATTITUDES TO HEALTH AND DISEASE

The nurse is concerned mainly with a short episode in the life of a patient, and possibly one aspect of care leading to his recovery, but the health visitor, by contrast, is concerned with the individual at many different phases of the life cycle. She learns to see birth, growing up, ageing and death as normal episodes and processes in the total fabric of the life span rather than isolated episodes which snatch the individual from home and family. In just the same way she recognizes that the common cold, measles, a road accident or a depressive illness can happen to any individual in any family, at any time. It is helpful, however, if some information is available about the frequency with which whese incidents can be expected to occur in the course of the health visitor's work, whether they are more likely to occur in some families or localities than others, what the causes are and whether the situations can be prevented.

THE USE OF FACTUAL INFORMATION

Factual information about health and disease can be useful in a number of ways.

1. The *national patterns* of the *incidence* of disease are vital to give an indication of the kind of health care services required, and when and where they are likely to be most needed. Such patterns also show where the greatest problems lie, or where preventive measures can be taken, so that health teaching and preventive services can be used effectively. Information of this kind also highlights the most vulnerable and underprivileged groups in society.

2. Locally, *current trends* can be compared with the national patterns and adjustments made in the provision of services and health education. Such knowledge is essential for the health visitor when planning her own priorities and assessing the problems she can anticipate in certain families or areas.

3. When seen in the context of *local population structure* or the *social class distribution*, it is possible to get some idea of the kind of problems which are likely to appear most frequently. For example, greater provisions must be made for services for the young child in new towns where the population consists largely of young families. Another example is the knowledge of the increased risk of death in the perinatal period for infants whose parents come from social class

V. Health visitors and midwives aware of this risk will be alert for all the possible opportunities for preventive measures.

4. *Changing patterns* of health and disease are of interest when seen in the context of social change. Schofield (1964) points out that as communicable diseases disappear they are being replaced by new types of illness such as chronic degenerative diseases or those linked with social problems, and neither of these responds to immunization and legislation, but must be dealt with by preventive methods. Many present disorders are, he says, brought about by infection, not from individuals, but from society. Such trends are important to recognize, demanding as they do quite a different approach.

5. Patterns of health and disease cannot be studied without a growing awareness of the influence of environment, both physical and social and therefore it is essential to know where environmental conditions can be improved with advantages in terms of health. It is interesting to note that while many environmental hazards have been eradicated with consequent health improvements, others, such as pollution, are increasing.

APPROACHING THE STUDY OF SOCIAL ASPECTS OF HEALTH AND DISEASE

All these aspects will be included in the health visitor's course but it would not be useful to enlarge here in detail on any specific trends as these patterns are constantly changing. The most useful way for health visitors to keep up to date with events is to be aware of the sources of information available and to know how to use them intelligently. Articles in journals will give current information on specific diseases, their aetiology, treatment and preventive measures, and research in areas such as genetic influence is constantly pushing forward the frontiers of knowledge. Suggested journals will be found in the Appendix at the end of this chapter.

The other sources of information available are the many reports and documents, official and otherwise, containing statistical data. Many health visitors find the approach to the study of such documents a formidable one, thinking that statistics are just dull figures and difficult to understand anyhow. This is, however, a very vital aspect of the knowledge needed by the health visitor in order to carry out her work efficiently, so it is important for this subject to be made interesting and relevant to the job at all points. Statistics unrelated to any specific topic *can* be boring but when used intelligently and presented with enthusiasm can become highly absorbing and fascinating. Health visitors themselves are constantly involved in record keeping and presenting returns which form part of the national sources of information about health and disease and it helps to appreciate the importance of the contribution made.

For these reasons the remainder of this chapter will concentrate on the areas of health and vital statistics that are basic for an understanding of the subject and fundamental to the use of source material. The chapter will conclude with a useful list of material which is likely to provide a permanent source of reference. Students will also find it helpful to develop a research-orientated approach to their study as research appreciation is an important aspect of any profession in the present day. This chapter should be useful in indicating the kinds of points to look for and the questions to ask when assessing the usefulness of any evidence presented.

SECTION II   RESEARCH AND VITAL HEALTH STATISTICS FOR THE HEALTH VISITOR

Sheila Jack

In the space available here, it is only possible to give a brief account of research and vital statistics, with some discussion on the presentation of statistics. Research methodology is obviously not within the scope of this section, nor can it provide current statistics, but the list of sources of published health and social statistics is fairly comprehensive and further reading is suggested at the end.

UNDERSTANDING RESEARCH

Two of several acceptable definitions of research are:

1. searching for information in a scientific manner;
2. an acquisition of knowledge by systematic enquiry.

Types of Research
Research may fall into one of the following categories.

1. *Retrospective*—looking back to try to discover reasons for a present situation or condition, e.g. most disease research.
2. *Longitudinal*—selecting a population and studying it from then on, over a period of time, e.g. National Child Development Surveys.
3. *Action research*—changing conditions as the research findings suggest, while continuing the research. For example, studies of the effects on people's health of living in high rise flats may be used to encourage action in the form of building different types of housing accommodation. The research into the effects on health continues for comparison (Wilkins 1964).

The Value of Statistics and Research to the Health Visitor
1. Unique to health visiting is one of its major principles—the *search for health needs*—unacknowledged or unrecognized by the individual or family or community. This search principle has implications for the health visitor's method and place of work and also for the knowledge she needs. The knowledge of *how* to search and *what* to look for has to come from her previous life experience and from several disciplines. Taking only one of these disciplines, it is possible to see how the knowledge from research and statistics helps. Firstly, it encourages an *attitude of mind*, a questioning of what appears on the surface, a continual seeking for answers. Secondly, it gives an *awareness of the need for rigour and honesty* in framing the questions asked and in assessing the answers. Thirdly, it gives a *knowledge of the techniques* that can be used to collect information and evaluate it. Fourthly, it gives *knowledge of national and local population and health trends* and where to find such information. For example, the health visitor starting work in a new area wants to know the possible health needs, unacknowledged or unrecognized as they may be. Before any attempt to assess these is made, it is necessary to find out the following information about the locality because these are the factors that influence health and provision and use of health services.

a. The composition of the local population—age groups, sex and social class.
b. The vital statistics. How they compare with the national ones. If they differ, why they do.

c. The employment rate and pattern.
d. Occupational hazards and diseases.
e. Local housing and other environmental factors.
f. Local statutory resources (social workers, GPs, hospitals, home help services and the like).
g. Local voluntary resources (mothers clubs, churches, WRVS and the like).

Most of this information is quantifiable and available, if not you can obtain your own information. (This will give only half the picture of course—information on the quality of local life is also needed and other information-gaining techniques are required to discover that, such as using one's senses, intelligence and intuition in combination with knowledge of the statistics.) It is also necessary to know why, and how, these factors influence health, as documented by research findings and commentary on published national statistics, as well as within one's own experience.

2. The health visitor's choice of present and future *priorities* and method of working should take into account specific research findings and the result of comparing the local indices and population with national indices and population data. For instance, research has been published on the work of the health visitor in London, and in Berkshire (Clark 1974, already discussed in Chapter 2), and also on the administrative setting for her work in primary health care teams (Gilmore et al. 1974). The findings of research into specific diseases and situations is available, e.g. alcoholism or family violence. Published routine statistics give considerable information on topics such as the following.

a. Regional differences in congenital abnormality rates (increased rate in South Wales, for example).
b. Social class differences in morbidity (e.g. bronchitis in the Registrar General's social classes IV and V is at a higher rate; social class I a decreased rate). (Definition of social class is given later.)
c. Cultural differences in morbidity, e.g. look at tuberculosis figures and nutritional deficiency diseases such as rickets.
d. Populations with different age compositions have different health service needs, for example geriatric health visiting service needed in seaside retirement towns; child health centres in new towns.

e. Differences in disease incidence over a period of time, e.g. the increase in mortality from coronary thrombosis as a proportion of the total death causes; the apparent increase in alcoholism within recent years amongst women.

3. The objective *evaluation* of past preventive work is made possible to some extent:

of the health visitor's own work by herself,
of an area's work, from the statistics provided by health visitors and others,
of the health visitor's work nationally.

The problem here, of course, lies in the multiplicity of variables that might have produced the results, and the difficulty of isolating only one factor, e.g. the health visitor, while holding the rest constant. We need also to devise measures of quality and particularly there is a great need for health visitors themselves to research into health visiting and health.

4. There is increasing *involvement* of the health visitor as a field-worker in research projects and she may well be asked to act as a data collector or interviewer. However, two things are essential, the first being to ensure that this data collection, for however worthy a cause, does not detract from her own work. The health visitor who takes in a survey questionnaire on her first or second meeting with a family has not grasped the first principle of her own method of work—that of initiating and establishing a relationship of confidence and trust. Secondly, health visitors as a group need to ensure that their contribution is acknowledged in the published research.

5. The personal *significance* of research for the health visitor should be recognized. To prove a point concerning such things as overwork, the necessity for a car allowance, or more clerical assistance, it helps to remember the prestige of statistical argument and its superiority over verbal communication (oral or written) in clarity, precision and easy comprehension.

The Significance of Research for Community Health

Research gives a factual, accurate basis for decision making; it is rational and without emotive and instructive elements or bias. It therefore gives a possible basis for decision making by:

1. *confirming* or refuting common knowledge;
2. *revealing* unsuspected facts or situations;

3. *publicizing* certain situations in a scientific manner, thus giving it respectability. For example publicity is used to exert pressure for social policy changes in situations relating to 'poverty in the welfare state' or 'living in high rise flats'.

Research also gives a basis for measuring existing policies and their effects, thus making evaluation more possible and rational. In addition it helps in *deciding* on future policies in the normal situation of scarcity of resources, for example in choosing between intensive care units *or* facilities for the disabled.

Common Arguments For and Against Research

It can be argued that research allows for the possibility of more adequate, informed and rational decisions; also that vital issues such as human survival depend on the increase of factual knowledge. On the other hand, some people fear the infringement of personal liberty and anything that looks like increasing the possibilities of state control. Research findings can also be used to delay action as well as to promote it and so divert scarce resources from remedying a situation into researching into it instead.

Other arguments concern the possibility of bias in the choice of subject, although research methodology itself is rigorous enough to ensure that the findings or statistics themselves are correct. Sometimes feelings of distrust are aroused by the false conclusions drawn from research and the misuse of statistics. Words, however, are just as likely to be misused as figures, but people are less suspicious of them because they are more familiar with their use. Questioning the use of both, however, is healthy, without a blanket rejection!

A common criticism is that research is a waste of time and money and just 'confirms what we already knew anyway'. This may be true for some projects but not all. All disciplines have their blind alleys in research and failure to produce positive results is inevitably inherent in the research process. Each enterprise therefore must be assessed on its own merits.

An example of this can be seen in the common assumption often made, that family violence only occurs in the lower social classes. Research done in the United States and by the National Society for the Prevention of Cruelty to Children (DHSS 1974) shows there is no social class difference at all. Common knowledge may be common myth.

VITAL STATISTICS

The Relevance of Vital Statistics for Health Services and Health Visitors' Work

Vital statistics are those concerned with population growth and health, e.g. birth rate, death rate, fertility rate, together with morbidity statistics.

Statistical rates provide stable, clearly defined, accepted and agreed measures which enable comparisons to be made over a period of time and between nations or regions. Although crude, they act as indicators of a nation's or region's health and of the effectiveness of its health and social services. Where rates are specific to vulnerable groups of the population, such as the very young or the old, they are more significant indicators of health.

Rates can be seen as the following.

1. *Diagnostic tools* to assess the community's health—nationally, locally or internationally.
2. *Planning tools* enabling allocation of resources where they are most needed, now and in the future. Note that the predictive value is questionable, where fertility and birth rates are concerned.
3. *Evaluation tools* enabling one to evaluate past action. Necessarily this is uncertain in that there are so many variables affecting health.
4. *Place measures* internationally or regionally. A country's place is important for prestige and national strength (economic and military) and a low international ranking by dispelling complacency may lead to more effective health and social policies. For example, our infant mortality record does not compare well with some other European countries.

The Birth Rate

The crude birth rate The crude birth rate is defined as the number of births per thousand of the population.

It is calculated as:

$$\frac{\text{No. of live births}}{\text{Population at risk}} \times 1000$$

The number of live births occurring in the calendar year is divided by the population *at risk*; in this case the entire population as it stands at the mid-year point. The result is then multiplied by 1000.

This 1000 is merely a factor of convenience. It is more convenient to express the final result as something 'per one thousand' rather than something 'per one hundred thousand' or 'per one hundred'. Most rates are expressed as per thousand. The exception that illustrates the point about convenience is the maternal mortality rate which is too low to mean much if expressed as per thousand. One gets a ridiculous statement about, for example, 0.17 of a woman per thousand dying. It means more to say 17 women per hundred thousand die as a result of childbirth. For actual up-to-date figures of maternal mortality look up the rates in *On the State of the Public Health* (DHSS).

For example:

$$\frac{850\ 000\ \text{live births in one year}}{48\ 000\ 000\ \text{mid-year population the same year}} \times 1000 = \frac{17.7\ \text{per}}{\text{thousand}}$$

The birth rate has been calculable with some degree of accuracy since the 1836 Registration of Births Act. Responsibility for notification of births and registration of midwives since the early 1900s has ensured increasing accuracy. The trend in the United Kingdom over the time since 1880 has been for a falling rate, with occasional peaks, as in the year 1945–6. Then the mid-50s to 1964 showed a rise, for which the explanations given were the earlier age of marriage and childbearing and more women marrying. From 1964 until 1977 the rate has fallen, followed by a slight rise (Table 3).

Table 3. Birth rate per thousand of the population in Great Britain, (1972–9)

Year	Birth rate
1972	14.8
1976	11.9
1977	11.6
1978	12.2
1979	13.0

Explanations given for the decline include: limitation of family size (no third child); more effective contraception more widely used; delay in having first child (perhaps caused by mortgage or housing situation; need for wife to work and an economic boom or vice versa).

No one can say, however, whether the number of births will stay low in the long term without a much better idea than we have at present of the reasons why people actually have children. The unpredictable higher rates for 1978 to 1980 have confounded plans to reduce the maternity services and primary education in the 1980s, but the planners may be comforted by the signs of a reversal of the trend in 1980 and 1981.

While it is possible to predict the current pool of potential parents from the birth rate of 20 years or so previously, prediction of actual birth rate trends has proved as uncertain on occasions as selecting Grand National winners. (For further discussion and information the student may refer to Kelsall 1967.)

Illegitimate births The percentage of illegitimate births rose from 6 per cent of all births in 1961 to 11 per cent in 1979 for England and Wales. A similar rise took place at the same time in Western Europe. Explanations advanced included changed social attitudes leading to less pressure to marry and also that, despite publicity, there is still considerable ignorance and/or unwillingness to use contraception among young women. One-third of illegitimate births in the United Kingdom are to women of 19 and under. Significance for health workers lies in the possibility of emotional, social, financial or physical deprivation of parent and children (see the Finer Report on the one-parent family, HMSO 1974). There is a higher infant mortality rate for this group of children than for those registered as legitimate.

The Death Rate

The crude death rate The crude death rate (CDR) is defined as the number of deaths per thousand of the population.

It is calculated as:

$$\frac{\text{No. of deaths}}{\text{Population at risk}} \times 1000$$

i.e.

$$\frac{\text{No. of deaths occurring in the calendar year}}{\text{The entire population as it stands at mid-year}} \times 1000$$

The rate has remained between 11 and 12 per thousand since 1920, rising slightly in 1972, but falling again to 11.9 for England and Wales in 1973 and 11.8 in 1974. The United Kingdom rate is similar, at 12.4 for men and 11.5 for women in 1978.

Comparability

The area comparability factor. To enable local figures to be compared with national ones, account has to be taken of the age and sex composition of the local population. An older population (e.g. Worthing or Bournemouth) will have a higher CDR than the national one. A younger population, e.g. new towns, will have a lower CDR than the national rate. More women aged 60 and under in an area will mean a lower death rate than for areas with more men, since women at all ages survive better than men. The Registrar General allows for these differences in population composition by means of the area comparability factor, thus allowing meaningful comparisons to be made between regions and towns.

The *standardized mortality ratio* (SMR) enables comparison to be made between groups of the population at the same time, or over a period of time. It is defined as the number of deaths registered in the year of experience as a percentage of those which would have been expected in that year had the age/sex mortality of the standard period operated on the age/sex population of the year of experience. Read it again, slowly. Basically 100 is taken as the standard. It is not a rate, or a hundred anything, or a hundred per anything! A ratio above 100 is a bad thing—the higher the figure, the worse the situation. A ratio below 100 is a *good* thing. Usually a period of three years is presented as the standard not just *one* year, in case the year chosen was atypical. The statistics in Table 4 tell us that over a period of nine years there has been an improvement in death chances overall, but there is indication of a trend that has continued to date—the increasing mortality amongst women from respiratory cancer. Since men and women have different illness and death experiences it is always more sensible to present SMRs for men and

Table 4. Standard mortality rate for females. Note that 1968 is taken as being the standard year. (Source: DHSS 1972.)

	1961	*1968*	*1969*
Deaths — all causes	108	100	98
Respiratory TB	169	100	85
Acute poliomyelitis	593	100	76
Cancer of lung, bronchus, trachea	72	100	102

women separately. Standard mortality rates for men and for women cannot be compared with each other.

Changing causes of death. The overall picture since the 1930s is as follows: acute illnesses and infections including TB, poliomyelitis, diphtheria have declined; ischaemic disease and cancer have increased as death causes. Cerebrovascular accidents, ischaemic disease, carcinoma and respiratory diseases were the main killers in the United Kingdom in 1980. Circulatory diseases accounted for almost half of all deaths (25 per cent of all deaths were due to ischaemic heart disease and 13 per cent of all deaths were due to cerebrovascular disorders). Cancer accounted for 22 per cent of all deaths (cancer of lung accounted for about 6 per cent of all deaths). Respiratory diseases generally account for about 15 per cent of all deaths (this varies slightly, dependent on influenza waves).

Life expectancy

1. More people are living into their 70s but there are not more living longer, that is into the 80s and 90s, than previously, and the trend is maintained until the present date.

2. The gap between men and women has increased—a six-year gap now exists. In 1840 men could expect to live to 40 years and women could expect to live to 42 years.

All social classes have improved absolutely in their length of life expectation (and in their morbidity experience) but there is still a substantial gap between the mortality and morbidity experience of social classes I and V, and this gap is widening despite a third of a century of the welfare state.

The Registrar General now divides the population into 16 socio-economic groups. The original five were:

social class I: higher professional and managerial;
social class II: intermediate non-manual, e.g. nurses, teachers;
social class III: skilled manual and routine non-manual;
social class IV: semi-skilled;
social class V: unskilled.

Since Groups IV and V include nearly one-third of the population there is considerable scope for this country to improve on its health record, especially in the inner city areas, where environmental factors, which could be improved, play such a part in poor health.

For comprehensive discussion of inequalities in health and health-care the reader is strongly recommended to read the report of the working party under the Chairmanship of Sir Douglas Black, *Inequalities in Health* (DHSS 1980), or forthcoming publications based on this report (see also Table 5).

The clear correlation of socioeconomic class with use and provision of health services, particularly preventive health services, is of great significance for the health visiting service, which exists uniquely to provide preventive health services for families in their own homes.

Table 5. Comparison between the standard mortality ratio of socioeconomic classes I and V. Note that the health experience of social class V was as unfavourable as social class I's was favourable. Source: Occupational Mortality Decennial supplement 1970–1972, England and Wales.

	Mortality of male children 1–4 years (England)
R.G's class	*1970–1972*
I	*61*
V	*129*

Infant Mortality Rate

The infant mortality rate (IMR) is defined as the number of deaths of infants under one year of age per thousand live births. It is calculated as:

$$\frac{\text{Number of deaths of infants under one year in any one calendar year}}{\text{Number of registered live births in that year, i.e. the population at risk}} \times 1000$$

This has been a falling rate since 1870 with the exception of the war years, particularly 1940–41. For example, the figures for 1978 and 1979 respectively were 13.1 and 12.8 (England).

The major age group in which there has been little improvement is in the 1–3 months group which is a group very vulnerable to environmental factors. During the first four weeks of life, asphyxia, atelectasis and immaturity are the commonest causes of death; congenital malformations being the most common. From then on until the age of one year, bronchitis and pneumonia kill as many babies as do gastrointestinal infections, other infections, congenital malformations and cot deaths put together.

The IMR shows a higher rate for the illegitimate than legitimate births.

Regional differences are still marked (DHSS, *On the State of the Public Health*). There are the usual more favourable rates in Southeast England and less favourable ones in Wales and Scotland, than the national average.

Significance for the health visitor's work

1. Respiratory and gastroenteric diseases can be affected by changes in the environment, including effective health education.
2. More attention and care are needed for the single parent, both in the antenatal period and immediately postnatal, especially after discharge from hospital.
3. A check on the local IMR against national figures, may require reflection on the difference, and some action.

Perinatal mortality rate The perinatal mortality rate is defined as the number of still births and deaths under one week per thousand registered live and still births. This is more valuable as an indicator of a country's health services, particularly of antenatal and maternity services, than the IMR on its own.

The rate has shown a decline in recent years: the figures for 1978 and 1979 were 15.4 and 14.6 respectively in England (see comments on IMR).

Maternal Mortality Rate

The maternal mortality rate is defined as the number of deaths of women ascribed to pregnancy and child-bearing per 100 000 live and still births (excluding abortion).

The rate has shown a marked fall since the beginning of this century, from 550 to under 20 during the last decade.

The Report on Confidential Enquiries into Maternal Deaths in England and Wales, 1973–1975 (DHSS 1973)

This enquiry was first instituted in 1950–51, the purpose being to analyse the causes of all maternal deaths and to ascertain what was done, or left undone, that might have contributed to the fatality. The presence of these 'avoidable' factors may not mean that death could have been prevented but does imply some lack of care for the mother. The Report stated that in 1973–5, avoidable factors were present in 59.6 per cent of the deaths. Half the avoidable factors occurred during the antenatal period and over two-thirds were the responsibility of the medical/ health service, the rest being the responsibility of the patient or her relatives.

For the first time since 1955, abortion was not the most frequent cause of maternal death. The commonest single cause was hypertensive disease of pregnancy (eclampsia and pre-eclampsia) and in nearly three-quarters of these deaths there were avoidable factors. The next most common causes of death were pulmonary embolism, then abortion and sepsis, then, equally ranked, ectopic pregnancy and uterine haemorrhage.

The maternal mortality rate for the three year period 1973–5 was 11.35 per 100 000 live and still births (excluding abortion) nationally for England and Wales. However, there was considerable regional variation, the lowest figure being 4.38 for the Oxford region and the highest being 18.64 in the North East Thames region.

The significance of these statistics for the health visitor's work

1. In terms of health education, this factual knowledge is essential to the health visitor, who must take into account the difference in attitudes and approach required for different groups and situations.
2. The social class variation in contraceptive use is important to remember and the effect of different cultures and religions needs to be considered.
3. The regional variations in the maternal mortality rate should provoke some thought when health visiting.

Barriers to Acceptance of Statistical Data

It is important to recognize the form of the barriers that exist against information in statistical form, so that they may be taken into account when presentation of material is required. Many people have an instinctive fear of figures and therefore have a 'block' when it comes to studying them for any purpose. Some have prejudices against statistics and are sceptical of their value, being well aware that they can be misinterpreted or misused. Again it is often felt that they are a waste of time as they confirm common knowledge and sometimes it is difficult to check their validity anyhow. (This is why it is important to be able to question the validity of a research project when examining the use of statistical data included.)

PRESENTATION OF MATERIAL

It follows that where such formidable barriers exist, presentation of material for general use is a point to be considered carefully if the work is to be credible and acceptable. Health visitors may from time to time be involved in this way, particularly if they wish to back up a statement by factual evidence, or use statistics for health-teaching purposes.

Clarity, brevity and liveliness of presentation will help to overcome a disinclination to consider material presented in statistical form. If you happen to have a mathematical 'block' yourself it helps because what makes sense and interests you is likely to make sense and interest other people.

Disbelief is interesting. People who accept unquestioningly your verbal and written statements will question your statistics. A questioning attitude is reasonable anyway in view of the fact that most people have been producers of statistics, but continuing total rejection reduces one's potential information unnecessarily. If the material is quantifiable, given well-established methods honestly applied it is at least as trustworthy as verbal or visual information, in fact arguably more so, since it can be less subjective, its definitions and boundaries stable and may be replicated by other researchers.

There are certain frequently used types of presentation which can make the material more acceptable, examples of these being:

1. tables
2. graphs
3. bar charts (Fig. 13)
4. pictograms
5. maps (Fig. 14)
6. pie charts (Fig. 15).

Some more examples can be found in the consultative document produced by the Health Departments of Great Britain and Northern Ireland (1976). It is important to remember, however, that such pictorial presentations are open to abuse as it is quite easy to vary the proportions shown in a manner that emphasizes a particular point unduly. Accuracy and simplicity are vital; and all relevant information such as percentages or ratios used must be included and the source of data clearly acknowledged. This is an area where the uninitiated could easily be misled if, for example, this kind of presentation is used in the mass media.

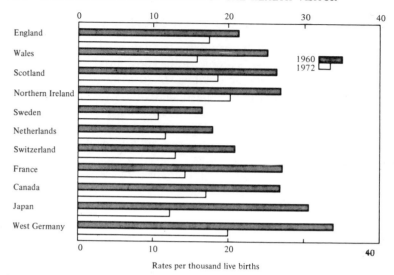

Fig. 13. A bar chart showing infant mortality rates in selected countries, 1960 and 1972 (Health Departments of Great Britain and Northern Ireland 1976).

The following are three statistical concepts commonly used in presentation.

1. *The standardized mortality ratio*, which has already been introduced.

2. *The normal curve of distribution*. Draw a bell shape. That is what the normal curve of distribution of such factors as intelligence, height, weight and other biological attributes, looks like in any population. Using the curve of distribution of intelligence as an example, most people are in the middle, with a symmetrical curving away downwards on one side towards the very few who have the lowest intelligence and on the other towards the very few who have the highest.

The fact that it is possible to take a sample survey instead of having to use the whole population and knowing that the findings from the sample (given the use of correct sampling technique) will truly represent the whole, stems from the existence of the normal curve of distribution.

3. *Correlation*. It is possible to show the correlation or lack of correlation between two factors. For example, there is likely to be a strong positive correlation between bedroom walls running with

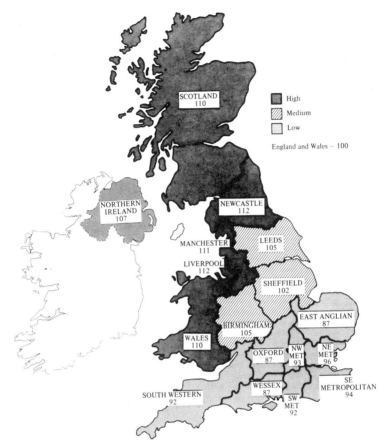

Fig. 14. A map showing standardized mortality ratios in the United Kingdom 1972 (Health Departments of Great Britain and Northern Ireland 1976).

water, and infant bronchitis. Given the relevant statistics we can test whether this correlation does exist and express the strength of the correlation numerically. Less obvious and more useful examples might be to see whether there is any correlation between the increased number of buses using the High Street and the number of road accidents, or the use of general practitioner premises for a well-baby clinic and the number of attenders.

Correlation can be negative as well as positive. It is possible that the number of road accidents has decreased in direct ratio to the increase in the bus service, since fewer people walk or cycle, i.e. the

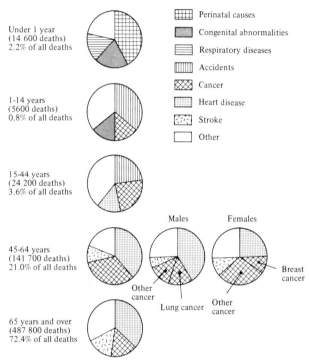

Fig. 15. A pie chart showing the main causes of death in various age groups in the United Kingdom 1972 (Health Departments of Great Britain and Northern Ireland 1976).

more buses, the fewer accidents. But in the first example the more damp walls, the more attacks of bronchitis.

There may be no correlation between two factors. It is possible that the number of road accidents has remained the same, however few or many the buses are, in which case the local accident prevention team will have to start again in investigating possible relevant factors. (The suggested reading list gives sources for further information in these topics.)

Credibility and Acceptability

Professional workers rarely understand that what is common knowledge to them is *not* common knowledge to the lay public, including politicians and other professionals, and that statistics may be unacceptable because they expose weaknesses. The international comparisons of infant mortality to our disadvantage has taken a long time to be accepted by health workers and is only recently (if now) becoming common knowledge as far as the general public is concerned.

Available data are limited. There is a problem of definition to be solved before morbidity figures are likely to be adequate and not all relevant information is quantifiable. Since we are human, and dealing with human beings, some of the most important things in health are likely to remain unmeasurable. But health visiting in particular has overdeveloped its art at the expense of its science. More attention to assessment before action and evaluation after using appropriate statistical information and techniques would be both a more intelligent and productive way of working and also more politic in the NHS, which is formed in a classic organizational mode which demands quantifiable accountability, and is beginning to discover preventive health in a climate of economic stringency.

SUMMARY

In this chapter the student is introduced to the value and place of relevant statistical information in health visiting practice. Definitions are given, with explanations of common indices and terminologies, showing their importance and giving examples of pictorial presentation of figures. The appendix following is intended as a useful source of reference material for current information and specific topics of interest.

QUESTIONS FOR ESSAY OR DISCUSSION

1. How has the changing pattern of disease in this country affected the content and provision of health care?
2. To what extent are class differentials reflected in patterns of health and disease and use of the health services?
3. Discuss the importance of research into health visiting. Describe any research study with which you are familiar, indicating how the findings may be of value for health visiting practice.
4. Compare the health problems of children from socially deprived and affluent families.
5. Discuss the value of routine screening. Outline the main arguments for a screening programme for the elderly.
6. Discuss the problem of obesity and its prevention.
7. Outline the data currently available to assist a health care planning team

considering services for the mentally handicapped in their area health authority.

8. Outline and comment on some of the significant population changes that have taken place in Britain this century. Discuss the significance of these changes for the provision of nursing care in the hospital and community.

9. In the light of demographic trends discuss the community provision of services, including health education, for the aged. Illustrate your discussion by reference to a common major health problem in old age.

10. Discuss the main causes of death in the first year of life. What contribution can the health visitor make to reducing the infant mortality rate in her own area?

11. 'The most prevalent disorders in the present day are due not to infection from individuals, but society' (see Schofield). To what extent do you agree and why do you think this has occurred?

12. What are the main statistical indices of infant and child health? Define these and discuss the recent trends at national level, comparing them with those of your own area.

REFERENCES

Clark, J. (1974) *A Family Visitor*. London: Royal College of Nursing.

DHSS. *On the State of the Public Health. Registrar General's Annual Report*. London: HMSO.

DHSS (1974) *Lane Report. Report of the Committee on the Working of the Abortion Act*. London: HMSO.

DHSS (1976) *Report on Confidential Enquiries into Maternal Deaths in England and Wales 1973–75*. London: HMSO.

Gilmore, M., Bruce, N. & Hunt, M. (1974) *The Nursing Team in General Practice*. London: Council for the Education and Training of Health Visitors.

Health Departments of Great Britain and Northern Ireland (1976) *Prevention and Health: Everybody's Business. A Consultative Document*. London: HMSO.

HMSO (1974) *Finer Report. Report of the Committee on One-Parent Families*. London.

Kelsall, R.K. (1967) *Population*. Harlow: Longman.

Schofield, M. (1964) The sociological contribution to health education. *Health Education Journal*, XXII, 1 (March).

Wilkins, L.T. (1964) *Social Policy, Action and Research*. Social Science Paperbacks. London: Tavistock.

FURTHER READING

DHSS (1980) *Inequalities in Health*. London: HMSO. (And forthcoming commercial publications.)

Harper, W.M. (1973) *Statistics*. London: Macdonald & Evans. Gives the basis of statistical techniques and presentation in detail but as concisely as possible.

Huff, D. (1962) *How to Lie with Statistics*. Harmondsworth: Penguin. Well worth reading as light relief with a serious intent. The only humorous book on statistics.

Moser, C. & Kalton, G. (1973) *Survey Methods in Social Investigation*. London: Heinemann Educational. The textbook for those interested in research and research technique. Illustrated by reference to various research into health.

Smith, Alwyn (1968) *The Science of Social Medicine*, London: Staples.

The Consumer Association (1975) NHS. How well does it work? *Which* (August).

* Journals giving current articles on specific aspects of health and disease:

British Medical Journal
The Lancet
Community Health
Child Care and Child Development
The Midwife, Health Visitor and Community Nurse
British Journal of Preventive and Social Medicine
Mother and Child
Royal Society of Health Journal
The General Practice Team
The Health and Social Services Journal.

Appendix to Chapter 7

SOURCES OF PUBLISHED HEALTH AND WELFARE STATISTICS

This list will save wasting time and energy in searching for sources, when information is needed during the health visitor's course or when working as a health visitor. The basic, vital publications which should be read annually are starred *.

International Sources

World Health Organisation WHO has major responsibility for a wide range of medical and health statistics. It publishes an *annual report* and *monthly summaries* on epidemiological and vital statistics.

United Nations Statistical Office This has a major responsibility for international collation of social, population and vital statistics via member governments or its own ad hoc research. The UN publishes a *Demographic Year Book* annually and quarterly population and vital statistics reports.

National Sources in England and Wales

Central government sources

1. *Registrar General's Annual Statistical Review*—three volumes, on population, on medical statistics, and of commentary respectively; based on the Census and the routine collection of vital statistics. Also weekly and quarterly returns of infectious diseases are published.

2.* *The Annual Report of the Chief Medical Officer of Health, On the State of the Public Health* to the Secretary of State for Health. This is based on the following.

    a. Routinely collected statistics, via other government departments, the Registrar General's Office and the Department of Health and Social Security itself.

    b. Ad hoc data, i.e. special surveys and research.

    c. International Statistics

3. The *biennial report* to the *Secretary of State for Education from the Chief Medical Officer of the School Health Service on The Health of the School Child.* Since 1972 when the School Health Service became part of the National Health Service, a similar report may be published by the Department of Health and Social Security, or the information included in the annual report *On the State of the Public Health.*

4. Similar annual or biennial reports from other government departments, e.g. the annual report of the social security branch of the DHSS includes statistics on absence from work due to illness. The annual report from the housing and local government branch of the Department of the Environment includes housing statistics.

5.* *Digest of Health Statistics for England and Wales* by DHSS. A very useful abstract of statistics from various sources published by HMSO.

Other official sources

1. Research departments/units, and individual researchers in universities, further education establishments and the National Health Service, for example the Department of Health and Social Security sponsors some nurses researching into nursing.

2. The Medical Research Council Units, e.g. air pollution research unit at St Bartholomew's Hospital; common cold unit at Salisbury; genetics units at the Institute of Child Health; child nutrition unit in Uganda. In view of international changes and shifts of emphasis in research, the Medical Research Council should be consulted for correct current information.

3. Organizations concerned with specific subjects and problems, e.g. The Race Relations Board.

4. Reports of Royal Commissions and Government Committees may include useful statistical and other information on specific subjects, e.g. abortion—Lane Committee, one-parent families—Finer Committee (full titles below).

Voluntary organizations

1. Societies concerned with specific diseases finance research and publish annual reports, e.g. Spina-Bifida Society, Multiple Sclerosis Society, Chest and Heart Association, Arthritis and Rheumatism Council.

2. Societies concerned with specific problems, e.g. Shelter, Disablement Income Group.

3. Research departments of interested professions, e.g. General Nursing Council Research Unit, The Royal College of Physicians.

4. Privately financed research undertaken by individuals not in research posts in the National Health Service or universities. Research may be financed by, among others, the Nuffield Foundation, Rowntree Trust, National Institute of Economic and Social Research (NIESR), Political and Economic Planning (PEP), Consumers Association (*Which*).

Local Sources

Local official sources

1.* Registrar General's local data, particularly births and deaths.

2.* National Health Service:

a. Up to 1972 the local authority medical officer of health's annual report which included statistics on personal and public health—including mental health, the health of mothers and young children, of the old, the disabled and handicapped. Also included were statistics from the local chest clinic and school health service. From 1972 look for information about personal health, school and communal health from the NHS community physician, and for environmental health from the local authority chief public health inspector.

b. Regional and area health authorities' research departments are being initiated and research officers appointed. Functions and appointments vary considerably in these early stages of the reorganized Health Service. Two major potential sources of information for the health visitor are the community physician, and any nursing research department which may be established. For example the South East Regional Health Authority has appointed a research nursing officer. Other regional nursing officers have made similar arrangements. Enquire in your area and region.

3. Local Government. Annual reports by the chief officers of

local authority departments, e.g. social services, education, housing, and vitally,* the report of the chief public health inspector.

4. Other official and semi-official sources. Local research may be undertaken by universities and hospitals. Enquire.

Local voluntary organizations or branches of national organizations

1. Societies concerned with specific diseases, e.g. the Mentally Handicapped, the Horder Society (arthritis).

2. Organizations concerned with specific problems or services, e.g. Housing Associations, Red Cross Society, WRVS.

SOURCES FOR SPECIFIC TOPICS ON AREAS OF INTEREST

Statistics on General Population Trends

The ten-yearly Census of Population and mid-term sample Census, e.g. The Registrar General's *Census of Population 1971* and *Census of Population 1966* (both HMSO). Also the following.

Central Statistical Office. *The Annual Abstract of Statistics*. London: HMSO.

Central Statistical Office. *The Monthly Digest of Statistics*. London: HMSO.

Central Statistical Office. *Social Trends*. London: HMSO. (Published annually.)

Registrar General. *The Annual Statistical Review* (3 volumes). London: HMSO.

The Office of Population Censuses and Surveys. *Population Trends*. (A quarterly journal.)

The Office of Population Censuses and Surveys. *General Household Survey*. (Published annually.)

The Office of Population Censuses and Surveys also publishes various population, family and mortality statistics at weekly, monthly or yearly intervals.

Health

Cartwright, A. (1964) *Human Relations and Hospital Care*. London: Routledge & Kegan Paul.

Cartwright, A. (1967) *Patients and Their Doctors*. London: Routledge & Kegan Paul.

DES. *Biennial Reports of the Chief Medical Officer*. Since 1974 responsibility for these has been taken over by the NHS.

DHSS. *Health Trends*. A quarterly journal.

HMSO. *Annual Reports of the DHSS*. London.

HMSO. *Digest of Health Statistics*. An annual publication.

HMSO. *Health and Personal Social Services Statistics for England* (plus Great Britain). An annual report.

HMSO (1974) *Lane Report. The Report of the Committee on the Working of the Abortion Act*. London.

HMSO. *On the State of the Public Health*. The annual report of the chief medical officer of the DHSS.

HMSO (1975) *Report on Confidential Enquiries into Maternal Deaths in England and Wales 1970–72*. London.

Royal Geographical Society (1975) *Regional Atlas of Morbidity*. London.

Statistics on Child Development and Child Health

Butler, N.R. & Bonham, E.D. (1963) *Perinatal Mortality*. Edinburgh: National Birthday Trust Fund.

DHSS (1975) *The School Health Service 1908–1974*. London: HMSO.

Douglas, J.W. (1964) *The Home and the School*. London: McGibbon & Gee.

Douglas, J.W. & Blomfield, J.M. (1958) *Children Under Five*. London: National Children's Bureau.

Douglas, J.W., Ross, J.M. & Simpson, H.R. (1968) *All Our Future*. London: Davies.

HMSO (1966) *Regional and Social Factors in Infant Mortality*. London.

HMSO (1974) *Finer Report. Report of the Committee on One-Parent Families*. London.

Newson, J. & Newson, E. (1963) *Patterns of Infant Care in an Urban Community*. Harmondsworth: Penguin.

Newson, J. & Newson, E. (1968) *Four Years Old in an Urban Community*. Harmondsworth: Penguin.

Pringle, M.L. Kellmer (1967) *Eleven Thousand Seven Year Olds*. Harlow: Longman.

USE OF THE PRESS

The national, local, and professional press offers summaries of extracts from officially published statistical material, House of

Commons answers, and original material hitherto unpublished. Bear in mind the vested interest/political slant of the newspaper or magazine. Even an apparently factual report without comment can distort the evidence, both because of the need for compression/summary, and by the selection of the material to be publicized. This applies to government and other official sources as well, of course.

The Nursing Mirror
Midwife and Health Visitor
The Health Visitors Association Journal
The Nursing Times
The British Medical Journal
The Lancet
New Society
Nature
Daily Times, Telegraph, Guardian
Sunday Times, Observer
The Times Health Supplement.

8. The Practice of Health Visiting

SECTION I   THE SKILLS OF HEALTH VISITING

Elizabeth Raymond

Any discussion of the skills of health visiting is inevitably interwoven with an attempt to specify the role of the health visitor. For the worker involved in the day-to-day practice of health visiting this is no mere academic debate, for if he or she is to be effective in the primary health care team there needs to be a clear concept of what is expected of the health visitor and of the skills required in order to fulfil these expectations in practice.

From the beginning, the role of the health visitor has been that of the promotion of health and the prevention of ill health. Over the years society has had changing health needs, and so the way in which the health visitor's role is interpreted has to be adapted to the specific needs at a given time and in a given place. Nevertheless, the health visitor's continuing responsibility is to promote a positive state of well-being of whole people. She can never consider the physical, mental or spiritual needs of a person in isolation from each other, and because man is a social animal, she cannot consider the needs of the individual without reference to the community and society in which he is placed. A consideration of the way in which the health visitor's responsibility as outlined above can be discharged will give an indication of those skills which a competent worker will need to develop (see Chapter 2).

The dictionary defines skill as *expertness*, *practised ability*, *facility in doing something*, or *dexterity*. Skills are not limited to any one sphere of human ability and include equally the *practical* and the *intellectual* aspects of an individual's functioning. In health visiting, psychological skills are of major importance. However, in considering and specifying the skills of health visiting it is important to bear in mind the statement made in paragraph 12 of *The Role of the Health Visitor* (1972):

> The individual skills of the health visitor are not peculiar to health visiting; it is the combination which is unique.

A skill then is something which may be developed with practice. In many respects the newly qualified health visitor is like a driver who has just passed her test. It is when she is responsible and on her own that she really begins to learn. However, unlike the car driver, she already possesses competence in some relevant skills gained during her previous nursing experience and in many instances she has also developed skills simply through circumstances in which she has been placed from birth. She has also begun to develop new skills as a result of her health visitor training. Perhaps the key factor in the development of a skilled, competent and effective health visitor is her recognition of the fact that she will be a learner throughout her professional life, and that the day will *never* come when she has all the answers in areas of human need. The almost universal reaction of the student health visitor, whether spoken or unspoken, is 'What do I do when I am visiting alone, and am asked a question to which I don't know the answer?' Consequently, it needs to be clearly stated from the outset that the health visitor does not stand in the same relationship to those she visits as does the nurse in uniform whether in hospital or the home. The uniformed nurse is there in a position of authority and responsibility, performing for the sick those tasks which they cannot perform for themselves. The health visitor is far more in the position of one who comes alongside the individual and family, to share her skills with them. Her aim is that by her professional expertise she will help them to become as independent of her as possible, as they face the problems that make up normal living, whilst recognizing the moment when her intervention is necessary.

What then are the skills of health visiting? The Council for the Education and Training of Health Visitors (1967) divides them into four groups.

1. Observational skills.
2. Skills in teaching individuals and groups.
3. Skills in developing interpersonal relationships.
4. Skills in organization and planning in her own sphere.

These skills are drawn from the health visitor's nursing background and from the additional preparation in the health visitor's course. Their development is based on the *knowledge* she has acquired, firstly during nurse education in human biology, principles of bacteriology, processes of disease, and therapeutic methods; secondly, from her obstetric course or midwifery training in prenatal development, factors influencing the subsequent health of the child, care of mother and baby during and following delivery and emotional factors associated with pregnancy and childbirth; thirdly, from the health visiting course. The five areas considered in the health visiting syllabus are as follows.

1. The development of the individual at all stages in the life cycle.
2. The development of the individual in relation to his social and cultural group.
3. The development of social policy.
4. The changing patterns of health and disease and the methods used to determine priorities in the service.
5. The principles and practice of health visiting.

While the role of the health visitor has received consideration at intervals (Marris 1969; The Role of the Health Visitor 1972; Clark 1976), there is very little material published which identifies the skills she needs to possess and develop, and virtually nothing which discusses these skills in detail with specific relation to health visiting.

SKILLS IN INTERPERSONAL RELATIONSHIPS

In terms of priority perhaps skills in developing *interpersonal relationships* come first. Without these skills the health visitor could hardly hope to carry out her preventive work, to be effective in health teaching or to mobilize others to meet identified needs. Of all health workers, perhaps the health visitor has the greatest difficulty in explaining her role to clients, to her medical and paramedical colleagues and even to her nursing colleagues. Experience teaches that the understanding she seeks will come on a personal level as she builds relationships and so often the challenge is to the health visitor to be the initiator of relationships even in the primary health care team.

Caring for the Whole Person
The foundation of any constructive relationship must be that of

mutual respect between those concerned. In dealing with clients, the health visitor has to earn that respect, sometimes from individuals who have no concept, or even a negative concept, of her role and function. In some instances, too, she will have to make conscious effort to develop respect for her client. However unattractive, inadequate, or even hopeless a client may appear, if a health visitor is to fulfil her professional responsibility to that client she needs to seek for the thinking, feeling human being behind the facade, to question the reasons for the client's appearance and behaviour. In the nursing profession, the expression *total patient care* is used, but its implications are often obscure and there are wide variations in its interpretation in practice. In health visiting, the brief is to care for the total patient—the whole person. The word *care* has in itself emotional overtones, but without caring for and about her clients, the health visitor will be extremely limited in the contribution she can make to fulfilling their health needs. In this instance caring consists more in how she acts towards her clients than in how she feels.

Verbal and Non-verbal Communication

To develop respect and build relationships, the health visitor needs to understand and develop skills of *verbal* and *non-verbal communication*. In any new area in which she works she needs to learn the particular local significance of words which are part of our language. For example, to a client from Northern Ireland the word 'desperate' will usually signify the equivalent of 'quite bad' to a client from the home counties. To some clients in the North 'bairns', and in other areas the expression 'the kids' can refer to individuals literally of any age. The health visitor also needs to have a clear understanding of the jargon used in medicine, sociology and psychology and to be able to 'translate' this into terms capable of being understood by her clients, not only in terms of local word usage, but also bearing in mind the client's intellectual level.

The development of skill in non-verbal communication is closely allied to *observational skills*. When visiting a client the process literally begins as the health visitor approaches the dwelling, where especially if the property is owner-occupied, the apparent care or neglect of the building may indicate something of the personality of the client. However, in interpreting non-verbal clues, care must be taken not to arrive at hasty judgements based on initial and superficial impressions. The way in which the door is opened to the visitor, for example, will vary in its significance. The door that is opened slowly and cautiously may indicate many things: that the client is an elderly, frail person afraid of intruders; or a mother whose previous experience of health visitors has been unsatisfactory; or someone who is embarrassed or ashamed at the state of their home; or someone seeking to avoid the rent collector; or someone in a state of open hostility with their neighbours or even members of their own family.

In assessing non-verbal clues from the client the visitor needs to note the clothing of the client, bearing in mind its quality and style, its state of repair and cleanliness, whether it is in keeping with the usual mode of dress in the neighbourhood and the overall impression of colour tones. All these factors may give some indication of the financial status of the client, the social class, the personality, and the mental state.

The whole attitude of the client's body may convey a great deal of information. The skilled health visitor will be alerted by a client whose body is hunched and tense or stooping and dejected. She will notice any spasmodic nervous or irritable movements such as drumming of fingers, or tapping of feet, or clenched hands or tightly folded arms indicative of tension. She will also gain clues from furtive movements by the client, either attempting to tidy up or maybe apparently attempting to hide something. Alternatively, she may encounter (and frequently does) a client who is erect and relaxed, whose movements are expansive and welcoming.

The client's facial expression provides further clues, especially where either 'crow's feet' or frown lines have become predominant. The inability of a client to meet the visitor's gaze could indicate the client's dishonesty, but could also merely be due to shyness or fear.

In conversation, the visitor needs not only to note the content of the conversation, but also the tone of voice of the client. A hard tone may indicate underlying anger, or merely self-protectiveness. Negative tonelessness may be an indication of apathy and depression. A repetitive dry cough or slight stutter or stammer may indicate nervousness.

The skilled health visitor will be responding to non-verbal clues from a client throughout any encounter, and will be alert to any change in manner or reaction which may take place. Such changes could be indicative of an emotional reaction on the part of the client to some aspect of the conversation, or perhaps something far more basic such as the need to start preparing a meal.

All the factors discussed above relate not only to the non-verbal communication the health visitor may receive, but also to the way in which she herself, consciously or unconsciously, communicates to her client.

Acceptance and the Need for Change

If a client is to relate in a meaningful way to the health visitor, the need of the client to feel *accepted* as she is becomes paramount. At the same time, the skilled health visitor will be identifying areas where there is a need for change in order to promote total health. The health visitor needs to develop the ability to recognize her own motives in seeking to promote change. Learning is defined as a more or less permanent change in behaviour, and the desired learning will not take place where the emotional climate is wrong. Psychological insights with regard to health visiting practice are discussed in Chapter 4. However, it may be said here that to demonstrate acceptance of the client, one important ability the health visitor must develop is that of *listening*. On occasion this may require considerable stamina on the part of the visitor, when she has to concentrate for prolonged periods on the verbal flow of a client under stress. The very act of listening can in itself be therapeutic if at the end the visitor is able to demonstrate that she has understood and has been listening with compassion as a caring human being, rather than in a detached way as a professional worker paid to do so. Very real skill has to be developed as the visitor walks the tightrope between developing empathy and identifying with the client on the one hand, and unhealthy and unconstructive over-involvement on the other hand. Apart from the strain on the visitor of the latter, the client needing support through stress must be able to depend on the objectivity and stability of the visitor. *Empathy* in itself is a skill which comes only with experience, and could be described as the ability to identify with another in such a way as metaphorically to enter into their experience with them. Another aspect of the skill of listening is that of identifying the real need of the client as opposed to the problem which she presents. Not only careful listening but also skilled questioning may be needed to enable the client to put into words the true need. The statement, 'The baby is always hungry and won't stop crying' may be the presenting statement for underlying problems ranging from a blocked teat to serious marital disharmony and even a potential baby-battering environment. The health visitor does need to remember, however, that it is usual for comparatively small problems to cause a disproportionate amount of distress, especially to inexperienced young mothers.

Relating to Colleagues as well as Clients

The skills in interpersonal relationships which the health visitor uses in relationship to her clients are equally important when it comes to dealing with her medical, paramedical and other professional colleagues and voluntary agencies. If she is to be fully effective when acting as a referral agency to the appropriate service, then not only her clients, but her colleagues, need to be treated as whole people first. The role which they perform must be seen as second to this, though nonetheless important.

Self-knowledge

In all her relationships, the health visitor needs to develop insight, not only into the basis of the behaviour of others, but also her own behaviour. There will be times when she feels that she is the focus for anger or hostility, for example. It is possible that this could be due to her own personality but it is more likely and more commonly true that she is being used as a 'safe' outlet for anger or frustration arising from quite another cause. The mature health visitor also learns to accept that no single individual has the capacity to relate constructively to all her clients and that as part of a caring team she will on occasion need to allow another member to fulfil her role.

OBSERVATIONAL SKILLS

Some of the observational skills of the health visitor have already been mentioned. Such skills need to be developed to a very high degree if she is to carry out her function in early detection of disease or abnormality. For example, whilst visiting a young mother with young children, she will not merely be talking with the mother, but at the same time noting the specific activities of the children and relating them to their ages and respective expected development. When the children are present, she may rarely need to ask direct questions but may gain a great deal of information by watching and playing with the children.

TEACHING SKILLS

Preventive *health education* is a major aspect of the health visitor's work. By definition, this field of education consists more in *changing attitudes* than in simply teaching clinical facts. Health education is discussed elsewhere in this book (Chapter 11) but teaching skills are essential and need reference here. The health visitor's main teaching role is in one-to-one relationships and small informal groups and as such she needs to develop facility in discussion techniques. Her aim is to help clients to arrive at the answers to their problems themselves, with her help, rather than by her telling them what to do. She may use *questions* as part of her approach, and if so, they need to be open-ended questions such as those beginning 'when', 'where', 'how', 'why', 'what', which will stimulate clients to think through for themselves. Such questions will also help the health visitor to discover what is already known to her clients and can be used as the foundation on which to build her teaching (see pp. 240–242).

SKILLS IN ORGANIZATION AND PLANNING

Assessment of Priorities

As an independent worker the health visitor has the responsibility to develop skills in *organization*, *planning* and *referral*. When she comes newly to her area, she is presented with a pre-existing case load. She also finds herself in a specific neighbourhood which has its own distinct social class and possibly racial mix and its own history or lack of history. Her first task is to determine the priority health needs of her area and the resources available. Her skill in accomplishing this will largely depend on the theoretical knowledge gained during her training and the skill with which she is able to apply theory to her practical situation. A neighbourhood study is part of health visitor training and a student should realize that this is a very valuable tool in helping the qualified health visitor to determine her priorities. Particularly in an area where there are many needs and few resources, the health visitor needs to develop skill in mobilizing voluntary and lay groups, encouraging self-help through community action groups, promoting the development of activities such as mothers clubs, luncheon clubs and playgroups. Developing skills in *identifying health needs* born of a given environment may enable the health visitor to prevent ill health in many individuals by her promotion of community action.

Decision Making

The identification of a health need carries with it the implication that the health visitor must decide on what action can or should be taken. Often this *action* will need to take the form of skilled *guidance* of the client by the visitor until the client herself recognizes the need. Once this position has been reached the client may be able to use her own resources to resolve the situation. Even when this is not the case, the awareness of need promoted by the health visitor is going to make the client far more willing to accept help and participate in change than would be likely if the client regarded the health visitor as an agent of intervention external to herself. A nursing background can often lead to an almost instinctive reaction on the part of the health visitor that she should act for the client, even though as Henderson's definition suggests (1961), 'the unique function of the nurse is to assist the individual, sick or well, in the performance of those activities contributing to health . . . in such a way as to help him gain independence as rapidly as possible'. The emphasis for the health visitor should be on deciding *with* the client rather than *for* the client. However, there will be occasions when this is not possible and where even the health visitor is not in a position to reach a decision alone as to the action to be taken. An example would be a case of suspected child abuse and here the responsibility would rest with the health visitor, if she identified this possibility, to initiate a case discussion with the aim of arriving at a group decision as to appropriate action.

Planning of Daily Work

In *planning* her daily visiting the health visitor needs to be realistic. Caseloads vary widely in their size and content. Not every health problem can be solved in practice, and most soluble problems can be tackled only when time has been invested in building relationships. Consequently the health visitor needs to develop skill in allocating her time, realizing that if she spends insufficient time with clients, that time in itself may prove to have been wasted. Regular *routine visiting* is still ideally the backbone of health visiting however, since clients are unlikely to turn for help to strangers whom they have seen only once after the baby was born. Skill needs to be developed also in determining the frequency of visiting appropriate to any given family. In allocating her time the health visitor must always allow for the unexpected, so that if some urgent demand on her services occurs, she has included in her day's timetable some routine work which can be postponed without much difficulty. Skilled health visiting requires considerable self-discipline combined with flexibility, not least in allowing for prompt *recording of visits* and action taken. Where economic resources allow, the quality and quantity of a health visitor's work can be enhanced if she has the use of a pocket cassette recorder and the services of an audiotypist. Immediate verbal recording of a visit, once the health visitor has mastered the use of the machine, can ensure that important details are not overlooked.

Recording and Reporting

As part of her training, the student should have gained a clear understanding of the roles of colleagues to whom she would commonly need to refer clients. When making reports, keeping records, or making referrals to such colleagues, it is essential that the qualified health visitor develops skill in writing relevant information clearly, concisely, and legibly, always signing anything she writes. It is of no use to anyone if a health visitor establishes ideal rapport with a client, identifies a need or needs, makes no record of her work and then is, for example, taken ill and unable to communicate with anyone professionally. It is part of her responsibility, having identified need, to ensure that all possible action is taken to meet the need. In this respect two important factors can give rise to a measure of conflict calling for the development of discernment on the part of the health visitor. If the total health needs of individuals are to be met, this can only be achieved by the work of a cooperating team, since no single person will possess all the expertise needed. This means that in referral and report writing the health visitor must be willing to share necessary information. At the same time she may possess information given to her in confidence by the client which she is professionally obliged *not* to communicate without the client's knowledge and permission. Personal records should always be kept in a locked cabinet, to which only authorized staff have access.

Any verbal report or liaison should be followed up in writing and carbon copies of any written communication should be retained in the health visitor's records for two reasons. One is so that the records contain a complete and accurate source of reference to any given situation and the other is so that the health visitor has written evidence of her activity, which could in some instances even serve to safeguard her professionally.

A consideration of record keeping is incomplete without reference to the use of a filing system. The health visitor may have to conform to an already existing system, or may be in a position to devise her own. In either instance experience teaches that any filing system must be meticulously adhered to in order to prevent a serious waste of time spent in locating misfiled records.

Evaluation

Finally, the health visitor needs to develop skill in *evaluating the effectiveness* of her work. This presents some difficulty, since it is impossible to prove conclusively that ill health has specifically been prevented by the work of the health visitor. However, local statistics can show, for example, a direct correlation between a health visitor's campaign to encourage immunization and a rise in uptake by the community of the immunizations offered. A change in the pattern of priority health needs in a given worker's area could also be an indicator that the particular health visitor was being effective in meeting those needs she originally accorded top priority.

The importance of skill in evaluation is highlighted in the Report of the Working Group of the Council for the Education and Training of Health Visitors on *An Investigation into the Principles of Health Visiting* (1977). In the Report four principles of health visiting are identified, including the principle of 'the search for health needs'. On page 28, paragraph 4.12, the statement is made that:

> The search for health needs by the health visitor is unique. Health visiting is the only profession whose primary aim is to promote personal health by searching for health needs.

In continuing to discuss the nature of this searching, the Report includes the following paragraph (page 30, paragraph 4.18)

> The expert nature of the search is apparent in the method used which consists of observation, interpretation, and deductions from data. Validation by collecting new facts to refute or confirm the hypothesis, follows. In reality this is generally the weak link in the practice of health visiting . . . It is, therefore, imperative to devise tools of evaluation in health visiting.

Current research in health visiting is beginning to seek to develop such tools. If the validity of the 'search principle' is accepted, with its uniqueness to health visiting, then skills in evaluation must have a very high priority in health visiting practice. Whether or not the health visitor can evaluate her work by methods which would satisfy research criteria, she needs to develop a constructively critical approach whereby she is constantly questioning her methods and her priorities. Society is constantly changing and in some areas environmental factors are such that the rate of change is greatly accelerated, in itself bringing new needs and problems, and new ways of communication to be discovered.

SECTION II THE SKILLS OF INTERVIEWING

Grace M. Owen

Interviewing is a very basic and essential skill for health visiting practice and therefore needs special consideration in some detail. It is fundamental to all health visiting in the one-to-one situation, in the home, health centre, a general practice unit, in fact, wherever the health visitor works with people in the process of carrying out her role and function. It involves a complex set of skills and includes a variety of different objectives. The following discussion might well apply to any professional interviewing, but it is the particular blend of skills and objectives needed in health visiting that calls for consideration here.

Benjamin (1974) defines an interview as 'a conversation between two people that is serious and purposeful'. Moser (1971) describes it as a *social process* involving two individuals, the *interviewer* and *respondent*, and the *interaction* between these two must be taken into account in any discussion. Benjamin goes on to describe two kinds of interview, one where the interviewer seeks help or information from the interviewee and another where the situation is reversed. The former kind includes such occasions as an interview for a post, or for purposes of a research project and is therefore not the *primary* concern of health visitors. The basic skills required are, however, similar, and health visitors are likely to be more frequently used in this kind of interview as they progress to management posts or become involved with research.

OBJECTIVES OF INTERVIEWING

There could be any combination of several different purposes in the interviewing situation.

1. *Information seeking*, examples of which can be seen in the research interview carried out for purposes of a sociological or health survey, or a fact-finding interview, when a doctor is recording a medical history. These both involve compiling records.

2. *Establishing relationships* is an important aspect of interviewing for professional workers and involves a number of skills of interaction, such as establishing contact and confidence, listening, questioning and reassuring.

3. *Information giving* may involve many kinds of professional work, including social advice, educational processes or health education.

4. *Counselling* involves a variety of therapeutic techniques: listening, assessing need, anticipatory guidance and attitude-change processes among others.

It becomes apparent immediately that the health visitor may use any one of these skills at any one time and different combinations of these skills, with different emphasis as occasion demands.

Benjamin's book *The Helping Interview* (1974) is particularly useful for health visitor students, giving a detailed approach for beginners. He defines *helping* as *enabling acts*, the interviewer enabling the interviewee to recognize, feel and know and to decide or choose whether to change. It demands considerable giving on the part of the interviewer—giving time, capacity to listen and understand; giving skill, knowledge and interest and, in fact, part of himself. This enabling act is a two-way process however and cannot exclude receiving and it takes place mainly by verbal interaction and, it is important to note, is not always successful. There is not a great deal of literature available on the practical aspects of interviewing for health visitors, but some of the wide range of American studies on counselling have some useful points to consider.

Shertzer and Stone suggest the term *helping relationship* means 'the endeavour by interaction with another, to contribute in a facilitating positive way to his improvement'. The helping professions engage in activities designed to help others to understand, modify or enrich their behaviour so that growth takes place. They are interested mainly in the behaviour of people living, feeling and knowing, and in attitudes, motives, ideas, responses and needs. One important point is that the helping person thinks not of individuals as 'behaviour problems, but as people seeking to discover the substance of life'.

Rogers (1961) defines the helping relationship as 'one where at least one party has the intent of promoting the growth, development, maturity, improved functioning, improved coping with life, of the other'.

Shertzer and Stone (1974) outline 10 useful characteristics of the helping relationship which may help in clarifying objectives in interviewing. Among these, they suggest it is a meaningful relationship which takes place by mutual consent of the individuals. It is also an affective relationship, with integrity, trust and respect present. It takes place because one individual needs the help and skill the other can offer. There is structure and purpose present, and collaborative effort, one objective being a change in behaviour. *Communication* and *interaction* take place and the helping person is approachable and accessible.

PRACTICAL CONSIDERATIONS IN INTERVIEWING

Interviewing skills are developed mainly through continual practice in the real situations of health visiting, and with the growth of confidence the student learns to gain the rewards and satisfactions of recognition of achievement in the process. A knowledge of certain principles relating to human behaviour and communication is, however, a great help in interpreting the process and some of these principles are discussed in Chapters 4 and 11. There are, however, in addition some very simple practical points, which, if observed carefully, go a long way towards facilitating the process for students when they are beginning to acquire these skills.

Health visitor students will already have certain basic skills acquired during nursing experience which are a valuable foundation upon which to build, and these can be used and modified as found useful, rather than discarded. The skills of observation, listening and establishing contact are particularly valuable and also the ability to measure and record. The student will also have opportunities to observe the fieldwork teacher's approach and may usefully discuss detail after the visit is completed. So often a skill which comes naturally to an experienced health visitor, while recognized, is not always understood by a student and it is helpful to go through an interview, discussing the objectives, the stages, the techniques used and the outcome, finally attempting to evaluate the extent to which the objectives are achieved.

Another useful way of practising these skills is through the use of *role play* as described in Chapter 11. This gives a valuable opportunity for students to practise without fear of making mistakes and to gain insight into what it feels like to be on the receiving end. Role play taken seriously, with the use of tape-recorded episodes, can be an excellent method of learning. Ultimately, however, it is in the real life situations that skills are acquired and confidence is gained, with the knowledge of the extent to which objectives are realized and subsequent satisfactions.

The following general suggestions may therefore be of use in application.

Setting
The interview may take place in the health visitor's office or health centre setting. This provides a neutral and professional environment free from interruptions from family or neighbours, particularly where confidentiality is important. It helps if the seating is arranged so that both health visitor and client are in comfortable chairs, preferably arranged at an angle of 90 degrees, so that while the health visitor can see the client's face, he or she does not always need to look straight at the health visitor and may look away without embarrassment. Some health visitors may prefer to remain seated behind a desk and while this may sometimes be useful, it can create artificial barriers and impose suggestions of an authoritative approach. A few professional files and papers could normally be found on the desk but too large a pile, or a cluttered appearance, can create an atmosphere of overwork, lack of time or inefficiency. Naturally any confidential material needs to be carefully locked away. It is also helpful to place chairs so that neither participant is looking straight into bright sunlight or worried by a brilliant lamp. If the interview takes place in the home, some of the same points apply, but naturally here the health visitor is the guest received into the home of the person to be interviewed.

The arrangement of the session depends much on the relationship already existing between the two persons concerned. A first visit may well be conducted under more formal circumstances but as relationships build up the health visitor often finds herself in a relaxed situation in the kitchen, while the mother watches the cooking. (This could of course create tensions as well!) Where it is at all possible to influence the situation, it helps if the health visitor can sit comfortably, again where both individuals can see each other. If possible avoid sinking into a deep armchair while the client remains poised on an upright one—or the reverse situation. Sometimes acceptance of the offer of tea or coffee will help to facilitate the early stages of an interview.

Interruptions

Sometimes it is absolutely impossible, or even unnecessary, to avoid these altogether, but if the nature of the interview demands peace, steps should be taken to minimize the disrupting effects of frequent phone calls or interruptions by other staff, particularly if confidentiality is important. In the home it is not always possible to avoid distractions from small children or neighbours but if a serious in-depth interview is required it is worth the effort of trying to make alternative arrangements to see the person concerned.

Timing

Timing is an often overlooked but very basic and elementary aspect of interviewing. The first priority is to arrange a time when both participants are most free from other possible commitments. For example, a mother who has to wait a few minutes for an interview mid-afternoon may well be getting agitated about meeting her children from school, or getting away in time to get the tea for the family. Alternatively, if visiting the home, it helps to become familiar with the family patterns, and avoid meal times if the husband or family is returning, or if it is likely to be a serious or lengthy interview. Conversely a call could be arranged just after a meal if it is necessary to see husband and wife together. One of the most difficult aspects of timing is terminating the interview. There are certain techniques helpful for the beginner and these are discussed later in this chapter.

Planning the Interview

The importance of objectives in the nature of interviewing has already been stressed and obviously it is essential for the health visitor to have consulted any previous records and noted the purpose of the present interview where it is a planned or routine visit. It is helpful to have some general objectives in view, even if these have to be abandoned because other more urgent matters arise. It may be helpful to make a note of the kind of interview likely, for example it could be *informative and educative*, or *therapeutic*, in which two cases the approach would be very different. In planning a whole day's work, it does help to avoid too many interviews of the same kind and intensity.

Recording the Interview

Recording the interview is a somewhat controversial issue and opinions differ as to the advisability of keeping records while interviewing. Many people are very disturbed at seeing someone taking records during an interview and this could inhibit the conversation. It would seem that unless the purpose of the interview is, for example, mostly fact finding, or completing a form of application, it is desirable for the health visitor to avoid note taking wherever possible during an interview and to practise the art of noting salient points to be recorded immediately on return to the office. This does, however, call for discipline and regularity in record keeping. Honesty and *confidentiality* are essential features of this aspect of interviewing and any questions about this are best dealt with sincerely if trust is to be achieved.

Personal Factors

There are a number of elementary but basic common sense factors that can be easily overlooked here, but establishing one's own code of behaviour can help towards successful interviewing. Many of these factors have already been discussed, such as the need to wear appropriate clothing or watching where one treads with muddy boots.

Some points, however, are specific to interviewing, such as the need to have a relaxed and friendly approach and the ability to initiate conversation. Sincerity and genuine interest are important attitudes which sometimes need to be cultivated. Small points, like noting the client's interests and talking about them, can be helpful in starting off an interview.

The personal *attitudes* and *prejudices* of the interviewer have great significance in terms of the ultimate success of the relationship. The interviewer needs to have knowledge and be aware of his or her own personal prejudices, biases or attitudes, if any of these are very strong, because they can have a significant effect on the outcome. They can be demonstrated so readily in facial expression or use of leading questions. Acceptance of oneself and one's personal limitations and aptitudes can be a valuable contribution in learning to accept the differences in people who are being helped and an atmosphere of acceptance is essential if teaching is to be successful, advice accepted or problems resolved.

Confidentiality and Ethical Considerations

The need for respect and trust of the professional worker has already been noted as an essential prerequisite for interviewing. The client may need assurances from time to time that confidences will be kept. Sometimes the health visitor may realize that certain information should be disclosed perhaps to a doctor or other professional and needs to be aware of the dangers of promising to keep confidences of this kind. Above all it is essential to remember and respect the rights of the individual to make his or her own decisions in the light of personal opinions and beliefs. It is not always easy to decide where responsibility begins and ends for the health visitor, who has developed considerable experience in the use of *manipulative skills* in the interviewing process. This can cause problems for many students working out their own approaches.

It helps to have in mind the ultimate goals already outlined earlier in the helping relationship, remembering that the essential thing is a sense of caring for the happiness and welfare of the individual who ultimately has to make the decisions, but may well do so in the light of the knowledge and experience gained in the interviewing processes.

THE STAGES OF THE INTERVIEW

The process of interviewing can be broken down into a pattern giving the interviewer a recognizable structure within which to work.

Planning, Preparation and Appointment

These aspects are important prerequisites, the practical details of which were discussed above.

Initiation of the Interviewing Process

It is the responsibility of the interviewer to put the client at ease and to facilitate the opening of the discussion. If it is a first encounter, it is particularly helpful for the health visitor to introduce herself, say where she comes from and give a general reason for visiting. Addressing the client by name is a valuable way of initiating contact, and visiting where there is a new baby can be relatively easy as there is always a ready-made topic for conversation, interest and shared admiration.

Development and Exploration

Once initial contact and trust have been established the interviewer can guide the discussion into the main field of the purpose of the visit. This stage is reached more rapidly where the two individuals know each other. It may be that one or several of the recognized techniques described later will be required here to gain information or to encourage expression of fears or difficulties. The role of the interviewer here is to guide and lead the conversation almost imperceptibly into appropriate channels, watching for leading points and picking up clues as the conversation develops. There may come a point when gaps in knowledge are revealed and questions asked, that allow for factual information and teaching to be given.

Closing the Interview

Closing the interview is often the most difficult part of the process, particularly for the beginner, but there are a few useful guidelines and techniques. A rough but useful guideline is that a period of 40–50 minutes is about the maximum for an interview. After this powers of concentration begin to deteriorate and the optimum period has passed. The interviewee needs some warning that the interviewer is drawing the proceedings to a close, and this can be achieved in a number of ways. A simple direct question such as, 'Now, have we covered all the points you were bothered about?' or a simple statement, 'I have to go in five minutes to catch the next bus back to the centre', will give due warning. Once this position has been clarified it is wise not to introduce new topics into the discussion but a good idea to reinforce any decisions made or practical information given. It often happens that the client will bring up a question or make a statement just when the health visitor is terminating the visit and this may reveal an underlying cause of conflict or anxiety or be a sign that a difficult decision has been reached. The health visitor may have to decide whether it merits dealing with at that point or make a note of the issue with which to open the discussion at the next interview—it may well be that having been stated, the problem will resolve itself in the intervening time.

With over-anxious people, or where the interviewing is of a supportive or therapeutic type, it is essential to make a further appointment before departing and if necessary to leave a telephone number for contact in an intervening emergency.

Recording the Interview
Some points have already been discussed but it should be noted that the recording of an interview forms an important part of the conclusion. The salient points need to be recorded, factual details on progress and issues to be pursued or clarified at the next visit.

Evaluation and Analysis
It is useful to cultivate the practice of attempting to assess what has been achieved. For the practising health visitor, it ensures a continuing critical analysis of work and progress in developing skills and an awareness of progress being made with each family. For the student a closer critical analysis is helpful, asking oneself questions such as, 'That point worked—why did it work?' or 'Where did I go wrong in my attempts to conclude that interview?' or 'Did I achieve my objectives?'

SOME USEFUL TECHNIQUES

Planning and Clarification of Objectives
Some reference has already been made to the importance of this in preparation for interviewing and it only remains to recapitulate here on the usefulness of deciding on the type and purpose of the interview and expressing the immediate objectives in view.

Style of Approach
The experienced health visitor will have an appreciation of the differences of approach required for each kind of interview; the purpose, the topic and the person's needs all being influential factors. Some of the principles outlined in Chapter 11 may well be of

use in determining the approach, for example a non-directive approach will be more useful for an intelligent-thinking person, whereas an immature or educationally subnormal person may respond more effectively to a more authoritarian approach. Personality differences, dress and cultural differences must all be considered. It is, however, important that the client retains his sense of participating, his responsibility and rights to make his own decisions and does not simply take a passive role.

If some change of behaviour is hoped for as a result of the interview, the process of *attitude change* may initially generate some aggression or hostility, as the faulty attitudes become apparent. It is wise to allow for some of this aggression to be worked off in discussion, bearing in mind that it is caused by the feeling of insecurity as the individual feels threatened. Once new attitudes begin to form they may be reinforced and encouraged. Here again the importance of acceptance of the individual is important, appreciating that opinions and expressions of feeling are worth listening to and respecting.

Listening

Listening is an art and often quite a difficult skill to achieve. It is more than simply hearing what is being said. It involves noticing the tone of voice, facial expressions and gestures, observing any changes of colour, or defence mechanisms used, or noting whether certain subjects are avoided. It may involve an occasional prompting from the interviewer, encouragement to proceed with the next point or a reminder to go back to a point that has been overlooked or avoided. The listener needs to be free of preoccupation with other things. A good listener will give the optimum amount of guidance to the interview, allowing the client to express feelings and apprehensions as they arise and often to work through problems and come to a decision. Sometimes the health visitor may feel she does rather a lot of listening and does not take enough action and yet on reflection may find that a number of people have talked through fears, asked questions and decided on action, confident that they have had expert advice!

Questions

The use of questions is often regarded as a basic tool for any interviewer but it requires a great deal of skill and restraint. Many interviewers feel it is their job to ask questions and get answers. They may, however, get the answers the client thinks they want and inhibit the free flow of conversation, in addition to which some people resent being questioned. While it is important for the health visitor to acquire a certain amount of basic information about the family background and environment to do her job effectively, this can often be obtained with the minimum of questioning in the ordinary run of conversation. She can encourage the client to talk about the home and family and while using her skills of observation can lead the conversation in the direction which supplies the necessary information.

The nature of the question needs to be carefully thought out, and should contribute to the sequence of thought and the process of the interview. Several types of questions have been described by various writers (Hale et al. 1968; Benjamin 1974) and these may be useful for health visitors. First of all it is important that any question used can be answered. A simple straightforward question will often help to establish contact, for example 'Did you have an easy journey today?' or 'Have you managed to see your mother since we last met?' These questions can easily be answered and may well give opportunities for building up a topic of conversation. These are often called *direct questions*, being straight enquiries. *Indirect questions* usually require no question mark but it is obvious an answer is required. 'I have been wondering whether you had managed to see your mother since we last met' or 'You must have had a difficult journey', will often trigger off the conversation quite well. Other types of questions are the open and closed types. The *open question* asks 'How' or 'What', for example 'How have you been feeling since your treatment?' and allows for a full description in reply, including thoughts, views and feelings. The *closed question* is sometimes called a *leading question* and presupposes the answer. For example 'You have been a lot better since your treatment, haven't you?' or 'You don't want to get mixed up with people like that, do you?' The respondent will often feel bound to agree. On the other hand, sometimes open-ended questions can be too confusing, especially in a group situation, when they can leave the respondent paralysed. An example of this is 'What do you think of the drug dependency problem?' This might be more suitably worded as 'Are you concerned about the problem of drug dependency in your daughter's school?'

One further question may be used by the skilled interviewer and that is the *probe* type of question. This needs to be used sparingly and with discretion, but can be very useful in the helping interview. When the health visitor has a well-established relationship with a mother, who has requested help with behavioural problems of her young child, the mother may need help with clarifying her worry. For example, the health visitor may have been listening to an account of the problems as stated and have been asking questions such as, 'How have you been handling the problem?' This could be followed by, 'What has made you handle him this way?' and 'How would you think he should be behaving?' These questions lead into the problem in greater depth and help in its definition and solution. They should not develop into a cross-examination, but rather be used to help the respondent solve the problem.

Anticipatory Guidance
Anticipatory guidance as outlined by Caplan (1961) is a skill used by many health visitors during the interviewing process. This is a technique which aims to lower the individual's anxiety level at a time of crisis by helping him or her to talk through and thus live through a situation before it happens. An example of this is used in the psychoprophylactic approach to childbirth which allows the expectant mother to work through the stages of childbirth, talking about her fears and anticipating the experience, expressing her feelings with someone who has expert knowledge of the process.

Counselling
Counselling is a term which is used increasingly these days to describe a process used by the welfare professions, often in the interviewing situation. It involves most of the skills already discussed and refers to a relationship which helps the client to become aware of alternative courses of behaviour and may provide for some element of intervention on the part of the counsellor. Reference to this is included in this discussion because much of the literature useful to the health visitor comes under the subject title of counselling as currently used today.

Health visitors who find they have an aptitude for counselling may wish to acquire further skills. Certain personal qualities are necessary, particularly a degree of self-awareness and insight into one's own reactions and attitudes (Nurse 1980; Tschudin 1982). Many local colleges now provide part-time counselling courses, and such training can add a useful dimension to health visiting skills. It could be especially valuable for managers or teachers, or those seeking to establish support groups of any kind for staff or for groups with special needs in the community. Support groups are being used much more frequently today as a means of helping individuals to share and understand their problems, and gain support in exploring possible action, or simply expressing feeling.

Other Techniques

There are, of course, other techniques which are also involved in the process of interviewing, particularly communication skills and health education techniques which are fully discussed in Chapter 11 and this current chapter should be understood in that context. Interviewing for the health visitor becomes such an integral part of her work, her role and function, that once the skills are acquired, it may well be difficult to separate them out for consideration and evaluation; but for the student it is essential to look at the process analytically and understand each step in context of the whole situation.

SUMMARY

The skills of health visiting practice could be summed up as being those skills required to identify the health needs of the individual and his family and the ability to mobilize the appropriate statutory and voluntary services necessary to meet those needs. In addition, the skills of health education, interviewing and interpersonal relationships are essential for working towards the prevention of ill health at all levels and for the promotion of the ideal situation of positive well-being in the individual and in society; skilled organization and management are also essential to facilitate the achievement of such objectives.

QUESTIONS FOR ESSAY OR DISCUSSION

1. How do you define a skill? What do we mean by the expression 'the skills of health visiting?'
2. Discuss the importance of verbal and non-verbal communication in health visiting.
3. How would you set about assessing priorities for visiting when starting work in a new area?

4. Discuss the value of keeping accurate records in health visiting. Outline some of the important features of good record keeping.
5. To what extent can the work of the health visitor be evaluated? What criteria would you like to use in evaluating your own work as a health visitor?
6. What are some of the practical points to take into consideration to develop effective interviewing techniques?
7. Discuss the use of questions as a technique in interviewing, indicating some of their value and limitations.
8. What do you understand by the term 'anticipatory guidance'? Discuss the value of this as a technique used in health visiting.
9. Discuss some of the ethical considerations involved in confidentiality in health visiting. Indicate some problems which can arise in this context in the process of record keeping.
10. To what extent are managerial and administrative skills part of the health visitor's work?
11. Discuss the importance of listening as a skill in health visiting.
12. It has been suggested that the health visitor could be called 'the nation's safety valve'. What do you think gives rise to this statement and is it justified?
13. What do you understand by the 'search process in health visiting'? How can a concept such as this help a health visitor in planning her work?

REFERENCES

An Investigation into the Principles of Health Visiting (1977) London: CETHV.

Benjamin, A. (1974) *The Helping Interview*, p. xii. Boston: Houghton Mifflin.

Caplan, G. (1961) *An Approach to Community Mental Health*. London: Tavistock.

Clark, J. (1976) The role of the health visitor—a study conducted in Berkshire. *Journal of Advanced Nursing, 1*.

Council for the Education and Training of Health Visitors (1967) *The Function of the Health Visitor*. London.

Hale, R., Loveland, M. & Owen, G.M. (1968) *Principles and Practice of Health Visiting*. London: Pergamon.

Henderson, V. (1961) *Basic Principles of Nursing Care*, p. 42. London: International Council of Nurses.

Marris, T. (1969) *The Work of the Health Visitor in London*. Research Report no. 12. London: GLC Department of Planning and Transportation.

Moser, C.A. (1971) *Survey Methods in Social Investigation*. London: Heinemann Educational.

Nurse, G. (1980) *Counselling and the Nurse*. Aylesbury: HM & M Publishers.

Rogers, C.R. (1961) *On Becoming a Person*, pp. 39–40. Boston: Houghton Mifflin.

Shertzer, B. (1974) *Fundamentals of Counselling*. Boston: Houghton Mifflin.

The Role of the Health Visitor (1972). London: Royal College of Nursing and the National Council of Nurses of the UK.
Tschudin, V. (1982) *Counselling Skills for Nurses*. London: Baillière Tindall.

FURTHER READING

Argyle, M. (1981) *Social Skills and Health*. London: Methuen.
Berne, E. (1967) *Games People Play*. Harmondsworth: Penguin.
Bessel, R. (1971) *Interviewing and Counselling*. London: Batsford.
Douglas, T. (1978) *Basic Groupwork*. London: Tavistock.
Halmos, P. (1977) *The Faith of the Counsellors*. London: Constable.
Parkes, C.M. (1972) *Bereavement*. London: Tavistock

III. The Sphere of Work

9. Special Areas of Work

Margaret Kerr

The term *area of work*, as applied to health visiting, may refer to geographical concepts of *neighbourhoods*, *communities* and *districts* or to the scope of *professional functions*: both these definitions must be considered when looking at the special duties of the health visitor.

Three essential qualities needed by the health visitor are versatility, adaptability and responsiveness to needs as they arise. These very qualities may lead to a dissipation of her skills unless she specifies her areas of work so that she may:

1. carry out her responsibilities as a home visitor and health counsellor;
2. establish preventive work and promotion of good health as priorities;
3. function as a practitioner in her own right within the context of the primary care team, working with colleagues and members of the community in response to health needs.

THE NEIGHBOURHOOD

To organize her work, the health visitor must first outline a picture of the community she is to serve. The exercise provided by the neighbourhood study forms an adaptable basis for her approach, including an analysis of demographic and sociological factors, services and facilities in the community.

Here it is useful to examine definitions of *community*, which does not simply imply a place, neighbourhood, village or town, but embraces the concept of 'a group of people with certain ties, shared interests and concerns'. The mental and social health of the individual in the community depends on this sense of neighbourliness, belonging and being accepted, within a certain locale (Wiseman & Aron 1972).

All these aspects must be considered by the health visitor, who may be working in a primary care team which covers, to a greater or lesser extent, a range of communities without immediately definable neighbourhood structures and served by more than one health authority.

The health visitor may be starting work in a rural community where life is centred on village activities, though many people now commute to nearby towns to work. Many young people leave very isolated villages altogether, which creates problems of an ageing resident population for the health and welfare services.

Many industrialized areas have their own traditions of cooperative support and neighbourliness, fostered in times of depression and hardship. Just as in the country, local dialect, folklore and customs may still express a common philosophy, affecting patterns of family life in the community.

New developments, in towns or suburbia, frequently present problems, with the break-up of old and the creation of new communities. A study of the neighbourhood to be served may reveal ways in which the health visitor can cooperate with people in new estates to foster neighbourliness and a sense of corporate life.

Immigrant communities with their own, sometimes exotic, customs, religions and ways of life, exist in many of our towns. Much patience, perception and sensitivity are often required to establish real communication with these people and to accept and learn from their different attitudes and customs. Health visitors who have developed an understanding and respect for immigrant peoples may have many opportunities to break down barriers of prejudice and mistrust between individuals and groups of the immigrant and indigenous population. Before commencing work among such communities, the health visitor would be wise to consult their leaders, to seek guidance and support. Often rules of social intercourse, hygiene, diet, child management and family life are based on religious beliefs and customs and it is impossible to achieve any relationships on which to develop health work with many immigrant communities unless their customs are known and respected.

From all this, it may be seen that the community study of the practising health visitor is never complete, but an organic and continuing venture with many possibilities for learning and teaching. To be professionally sound it must surely be *research orientated*. In this way the health visitor and other members of the primary care team may become involved with the people they serve in projects which have real value and meaning in the community. But before this can happen they must be functioning effectively as a team.

THE PRIMARY HEALTH CARE TEAM

A team has been defined as 'a group of people who make different contributions towards the achievement of a common goal'. Members of the *primary care* or *community health* team contribute different knowledge and skills which are pooled and utilized in the provision of preventive and curative services (Gilmore et al. 1974).

To define her special areas of work within the team, the health visitor needs to:

1. clarify concepts of her function;
2. translate concepts of her role to her colleagues and clients;
3. consider her own special skills and interests in relation to the needs of the community and services available.

The period of introduction to the health team may present difficulties for the health visitor as it may be associated with feelings of conflict regarding her autonomy. Studies have shown that team members frequently express the view that general practitioners should be involved in choosing the people they work with. This implies the doctor's right to define team members' areas of work and is a view more commonly held by general practitioners and district nurses than by health visitors (Gilmore *et al.* 1974). For the health visitor who is developing her listening, supportive and counselling role, in contrast with her more easily appreciated previous nursing and curative functions, doubts about her own health visiting abilities and priorities may be aggravated. Progress in health visiting is difficult to assess: the paradox that acceptance by clients may sometimes be expressed in the form of venting anxieties, anger, even hostility, on the health visitor is often hard to appreciate. Under these circumstances, the more obvious practical challenges offered by secondary and tertiary prevention in a diffuse range of situations may be more easily appreciated by clients, colleagues and the health visitor herself (Clark 1974). Inevitably, this will lead to less *routine* home visiting and promotion of health with families where there are young children. Consultative support from experienced health visitors with a firm commitment to health promotion and primary preventive work may be crucial to steer less experienced colleagues towards these long-term objectives.

The loss of a clearly defined geographical area, where the health visitor is generally known and can organize her work effectively from the travel point of view, is sometimes cited as one of the most considerable drawbacks to practice-based team work. The fact that the health visitor's caseload and geographical range of travel are largely determined by the doctor's practice area may reinforce a view of the doctor as the arbiter of work priorities and decision maker. However, when work is based on a health centre where there is a group of doctors and more than one health visitor, there should be possibilities for organizing areas of work on a logical semi-geographical basis (Gilmore et al. 1974).

There may also be scope for the health visitor to develop specialized knowledge and skills and act in consultative capacities, not only within her own team, but in liaison with members of other disciplines. For example, this may be particularly helpful in an area where there is a large immigrant community and where the health visitor has a special knowledge of the language and customs.

What is crucial is that the health visitor is able to retain and develop previously acquired knowledge and skills in the context of health visiting priorities. Even allowing for the fact that her role cannot be absolutely defined, if her real aim is her clients' healthy autonomy and her counselling fosters their decision making, not dependency, she will surely be able to move towards developing her own, her clients' and her colleagues' concepts of her work. Attitudes more appropriate to a nursing function or to a social worker may thus be avoided and with them a tendency to concentrate on individuals and families whose autonomy has broken down.

The circumstances surrounding the work of the primary care team are so varied that precise formulae for members' ideal functioning are inappropriate: what appears essential is a positive attitude to the benefit of team work and cooperation, 'a realization that it does not just "happen" because people are based on the same premises, or have been directed to liaise' (Gilmore et al. 1974); that standards of service to individual clients must be the measure of the team's success or failure. Versatility, adaptability and responsiveness to needs, as they arise, must be in answer to the needs of clients who may be in danger of falling through the protective net of health services, perhaps because they are not registered with a doctor or do not fall into any easily definable category.

THE REORGANIZED NATIONAL HEALTH SERVICE AND NURSING EDUCATION TRENDS

Inevitably the reorganized National Health Service affected health visiting practice and created problems and opportunities in many areas of work. The reorganization of the health service, which brought hospital and community administration into the same hierarchical structure, was part of a logical sequence of events. The growth of community health teams, from the concept of group attachment, recommended in the Jameson Report of 1956 (Ministry of Health 1964) is but one example of attempts to work for an effective integration of services in the health field. Parallels of development between hospital and community services were drawn when the recommendations of the Salmon Report (Ministry of Health and Scottish Home and Health Department 1966) were implemented and Mayston (DHSS 1970) followed suit with adaptations which altered the structure of nursing and health visiting administration in the community.

The need for a new approach was also reflected in some of the recommendations of the Report of the Committee on Nursing (HMSO 1972) which advocated changes in nursing training which would enable nurses to move more easily than at present from one area of nursing to another. The Report also examined the possibility of a wider range of nursing skills and levels of responsibility within the community nursing team. This could well create a structure where the qualified health visitor would have special responsibilities for organizing and relegating some areas of her work to other, less senior, members of the community health team.

SPECIAL RESPONSIBILITIES OF THE HEALTH VISITOR

The Briggs Report was seen by many health visitors as a challenge for them to define their special areas of responsibility and the publication of *Health visiting in the seventies* (Health Visitors Association 1975) was one result of a concentrated effort by members of the profession to clarify and reassess their role in the community today. The study emphasized that the health visitor's duties remained essentially unchanged in the reorganized National Health Service, but the removal of a number of services, such as supervision of daily minders and organization of home helps, from the health to the social services departments was seen as creating problems where the priorities of social workers were not those of health visitors.

Factors which may have contributed to overwhelming pressures and uncertainties in some social services departments must be considered. These included shortages of staff, lack of funds and facilities.

The conclusion may be drawn that, where the health visitor no longer has a direct responsibility for a service, her special area of work moves from the field of organization to an emphasis on communication, liaison and cooperation. Nursing officers in the NHS have an advisory and monitoring role which should ensure their help and support for the health visitor in her effort to cooperate with other workers and secure services for clients.

The health visitor's study of some of the principles of psychology and group dynamics should give her some insight into the frustrations, conflicts and difficulties she may encounter and help her to cope with her own reactions and work towards a mature and professional approach to problems.

THE CASELOAD

The effective organization of the health visitor's special areas of work will also obviously be influenced by the size of her caseload. For all practical purposes, this is the number of families or individuals for whom she holds cards recording visits or the provision of other services and for whom she consequently considers herself responsible.

For administrative purposes the need for health visitors is calculated in relation to population size. The DHSS advised local health authorities that in areas with a highly developed system of attachment to general practice or with a high immigrant population, a ratio of 1 health visitor to every 3000 of the population may be desirable, rather than the Jameson Report's recommended national average of 1 health visitor to every 4300 of the population. In practice even this ratio may not be achieved.

The type and degree of the health visitor's involvement with the primary care team will also affect the nature of her actual caseload. In areas where there are staff shortages, with a plethora of secondary and tertiary health and social problems, time for truly preventive work is curtailed. When working under severe pressure, it appears inevitable that the health visitor's attention is concentrated on new births, antenatal mothers, request visits and referrals. This is demonstrated by an amalgam of priorities put forward by health visitors and documented in the article *Health visiting in the seventies* (Health Visitors Association 1975). However, it may well be argued that *routine home visiting* of all families where there are young children is one of the cardinal features of health visiting and that, when pressure of work prevents this, the most important professional function of the health visitor, is not being fulfilled.

Caseloads are built up as follows.

Antenatal Mothers
Notification through the doctor, hospital, clinic, or the mother herself.

New Births
The local health authority has the responsibility of informing the health visitor of any new births in her practice. They will remain on her books until the age of five years.

Removals-In
Notes may be sent through the local health authority or the health visitor herself may request these when new clients are registered. They should never, under any circumstances, be given to the clients themselves.

The Age–Sex Register
The age–sex register is an important record of clients which is kept in many group practices. This enables the health visitor to identify and visit a number of clients, particularly the aged, who might otherwise be missed.

Referrals
Referrals may be from a variety of sources: health visitors' colleagues; hospital staff; social workers; or members of the public.

Through these sources the health visitor may become aware of need, particularly for aftercare and rehabilitation after hospitalization or illness. The health visitor herself may encounter people who have not registered with a doctor and who are very much in need of health and welfare services.

HOME VISITING

The special contribution the health visitor has to make and a cardinal feature of health visiting, is based on direct observations of her clients' normal mental, physical and social states within the context of their own environment. This gives her the opportunity to develop a unique professional understanding of their needs, based on environmental rather than clinical observations, and remains the basis for health visiting. By placing herself in the position of a guest in homes, the health visitor also emphasizes her regard and support for her clients' autonomy. The right and ability to make decisions are crucial to mental and social health and development.

The health visitor has no *statutory right of entry* into homes. Sometimes the first visit to a new baby is mistakenly referred to as a 'statutory' visit. In actual fact it is the provision of the health visitor *service* that is required by statute, and not any particular visit. Frequently visiting in situations where no specific problem is known to exist, and where the reason for her visit may not be immediately obvious to the client, the health visitor needs to think very carefully about her aims. For the newly qualified health visitor, whose previous experience has been largely of direct nursing care and instruction of patients, this will help to develop the tenets of her health visitor training and give purpose to a situation where direct activity on her part is inappropriate. To define her aims she must consider the whole context of her clients' needs and what is required in the home environment to ensure that these needs are met. To make sure that her purposes are achieved, she must then plan her visit. Here it must be stressed that the basic analysis and plan of home visiting are the vital structures on which the health visitor can develop her skills. The same essential plan of work must be interpreted and expressed in widely different ways to suit a great variety of home situations. The health visitor cannot afford to make vague subjective judgements of situations, but must be able to discipline and structure her observation techniques to ensure, as much as is in her power, that she has a complete and accurate record. This is especially important where the safety and well-being of her most vulnerable clients are concerned and where, to a superficial and unanalytical observer 'all is well'. The experienced health visitor, working under pressure, may seem to be functioning intuitively, but those less experienced must base their observations on a consciously systemized plan. This is particularly important in the special area of home visiting where objectives may be difficult to achieve and clients may misinterpret the health visitor's role. This professional approach, with clearly defined, client-centred purposes, differentiates the sometimes apparently casual home interview of the health visitor from social discussion. Obviously, a very careful study of any previous records available is vital, so that the health visitor has a background of information to work on and unnecessary duplication of questions is avoided (see Chapter 8).

Some essential considerations are listed under the following four headings. Individual items such as literacy, are obviously not appropriate to all age groups, but are important when considering the function in society of the family as an autonomous unit.

Environmental factors Environmental factors include such elements as: type of area, housing, safety, heating, ventilation, hygiene, food, clothing, exercise, routine, amenities and overcrowding. Where conditions are poor, it is especially important to look at facilities such as lavatory, bathroom and kitchen accommodation. This may help when writing reports with the objective of furthering the case for rehousing. Where the safety of a baby is concerned, the immediate environment of the cot, fit of mattress, type of clothing must be checked. Sterilization of equipment is often poorly understood and needs to be carefully discussed, especially when babies are artificially fed. Accuracy of mixing feeds is also vitally important. Where the very young and old are concerned, maintenance of environmental temperature and safety of equipment and surroundings are especially important.

Physical conditions Physical conditions include general appearance and care concerning vital functions (vision, hearing and the like). Of particular importance regarding children and old people are muscle tone, coordination, large and fine movements. For postnatal mothers, observations or inquiries must include noting the condition of the breasts, amount of lochia and the state of the perineum.

Mental and emotional conditions For babies this would cover their responses, e.g. degree of alertness, time of smiling and vocalizing. At other stages in the life cycle the mental and emotional state, introversion–extraversion, understanding, language, verbal and non-verbal modes of communication and literacy are considered. Attitudes must also be assessed, e.g. that of new parents to their babies, and to such factors as birth control.

Social factors Social factors to be considered are family relationships (nuclear and extended), native or immigrant cultural patterns, beliefs, participation in the community, knowledge of the community and ability to use the services available.

This list is very basic, general and incomplete, but may be developed by further analysis of possible examples of visits.

The Antenatal Period

The health visitor has a very special responsibility to help parents use, and not be overwhelmed by, the advice and services available to them. The antenatal period is a crucial preparatory time. Clients may be very vulnerable to fears and phobias but equally susceptible to encouragement. A healthy attitude to parenthood may be fostered during home visits. Some may be advised to attend parentcraft classes where an emphasis on skilfully led group discussion helps to foster autonomy and confidence. It is important to note that some clients are overwhelmed by words such as 'group discussion' but will respond to the idea of 'a chat and a cup of tea'. Thus, various approaches, tuned to the needs of individual clients can help to relieve the tensions and anxieties which can inhibit the formation of early parent–child relationships. Both health visitor and clients can also learn a great deal about each other and lay the foundations for a useful working partnership. The expectant mother is particularly receptive to most areas of health education and home visiting presents many opportunities.

First Visit to a Family with a New Baby

It might be helpful to take an example for analysis of an apparently prosperous middle-class suburban family where there is a new baby girl. The notification of birth indicates that the mother is multiparous, further enquiry that the family has only recently moved into the district and that they have a two-year-old boy. Both parents are in their late twenties and the husband appears to have a well-paid managerial position. A note on the records indicates that the mother is a State Registered Nurse.

This family may seem a daunting proposition as clients for a newly qualified health visitor. It may be too easy to assume that they will cope without much support. The health visitor needs to examine her own feelings and motives before visiting such families. It is easy to be preoccupied with worries about coping with a professionally qualified and experienced mother, or to be more concerned with clients in very obvious need of help. This may be understandable in the early stages of health visiting but may lead to a reliance on superficial reassurances that 'all is well'. Care must be taken to look beyond the façade of competence likely to be presented in such cases, whatever the real problems.

Time of the visit. The mother normally is visited as soon as possible after the tenth day. In some areas the midwife visits the family for the first month after the birth of the baby. Close liaison by members of the health team is required to ensure a continuum of care and that the timing of the health visitor's first visit suits the family.

The introduction. Initially the health visitor should give her name and designation. In fairness to clients, she should also make a point of presenting some official form of *identification*, such as a visiting card. It is also important to be sure of addressing clients by their correct name. Meanwhile the health visitor's dress, manner, tone of voice, accent and expression will all carry messages. To be sure they are the ones intended, she needs to think about all these factors before embarking on any visiting.

The environment. The house, in a pleasant suburb, may have every convenience but may also be heavily mortgaged. Consideration should be given to the strain this puts on a young family, whether the husband's job is secure and how budgeting for items such as food is managed. While it may be assumed that the mother, a trained nurse, understands many principles relating to child care, she may, for this very reason, be particularly aware of gaps in her knowledge. She is also likely to be as concerned as anyone about such items as the cost of food and heating.

Infant-feeding. If the records indicate a previous history of successful breast-feeding, it may be falsely assumed that there will be little need to discuss the subject with an experienced mother. However, careful consideration of other information available already shows a completely different situation; a new move and the presence of a toddler in the house are two factors which raise the possibility of new difficulties. Also, no two babies are alike and this may affect the mother's—and father's—attitudes. Equally, problems may arise if the baby is bottle-fed. With the present debate on infant-feeding, parents may have many anxieties whatever their previous knowledge and experience.

The mother. While the mother herself will usually be concerned with problems related to her family, it is important for the health visitor to demonstrate her primary concern with the mother's own needs. Her outward physical appearance will give the first impression and she may be willing to discuss her physical state as a prelude to talking about other matters.

The health visitor's initial concentration on the mother's needs, her concerns and condition, will also help to emphasize the priority of fostering and supporting her autonomy and key position in relation to her own family. The mother's mental and emotional states must be assessed, in this case, in relation to the upheaval of a recent move and the birth of the baby perhaps before the family has had time to make friends in the neighbourhood.

The father. The father's relationship to the mother is complementary to that of mother and children. Appreciation needs to be shown of his protective role and his own relationship with his children. He, too, is fundamentally concerned with the family's environment and his health and attitudes are therefore important. How he is coping with his work, his worries and other responsibilities may profoundly affect his relationship with his wife and children.

If the father is present during the visit, he may be interested in joining in some of the discussion and will give the health visitor an opportunity to show recognition of his role and for him to express some of his own thoughts and concerns about his family. It may become obvious that he has health problems associated with pressures of work, and the health visitor may make a mental note to encourage further discussion during future visits. She must make it clear that she sees the family as a whole and is really concerned with each one of them as individuals.

If the mother is rather depressed, she may appear aloof and unresponsive but be in great need of help and understanding. The husband's own state of health may be crucial in his support of the mother and cooperation with the community health team. An opportune moment may be found to introduce the topic of family planning if the need is apparent.

The toddler. The toddler may be demanding more attention than the baby and will certainly be aware of the health visitor's prior interest when she visits. Means of assessing development and behaviour are discussed in Chapter 10. It should also be remembered that if the health visitor avoids staring at, or directly approaching the child, he will have a chance to become accustomed to her presence and make his own overtures.

Parents are usually very interested in discussing a toddler's progress and adjustment to the new baby and this will give the health visitor a chance to assess their knowledge, attitudes and relationships as well as to observe the toddler's developmental progress.

Jealousy and resentment of the mother's relationship with the new baby are common. Disturbance may be overt, taking the form of disruptive behaviour, particularly when the baby is being fed. Aggression may be expressed physically towards the mother or baby. Covert jealousy may be expressed in the form of regression to previous behaviour such as refusal to cooperate with toileting procedures, demanding the baby's bottle for drinks or refusing to eat solids. Sleep patterns may also be very disturbed. Some symptoms, such as listlessness or lack of appetite, may be aggravated by physical problems such as infections or pain from teething or constipation.

Counselling of parents should include a consideration of all the emotional, mental and physical development factors that may be involved. The father may be particularly interested in discussing his son's development and needs reassurance that regression to babyish behaviour is not an uncommon reaction at this stage. The growth of a happy father–son relationship, which forms the basis for the child's healthy emotional development, will be fostered if the father is able to demonstrate plenty of reassurance, warmth and love. A feeling of security will also help the toddler to accept the baby.

The baby. The health visitor has an important responsibility to check the baby's condition and care, which should always be observed as they are fundamental in obtaining a reliable picture of the infant in his home environment. The skills of health visiting should be exercised so that the mother will volunteer to show the baby to the health visitor and allow her to examine it. Obviously, if a previously fretful infant has just gone to sleep, it may be diplomacy to call again later when it is likely to be awake. But generally, if a visit is well conducted and the health visitor demonstrates a helpful and understanding attitude to the family, the mother will offer to show her the baby and give her every opportunity to make an examination. This should, of course, be done with the absolute minimum of fuss and only sufficient comment to make the health visitor's purpose clear.

When the baby is examined the following should be systematically noted: general appearance and responsiveness, state of the scalp, width and tension of fontanelles (checked when the baby is lying down), eyes, for signs of infection and reactions to light, mouth for any traces of *Monilia albicans*, skin condition, particularly skinfolds, umbilicus and buttocks, type and frequency of stools and urine passed should also be discussed and posseting distinguished from vomiting. Muscle tone and reflexes such as grasp, Moro and Babinski, should be noted; and the health visitor needs to be alert to any abnormalities that could have been overlooked. Reaction to sound may be demonstrated but is not necessarily indicative of unimpaired hearing.

Terminating the visit. Often, if ending a visit is tactfully mentioned, but no immediate move to go is made, clients will gain the confidence to bring up points they have been hesitating to discuss. This has been referred to as *the doorknob syndrome* (see Chapter 8) and marks a point when the health visitor can check over important factors that should have been covered during the visit and make a mental note of points to be discussed in future.

Before leaving she must be sure that her client has the necessary information regarding such matters as her postnatal check, times of the child welfare clinic, and knows where to contact her in case of need. This does not mean that another visit will not be necessary if the client makes no contact. The health visitor should follow up her initial visit, if possible, after not more than a day or two. This is to emphasize her continued concern and interest and make sure of her assessment of the family's situation during a vulnerable period.

Length of visit. Generalizations are difficult but it should be remembered that: both the client and health visitor may have a busy schedule; there is a limit to the amount of new information that can be absorbed and remembered accurately by either party; setting a mental time limit to the length of a visit may help to discipline the interview and still allow the client time to discuss problems. A time limit, perhaps half an hour, can always be extended if a vital discussion develops (see Chapter 8).

Records. Notes should be made as soon as the interview is over, preferably before other clients are visited. These should be a succinct and factual account of what was observed or discussed. Subjective interpretations and speculation should be avoided. Records should be made up daily on the health visitor's return to her office and a careful note made of points to be followed up when the family is next visited.

Legality Avoidance of subjective and emotive remarks also helps to form the basis of legally acceptable records (Fisher 1972). A defence for clients, as well as the health visitor. For example: the recording of markedly aggressive behaviour from a parent and bruising on a child would sensibly be accompanied by notes regarding any discussion with senior colleagues, copies of letters written, and record of any further action. There would be no need for subjective comment. But it must be shown, if a situation like this develops, that the health visitor is aware of the limitations of her role.

Where a situation deteriorates and support and observing become stressful, and in danger of being seen as policing, communication between client and health visitor may be lost. Other therapeutic agencies, such as social workers and NSPCC, might be acceptable to the client and valuable in supporting and advising the health visitor.

The law is often seen as authoritarian and punitive; but firm action *does* sometimes need to be taken to protect life. However, it should be remembered that, if the police do become involved, they do have discretionary powers as to whether or not to bring criminal proceedings (Godber 1980).

If a situation arises where a health visitor is asked to make a statement for the police, she should always ask for the support of her supervisors, and legal advice, before involving herself, either verbally, or in writing. This support and informed advice will be necessary if legal proceedings develop. Here again, well-kept

records, succinct and to the point, will be an excellent basis for the
health visitor's evidence.

HEALTH CENTRES

The National Health Service Act of 1946 envisaged the development of health centres where professionals in the community health
service could work together under one roof. This was to foster
cooperation and efficiency in care of clients, use of specialist and
ancillary services, facilities and equipment.

The centres vary in size and scope, the largest offering a range of
services with general practitioner, nursing and health visiting teams,
dentists, chiropodists, speech therapists and social workers among
those based at the centre. Many centres not only cater for clients, but
also a range of students intending to work in the health service. The
health visitor may become involved in teaching them about all
aspects of her work and passing on some of her skills.

Centres of particular architectural merit may also attract architects, planners and others interested in their design and function, all
this creating a hub of activity which may be rather overwhelming for
some clients. The health visitor in this situation will have a particular
responsibility to cooperate with other workers at the centre to
ensure that their primary concern remains the care of clients as
individuals and that this is clear to everyone coming to the centre.

The health visitor's special contribution to the work done will be
based on her concern with observing normal development, identifying problems at an early stage and promoting optimum health. Her
knowledge of individuals and families, gained by regular home
visiting, will enable her to reinforce, interpret and develop advice
given by other colleagues in ways which are acceptable to individual
clients. By liaising and cooperating with other workers at the centre
she will be able to develop her role as an intermediary between them
and her clients and make her special contribution as a generalist
interested in the promotion of health. The health visitor's interviewing skills and knowledge of families should enable her to contribute
valuable help to research projects and eventually, to build up
material for her own research, keeping accurate records on which to
base her work.

The centre will also present many opportunities for health education activities with all age groups, during individual interviews, in

clinic sessions and classes. The interest and value of health education projects will be enhanced by the opportunities for cooperation with other workers and the use of a variety of media.

Through her work and imaginative interest in a wide range of community activities, the health visitor will participate in helping members of the community to join in using the health centre to promote better health for themselves and their families. In this way the centre will be really serving the community and become part of its life.

CHILD HEALTH CLINICS

Health visitors encourage parents to bring fit babies and young children to child health clinics so that routine medical checks, tests, developmental assessment and immunizations may be carried out and all aspects of families' and children's health discussed.

Clinics may be held in purpose-built medical centres, church halls, or general practitioners' premises. Wherever they are held, standards of cleanliness, warmth and safety must be maintained and, at the same time, a friendly, caring atmosphere fostered.

Ancillary staff may be responsible for clerical work, preparation of the clinic, laying out of equipment and organization of medical supplies. However, as the health visitor encourages parents to bring their children to the clinic, she has a responsibility to them to see that high standards are observed. This requires skill and diplomacy, as it may be necessary for her to instruct staff on such matters as care of vaccines, explaining the principles underlying their safe storage, supply and administration.

An important aspect of the health visitor's work in the clinic is her teaching and advisory role which should complement that of the clinic doctor in supporting parents. Inevitably roles will overlap in some instances and the health visitor should discuss particular areas of responsibility with the doctor. It should be remembered that she has had special training in all aspects of child development and care. The doctor is the trained diagnostician and has a responsibility to carry out the immunization programmes. He may be assisted in carrying out injections by a clinic nurse.

Health education may be carried out with individual parents, in the interview situation, or by using opportunities for informal group discussion. If facilities are available for serving refreshments, spontaneous discussion may take place in a friendly atmosphere over a cup of tea. This could also provide a much needed break and chance to make friends for parents who may be suffering from stress and loneliness.

The fact that the health visitor is concerned with all aspects of the family's well-being and children's health should be clearly demonstrated. Common problems associated with malnutrition, such as obesity and dental caries, cannot be divorced from social, emotional and mental aspects of health.

It may be possible to provide toys and play facilities for children waiting in the clinic, which will show an understanding of their needs and the importance that is attached to their activities. Perhaps voluntary workers, with a particular interest in the socialization of children, could participate by helping to occupy the time of these children. This could also be of value to some parents by giving them ideas for children's activities.

Whatever developments are possible, it is the health visitor's responsibility to see that they are in response to the real needs of the families the child welfare clinic serves; that her priority is to be free for consultation with parents and not preoccupied with other duties and that highest standards are maintained (HMSO 1976).

VOLUNTARY WORKERS AND ORGANIZATIONS

A sense of personal responsibility has traditionally prompted individuals and groups to voluntary work in the community. These activities may be in response to need where no state service exists, as in the case of hospitals run by charitable organizations before the National Health Service; to complement and cooperate with state services, as in the case of the meals-on-wheels service often supplied by the Women's Royal Voluntary Service, with the backing of the social services departments; or to give service where state provisions are inadequate, as in the case of the activities of the Pre-School Playgroups Association.

The health visitor's responsibility to clients may involve her with a number of voluntary organizations: through liaison activities to secure their cooperation to help with individual clients or with projects; through consultative work, where her professional expertise is sought; by identifying the need for a service and following this through, by bringing together individuals who can help in, and be helped by, participation in providing that service.

Where working in conjunction with voluntary organizations is concerned, the health visitor needs to identify areas where she still has a professional responsibility. This may be illustrated by her involvement with the activities of the Pre-School Playgroups Association. Her professional responsibility towards pre-school children and their parents means that she should be available to discuss all aspects of their health and developmental needs with playgroup leaders and, where problems arise, liaise with parents or others concerned with the care of the children.

Other groups, such as slimmers' clubs, may ask her to participate directly in their health education activities by giving talks, leading discussion groups, or taking part on *brains trusts* or panels. In this way she may meet, and help, people not generally encountered during the routine course of her work. This might include adolescents who have left school or single adults and middle-aged people, towards whom she has an important responsibility as a counsellor and health educator.

DAY NURSERIES

Day nurseries come under the jurisdiction of the social services departments, but the health visitor often has a valuable role to play in helping their staff to ensure a continuum of care for the children and families they serve.

Because of the acute shortage of day nursery places in many areas, there is a tendency for the children placed in them to come from domestic environments where there are many problems.

The children may come from single-parent families where the mother or father is out at work all day. This means that health visiting support and advice on child care and development may be minimal or non-existent if special efforts to meet these parents are not made. Yet the families concerned may be under great stress and in acute need of help.

Day nursery staff are often grateful for means of liaising with health visitors and cooperating with them to secure help for the children and their parents. When leaving or collecting their children, parents are often too rushed to really talk to the nursery staff.

The home circumstances may often be such that there is a strong case for evening or weekend visiting, to ensure that contact is made and relationships developed with the families.

OTHER SPECIAL RESPONSIBILITIES OF
THE HEALTH VISITOR

Many of the health visitor's responsibilities are not easy to categorize: children of foreign students, temporarily fostered in this country; families who have not registered with any doctor; itinerant groups, such as gypsies, may all need, and have a right to, her special skills. Consideration of the needs of special groups is dealt with in Chapter 10.

Parents often need a continuum of skilled support and advice to help their developing children through the school years. This may be especially important at certain stages of development, particularly with handicapped children as they approach adolescence.

In many instances the health visitor's qualities of versatility and adaptability will be best expressed in an imaginative and open-minded response to individual needs as they arise. A sense of real responsibility will ensure her cooperation with members of the primary care team and the people she serves.

SUMMARY

This chapter introduces a new section by looking at the health visitor's sphere of work—in other words, the place in which the skills and knowledge are brought together in practice. First of all, the wider contexts of community, neighbourhood and primary care team are discussed, in the setting of the health service. Home visiting, health centres and clinics follow, with a brief reference to voluntary organizations and nurseries. This chapter forms an introduction to the next, which concentrates on the needs of the people in the sphere of work.

QUESTIONS FOR ESSAY OR DISCUSSION

1. How do you consider the role of the health visitor has changed over the last ten years? Discuss this in relation to the areas of need in the community.
2. Discuss the role of the health visitor in the primary health care team.
3. What are some of the advantages and disadvantages of health visitors working in attachment with general practitioner teams? Support your argument with evidence where possible.
4. What observations would you make on first visiting a mother with a new

baby? Discuss the importance of this visit in relation to your subsequent work with the family.

5. Discuss the value of the child health clinic in relation to present-day family needs in Britain. How do you see its role in the future?

6. What do you understand by the term 'routine visiting' and what is its value? To what extent is it possible for health visitors to achieve this in the present situation?

7. How would you set out your objectives in home visiting and how would you assess the achievement of these objectives?

8. How do you see the role of the health visitor during the antenatal period?

9. What part can the health visitor play in the life of any school in her area?

10. Discuss the role of the health visitor vis-à-vis that of the social worker in relation to care of the elderly.

REFERENCES

Clark, J. (1974) *A Family Visitor*. London: Royal College of Nursing.

DHSS (1970) *Mayston Report. Report of the Committee on the Management Structure of Local Authority Nursing Services*. London: HMSO.

Fisher, N.S. (1972) The health visitor and the courts. *Health Visitor, 45* (April).

Gilmore, M., Bruce, N. & Hunt, M. (1974) *The Work of the Nursing Team in General Practice*. London: Council for the Education and Training of Health Visitors.

Godber, Peter (1980) The health visitor in court. *Health Visitor, 53* (May).

Health Visitors Association (1975) Health visiting in the seventies. *Health Visitor, 48*, 9.

HMSO (1972) *Report of the Committee on Nursing*. Cmnd. 5115. London.

HMSO (1976) *The Sheldon Report on Child Welfare Centres*, p. 21, para. 74. London.

Ministry of Health and Scottish Home and Health Department (1966) *Salmon Report. Report of the Committee on Senior Nursing Staff Structure*. London: HMSO.

Ministry of Health, Department of Health for Scotland and Ministry of Education (1964) *An Enquiry into Health Visiting*. London: HMSO.

Wiseman, J.P. & Aron, M.S. (1972) *Field Projects in Sociology*, p. 126. London: Transworld.

FURTHER READING

Caplan, G. (1974) *An Approach to Mental Health*. London: Tavistock.

Matterson, E.M. (1970) *Play with Purpose for the Under-Sevens*. Harmondsworth: Pelican.

A booklet entitled *Organisations relating to the Health and Social Services* gives a list of addresses and is obtainable from: King's Fund Centre, 24 Nutford Place, London NW1 6AN.

10. The Needs of Specific Groups

Maureen Lahiff

The health visitor, being concerned with individuals within groups, needs to have a good background knowledge of the kinds of social groups to which people belong. Membership of some groups is by choice but in other instances it is thrust upon the individual. For example, one chooses a partner in life and, to some extent, to have or not to have children. It is unlikely that one chooses to be handicapped, or poor, or have overwhelming social problems.

To some extent then, it is possible to divide groups into desirable and less desirable or normal and abnormal. This does not mean that people cannot belong to more than one group or are themselves normal or abnormal. All such divisions are arbitrary and any individual working in a caring profession needs to use such words with care. Equally one must attempt to avoid using a *category* or *label* instead of being aware of the person. Sensitivity regarding the needs of the individual should remain a paramount attribute.

With these qualifications in mind, this chapter is divided into two basic areas. The first part is concerned with the ordinary *life cycle*, from its inception to its demise. The second part is about *minority groups* with special difficulties. In each section there will be a conclusion about the health visitor's role and function in relation to the groups discussed.

SECTION I   THE FAMILY LIFE CYCLE

To function effectively as a worker promoting health and preventing ill health, the health visitor needs a theoretical knowledge of the physical and emotional development of the individual. This will be obtained from her studies of Section I of the Council's Syllabus and will include factors affecting the growth and development of the fetus, infant, young child and adolescent. The changes that occur in pregnancy, menopause and old age will also be studied. The health visitor will also need knowledge and understanding of how social groups and individuals interact with one another. The relevance of this has been discussed in greater depth in Chapter 5.

To avoid unnecessary repetition, these points will not be discussed here but need to be borne in mind when reading this chapter.

WHEN DOES A FAMILY BEGIN?

This is a chicken-and-egg situation and probably best left to the philosophers. For the sake of simplicity it will be assumed that a family begins when two people form a close, stable relationship. They bring to this family situation their personalities with positive and negative qualities, their past experiences both remembered and forgotten, and their state of health, physical, mental, social and emotional. Much of this will be inherited and much of it learnt from their own families, while some may need to be changed or unlearned if some degree of harmony and stability is to be attained.

There is considerable debate in the media about the desirability of *family life*. *Marriage* and family life may be changing, but the majority of individuals enter into it, particularly if they plan to rear children. Fletcher (1966) summarizes the more important *functions* of the family as follows.

1. The family regulates sexual behaviour in relation to the satisfaction of both sexual needs and the achievement and maintenance of other desired qualities and relationships.
2. The family secures a legitimate and responsible basis for procreation and the rearing of children.
3. The family provides for the sustenance and care of its dependent members—whether children, aged, or those dependent for other reasons.
4. The family provides in a continuing and detailed fashion the earliest and most impressive education for the young. In so doing, it introduces the child to those values and modes of behaviour which are appropriate to all kinds of social activity both within and beyond the family. It accomplishes what is

usually called the *socialization* of the child. It thus serves as an important agency in the perpetuation of social tradition.

It is also important to recognize the part played by the family in the learning and reinforcement of gender roles, for children and adults alike. In recent years, as the women's liberation movement has gathered momentum, this aspect of family life has been the subject of considerable examination. Satisfactory solutions have not been easily found, although some parents have exchanged roles, while others have managed some kind of working partnership where both parents combine working with parenting. The nuclear family has the potential for the development of such experiments, while for others it is isolating and restricting.

For a minority of individuals there will be no ceremony of marriage. For them the stable relationship is sufficient and possibly works better. Human nature is such a variable and complex condition that it is unlikely everyone will be satisfied with the same thing.

ESTABLISHING A RELATIONSHIP

The period of establishing and maintaining a stable relationship is a time when individuals mainly manage their affairs without recourse to outsiders. The cultural myths concerned with falling in love perhaps have a contribution to this situation. For many couples this does not matter, since their personalities and their experiences and expectations regarding marriage will enable them to make the necessary adjustments.

For some, however, this will be very difficult and for others impossible without help. The problem is not only to accept that one needs help but also to discover where help is available.

There are a variety of agencies prepared to help couples anticipating marriage. They include the Marriage Guidance Service, youth advisory services, Family Planning Association, school and student counselling services, occupational health nurses, youth workers and various groups. This list is probably incomplete, but from the health visitor's point of view the important thing to ascertain is what these various bodies are prepared to do on this particular issue in her locality. She may discover an unmet need and her role may be to persuade someone to fill it. It is debatable whether she should aim to fill it herself, and this would need discussing in the light of other commitments.

The situation would be somewhat different, however, if some specific crisis presents such as termination of an unwanted pregnancy. Should individuals be in this position and not have recourse to any other agency, the health visitor should fulfil her counselling role.

SETTING UP HOME

Setting up home would appear to be the logical step to take after establishing a stable relationship. Since Section I of this chapter is concerned with normal family life, it will be assumed that the young couple are able to take this step. It is accepted that it is very difficult for some people and such problems are discussed in Section II.

Not infrequently, homes are acquired, decorated and furnished at great effort and expense to suit the needs of two adults. The arrival of a baby does not affect things much until the latter part of the first year when the baby's increasing mobility, attempts to feed himself, his need to play with messy materials and so on can lead to a considerable degree of conflict. A small child's needs in a home are very different from those of two adults who are out at work a good deal.

The health visitor's role here is to encourage teenagers and young adults to be realistic in their plans, and to do this they need knowledge of infant and child development. The concept that the child has a right to have his needs considered also requires thought and is probably more easily handled in an informal discussion group situation.

THE CHILDLESS COUPLE

Some couples decide against becoming parents. Until the present time this issue has not been discussed to any great extent outside the family circle. It has often been frowned upon and considered selfish and unnatural but present publicity for the childless marriage is opening up this facet of life for discussion. It is possible that girls being brought up to consider motherhood inevitable have great difficulties resolving the problems of sterility, conflicts between motherhood and career or even the possibility of being unsuitable as mothers. Health visitors are unlikely to have much connection with individuals actually making such a decision but it may well come into discussions with groups of mothers or adolescents.

This is not the place to consider the argument in detail but it serves as a reminder that health visitors need to think about this aspect of family life and examine their own attitudes towards it.

THE FIRST BABY

The anticipated arrival of the first baby is often the health visitor's initial introduction to a couple. Whilst there are local variations, it is usual for a health visitor to be notified when a woman books a hospital bed for a confinement.

The action the health visitor takes is variable depending on her selection of priorities. She may make contact as soon as possible or invite the mother-to-be to antenatal classes when she has ceased work. Either way, the sooner she makes contact the better, as most of the topics the health visitor can discuss usefully are important in the early months of pregnancy. It is also useful to begin establishing a relationship at a time when many initial queries are unanswered.

The roles of the health visitor and the midwife overlap here and it would be valuable if they arranged together at local level who is best suited to deal with the different aspects. The overall difference would seem to be that the midwife has a comparatively short-term responsibility for a mother and baby, albeit within a family setting. The health visitor on the other hand has a longer term responsibility for a family which is currently preparing for the arrival of a baby. Both professions have a commitment to the physical, mental and emotional well-being of all concerned. Both will work more effectively if they are able to spend time establishing a relationship with the individual family.

Whichever worker plays the more active role at this time, it is important that the expectant mother is not allowed to fall through the net while professional individuals quarrel. Caplan (1974) argues in favour of a health worker concerned with the promotion of the emotional health of pregnant women. The increase in the breakdown of mother–child relationships which is evident from cases of non-accidental injury shows that it is important for attention to be paid to this aspect of health. The decrease in the birth rate should ease the work load. Where resources are stretched it might be useful to perform some kind of selection at this early stage. Research by Frommer (1973) suggests that one group of women likely to have difficulties with early infant–mother relationships are those who suffered serious parental separation in their own childhood. Caplan (1974) discusses the value of encouraging pregnant women to describe their fantasies about their babies. He says that those who constantly describe a young child or an adult are likely to have difficulty relating to a real baby. Selection such as this must only be considered as second best. Caplan's definition of prevention has already been described in Chapter 4. He also stated that for primary prevention to be effective the whole group at risk should be surveyed.

Parentcraft Classes

Traditionally, both health visitors and midwives have conducted parentcraft classes during the antenatal period. They each have a good deal to contribute but bearing in mind the differing roles discussed in the preceding section, it should not be too difficult to resolve any difficulties.

The content of antenatal classes usually includes the facts about fetal and maternal development, nutritional needs and the details of labour and infant care including feeding. The emotional preparation is very important but variable and there is room for considerable improvement according to Rathbone (1973). For classes to be effective they would have to provide and maintain a group setting from the recognition of pregnancy through to the child's third birthday. To cover social needs adequately these groups would provide social and educational activities throughout pregnancy and the first three years. Such classes are more likely to be held in the community settings than the hospital.

Considerable discussion has taken place regarding the need to help parents learn about their own and their children's changing needs. Perhaps antenatal classes should be considered as the introductory course to parenthood with follow-up courses after the birth. The date for graduation is open to question. These later courses would definitely be in the health visitor's sphere of work.

Infant-feeding

Infant-feeding is an important aspect of child care which needs to be studied in depth by the health visitor. Apart from the facts available on the subject, amongst which there is disagreement anyway, she needs also to have some understanding of the psychology involved. According to Rice and Seacombe (1975), individual attitudes may be formulated before pregnancy begins. *Attitude formation*, then, is a subject which needs to be considered, both in relation to the professional person and the client.

There are three main areas which concern mothers about infant-feeding. These are the initial choice between breast-milk and cows' milk and the optimum time for weaning. Before considering these matters in detail the health visitor should look at the total situation and both short- and long-term objectives.

In the short term there are some basic principles which can usefully be applied in the majority of situations. Any method of *nutrition* should:

1. supply the necessary requirements for satisfactory growth and development;
2. be acceptable to the individuals concerned;
3. be free from infection and harmful additives.

Long-term objectives serve to remind everyone that what happens in infancy may affect later events. The significance of this is only just beginning to affect infant-feeding practices and is partly responsible for the present swing towards breast-feeding and late weaning. The available research (DHSS 1974) suggests a correlation between artificial feeding and early introduction of solids with obesity, increased number of fat cells in overweight infants, increased incidence of coronary artery disease in later life amongst those fed on cows' milk, excess solute load and brain and kidney damage.

Inevitably, perhaps, there is some disagreement about the conclusions since infant-feeding has only recently been considered an important topic for research. Whatever the outcome, in the long term, it seems unlikely that the evidence could come down against the value of human milk for human infants. Modern technology may need to work much harder to produce a product equal to that produced by mothers. Meanwhile efforts should be made to modify cows' milk and make it as safe as possible for those human infants whose lives are going to depend on it.

Whilst considering long-term objectives, health visitors should remember that about 12 months after birth the young child will be sharing family meals. She should thus help the mother consider family nutritional needs. This is particularly relevant during the first year of life of the first child, and a basis of healthy nutrition can be worked out over the year which could benefit the whole family.

Attitudes in infant-feeding Apart from the essential factual knowledge regarding nutrition, it is very important for health visitors to recognize that imparting information is not the only aspect of health education (see Chapter 11). Using this knowledge effectively requires, as stated earlier, a knowledge of attitude formation and change. The health visitor will need to give clients time, both in the one-to-one situation and in group discussion, to examine the knowledge in the light of their own feelings on the subject. An example of this can be given by considering the decision to breast-feed an expected infant. Both the parents may rarely have seen an infant being breast-fed. They are very likely to have seen an infant being bottle-fed. The available evidence may convince them both that breast-feeding is desirable and they agree on this. When the time comes, however, breast-feeding presents some difficulties, the baby perhaps cries a lot and sleeps for shorter periods. The parents' patience becomes exhausted. They resign themselves to the idea that the milk is unsuitable, that bottle-feeding is just as good, thereby resolving the conflict between their original attitude, that babies are bottle-fed, and their intellectual decision, that breast-milk is best. This situation could be improved by involving parents in discussion about the effects of previous experience on our present behaviour (see Chapter 4).

The health visitor's role in infant-feeding is clearly one of promoting health, by encouraging what nature intended and preventing ill health by making the alternative as safe as possible. She can also make a valuable contribution to family health through wise use of her knowledge of nutrition and her skills in spreading this knowledge.

THE EARLY MONTHS

The experiences of the first few months of parenthood may set the scene for a long time. Just how long is open to question, but Richards and Bernal (1974) have demonstrated that babies who cry a lot in the first few days of life are doing so weeks, months and years later. Why this should be is not clear, but it is evident from their work that health visitors and others should work very hard to help these parents in an unrewarding situation. It should not take detailed research to convince a caring profession that to care for a baby who cries a great deal is a demanding and often unsatisfying experience. The likelihood of this affecting subsequent parent–child relationships is high if psychological studies are recalled (see Chapter 4).

The health visitor's objective at this time should be a contented family which, for some couples, is achieved without much effort but which, for others, is like the rainbow's end. Much attention will be paid by all concerned to the baby's feeding, and whatever method has been chosen during the antenatal or immediate postnatal period will be high on the list for change if the baby does not settle down. The health visitor should use her knowledge of infant-feeding to help the mother avoid this pitfall. Changes do occasionally need to be made but should be done in the light of evidence that a baby is not thriving. Crying can be caused by such a wide range of things that it is doubtful if, in the very new baby, its origins can be clearly defined. The possible causes to be considered can include a history of birth trauma, temperature, clothing, noise, quiet, loneliness, thirstiness, as well as the discomfort of an empty or overfull stomach. Cultural patterns may be implicated: the western civilizations are much concerned with putting babies down to sleep in cots or prams which is in contrast to the practice of so-called primitive women, who keep their babies in constant touch with their own bodies. Perhaps it is not surprising that crying babies quieten when picked up.

Some of the studies referred to in Chapter 4 (p. 89) show how important it is for very young babies to be handled gently and confidently, and picked up, held and quietly talked with, rather than being left to cry for long periods without attention. It is not always easy for mothers to appreciate the importance of and reasons for this handling, and health visitors often need to use their knowledge of psychology to help a mother understand the child's emotional development and so learn to meet the baby's basic needs for love and security.

As the baby grows the mother may well require further help to accept her child's need for a warm affectionate relationship which can be established, particularly during such procedures as bathing and feeding, when it is essential to allow time for the baby to play and enjoy sensory stimuli. The importance of such handling in developing a warm and trusting relationship and providing consistency in caring for the child is discussed in Chapter 4 particularly in terms of its relevance for conscience formation and other aspects of personality development.

The new mother in our present nuclear family spends a good deal of her time alone in her own home with her new baby. A member of the family may provide help and support for a week or so after confinement. This is frequently the husband, using some of his annual leave, although maternity leave for men is slowly becoming a reality. The present emphasis on the physical aspects of childbirth convinces mothers that it is a normal physiological process. For medical reasons, early ambulation is the order of the day, but one wonders if it is desirable to carry this through to the extent we do at present. It is now quite the normal thing for a woman to be responsible for all her household chores and caring for the baby within two weeks of his arrival. Present-day standards of living carry their own demands. Clean houses, clean clothes, shopping and cooking all provide considerable scope for activity. Add to this feeding and general care of a baby which can often absorb 6 to 7 hours out of 24 and with a disturbed sleep pattern thrown in it is little wonder that many mothers are disillusioned by their early experiences of their new role.

The health visitor's role should be to help the woman to accept her dual role of responsibility for the baby and her own dependency on others. By discussion beforehand, any offers of help can be accepted and used constructively; female relatives are often willing and able to lend a hand and may be channelled towards the chores whilst the mother and baby get to know one another. One Nigerian group in its village setting does not allow nursing mothers to prepare food or see to the detailed care of any other children for six weeks after the delivery. This seems a sensible way to promote breast-feeding.

THE EARLY YEARS

Once over the first few months of parenthood, adults are tempted to relax and think they have got the worst period behind them. Towards the end of the first year, however, their cooing, friendly baby becomes mobile. Parents are just beginning to accept the effect of this event on their lives when the child begins to exercise his own will. The stage is now set for the next few years and can easily become a battleground where the adults grudgingly give in, inch by inch, over territory they had previously vowed they would defend for ever.

The topics which dominate these years are such things as *feeding*, *sleeping*, *toilet-training*, *temper tantrums*, *prevention of accidents* and *discipline*. The management of all these aspects of child care can be made a little easier if one has some understanding of the developmental sequence and of the child's needs (see Chapter 4). Parents have their needs too, but being the more experienced in the situation it is they who must develop new roles and face up to conflicts both with each other as well as with their children.

Facts alone do not appear to be a complete solution. The market for books on child care appears insatiable. Health visitors have helped by discussion with individuals at home and in clinics and there is a case for extending this into small group discussions which include fathers whenever possible. A real difficulty when trying a new approach with a child is having to convince one's partner of the value of other opinions or ideas. As suggested earlier, there is plenty of room for the expansion in provision of parentcraft classes.

Professor Titmuss (National Council of Social Services 1954) has this to say about the family:

> Society is in process of making parenthood a highly self-conscious, self-regarding affair. In so doing it is adding heavily to the sense of personal responsibility among parents. Their tasks are much harder and involve more risks of failure when children have to be brought up as individual successes in a supposedly mobile individualistic society rather than in a traditional and repetitious society. Bringing up children becomes less a matter of rule-of-thumb custom and tradition; more a matter of acquired knowledge, of expert advice. More decisions have to be made because there is so much more to be decided; and as the margin of felt responsibility extends, so does the scope for anxiety about one's children.

Decision Making

It is in these years when the children are very young that some far-reaching decisions frequently have to be made, bound up with such things as housing, finance and contraception. For example, a young couple with a baby a few months old, living in rented accommodation, embark on home ownership and commit a large proportion of their income so that it seems sensible for the wife to return to work to supplement it. After the move the wife discovers that care for her child, her own fares and other expenses for working must be met. Add to this anxiety her often unresolved feeling of guilt about her maternal role and her apparent rejection of it and there can be considerable stress in the situation. Failure of contraception at this point can trigger off a crisis of enormous proportions and may put the couple's relationship in jeopardy.

There are many possible permutations on this example which could have a similar effect. The health visitor with a responsibility towards the health of a family has an important counselling role here but needs to make it more widely known amongst her clients. She may also have to be available outside her accepted working hours if she is to reach husbands as well as wives.

Similarly, in the present climate of increasing independence for women, the dual claims of work and motherhood can cause stress and unhappiness for all concerned. There appears to be some considerable misunderstanding of Bowlby's work (1965) on maternal separation and maternal rejection. Whilst he stresses the importance of the early mother—child relationship, he does not say it should be the only one. As the child grows he widens his social circle and it seems unlikely that the small child will not benefit from the opportunity to develop loving, trusting relationships elsewhere. Many women would appreciate the opportunity to discuss this on an individual or group basis with an informed person such as a health visitor. Such work would come clearly into her function of promoting health. The discussion on women at work in Chapter 5 may be of help here. An understanding of both the psychological and sociological studies on socialization will be very helpful to the health visitor in assisting the parents to appreciate the need for maintaining the quality of their relationships with the young child where short periods of separation are inevitable (see Chapters 4 and 5).

EARLY SCHOOL YEARS

While some health visitors hold a dual appointment as school nurses, in other instances school nurses are employed on a full-time basis and are, increasingly, being given the opportunity to undertake the school nurses' course. In primary and junior schools the school nurse can follow the progress of children known to them since birth and have an excellent opportunity, through their knowledge of a particular school, to help parents prepare a child for starting school. Where there are children with special difficulties, the appropriate teacher can be helped to understand them more with some knowledge of their background. To perform this function well the health visitor needs knowledge and understanding of the education system, as well as the other areas she has studied. As with all situations where there is consultation with other professional groups she needs a balanced view of the ethical problems involved.

The health visitor's aim during these years should be to help a child adapt to the school situation so that he can benefit from what it has to offer. As well as *screening techniques* for deviations in physical performance, especially in the special senses of vision and hearing, the health visitor will need to be alert to signs of stress in children. This may take the form of antisocial behaviour such as stealing or destroying articles. It may be attention seeking or failure to settle to any activity or be accepted into a peer group; or a willingness to accept bullying. Occasionally, behaviour at school may not show any disturbance but is saved for the home situation where temper, tantrums, excessive jealousy, bed-wetting or some other change in behaviour may be the clue.

The health visitor is not necessarily the person to deal with such behaviour difficulties explicitly, any more than she prescribes glasses or hearing aids when they prove necessary. Her role is to help the parents take the necessary action, which may mean laying the necessary foundations for accepting the services of the child guidance clinic. To many people a sudden referral to such a service is unacceptable. The health visitor, with her counselling and assessment skills, may be able to defer the suggestion until it is likely to be accepted.

Such steps may not always be necessary. For example, a child of 10 who stole articles of little value from his parents was causing them great concern. Initial discussion revealed little to explain this until a chance remark about leisure activities in the family was made. It appeared that the parents were judo enthusiasts and included their eldest child in their interest. Before long, he was able to throw his mother in the accepted way. The health visitor suggested that this might prove disturbing to the young child who still needed confidence in his parents' strength to protect him. For the next few weeks the parents did not actively encourage the elder child to join them and he dropped out of the club. The stealing stopped.

In this situation the health visitor's knowledge of children's emotional needs enabled her to make a useful suggestion about management.

ADOLESCENCE

Adolescence is a period of life in which great changes occur as the child approaches adulthood. Parents will need all their ingenuity, imagination and patience if all are to emerge at the end with affection and respect for one another as individuals. Recourse to an outsider may be necessary, especially where a breakdown in communications produces deadlock where each side complains that their point of view is ignored.

The emerging adult has an overwhelming need to test himself out in new situations. He wants his opinion to be respected so that he can build up a working knowledge of himself and his judgements. He still needs love and security but expressed in different ways. While he may know that his parents' attempts to control him indicate their continuing love, it might seem to him more appropriate if they demonstrated it in other ways. Ultimately it has to be self-control which takes over from parental control and if a child has been allowed to develop this self-control from a young age, the test now is for parents to believe in their previous work.

In many families the situation is not helped because the parents are facing changes within themselves and their relationships. This aspect will be discussed later, but it needs to be restated that parenthood is a dynamic situation in which all the individuals have needs of their own. Problems are more likely to arise when these needs conflict with those of others; adolescence is such a time for many families.

To meet the challenge of adolescence a child needs confidence in himself and his achievements. The appearance of physical sex characteristics has an effect on the individual and on the group. According to Smith (1968):

> Despite the growing complexity of social roles in modern society the most important thing to be learned in adolescence is still how to behave as a man or a woman.

Health visitors should be aware of trends in statistics about venereal disease and abortion amongst adolescents. They should also consider the positive side of health teaching at this time (see Chapter 11).

Although during these years young people are only allowed limited roles and responsibilities, they are expected to sort out what they want to do and to enter upon the appropriate training programme in respect of their future work. There is at present no comparable emphasis on a training programme for other adult roles, particularly regarding relationships and parenthood. Society relies on past experiences, which may be unsatisfactory or distorted, followed by trial-and-error learning on the job. This can result in some bitter experiences not only for the adults but for the children who may have been born by then. A useful biography of the problems of maturing while being a wife and mother is *A Family 'Affair'* by Margaret Wilkins (1975).

The extent to which health visitors are involved specifically with this age group depends on such factors as the caseload, priorities, health education skills and interests. The role may be one of individual or family counselling or reference to and liaison with others such as the School Counselling Service, social worker, Youth Employment Service, youth leaders and child guidance centres.

THE MIDDLE YEARS

The phase of the life cycle referred to as the middle years often coincides, in family life, with that of adolescence. Awareness of one's own limitations, lost opportunities, decline of physical strength and appearance can produce envy, which appears as resentment of the increased opportunities, spending power and leisure activities available to many youngsters at present; equally, very successful parents may be hard to emulate. Besides envy, anxiety about the future is likely to be a factor affecting family relationships.

The eventual departure of the children can have a profound effect on the parents' lives and their own relationship. The time-lapse since they were last on their own will be something in the region of 20 years. The ability to maintain a live, working partnership is variable. Some couples will have prepared for this event and looked forward to the opportunities it presents. There is often less concern about family income. In her book on the subject, Wynn (1970) refers to this *plateau*. Money can be spent on the home or travel or hobbies on a level which may not have been possible before. The more negative side of this phase can be seen by considering the large amount of sedatives and stimulants taken by middle-aged women or by studying the number of consultations with general practitioners; equally, the rise in the number of male alcoholics or the number of suicides which occur. Social concern for the young and the old is expressed in the legislation directed towards them by the health and social services but there is little evidence of concern for the middle-age group.

Whether the problems of middle age can be attributed to physical changes or to a combination of these with environmental and personality factors is at present an unanswered question. For the health visitor there is a challenge to be met both on an individual and a group basis. People should be helped to find their own solutions to their particular difficulties within these opportunities.

This is also a time for laying the foundations of a healthy retirement. There is increasing interest in planning courses on the subject and these are held in a variety of places; industry, adult education and local voluntary and community organizations can all be interested. Health visitors can be involved at any stage from initiating and running a course at a health centre to advising or teaching in other places.

Physical health should not be neglected and teaching about specific screening schemes is a continuing part of the health visitor's function. These include cervical cytology and breast examination for women. There may be selected screening for individuals known to have worked in a high-risk occupation, for example screening for tumours of the bladder amongst rubber workers. While much of this is the role of the occupational nurse, the health visitor may be required to follow up those people who have left the industry.

It has been suggested that the middle aged are a neglected group in modern society. The health visitor has plenty to offer if she is working with a realistic size caseload which enables her to actively involve herself here without cost to other groups.

RETIREMENT

With increased life expectancy, retirement may cover a period of 20 to 30 years, depending on the age at which full-time employment ceases and when death intervenes. The beginning of retirement is often very different from the end. For this reason this phase is considered under the headings active and inactive retirement.

Active Retirement

Active retirement may commence between the ages of 50 and 65 and can be the result of individual or organizational decision. The most important aspects are the cessation of full-time employment and the possible consequent drop in income. The effect of these two events can be overwhelming for some people, whilst others manage the necessary adjustments and find new experiences to enjoy. The ability to make a happy transition probably stems back to personality development and past experiences.

Contact with the health visitor is limited unless she is involved with holding discussion groups or giving short talks on aspects of health which are of special concern. There is room for health promotion, encouraging people to remain active, have a balanced diet and pay special attention to accident prevention in the home. There can be considerable overlap here with the pre-retirement phase, especially amongst those who adjust smoothly to the new status.

Inactive Retirement

A leading geriatrician presenting a conference paper in 1976 has described four giants which affect the elderly. Since the elderly do not end life spectacularly, insufficient resources are allocated to them. The 'giants' are *immobility*, *instability*, *incontinence* and *intellectual impairment*. They affect the quality of personal life dramatically, forcing people to adopt a *dependency role* which many find extremely difficult. This is not surprising when one considers society's emphasis on independence once adulthood is reached. In the words of Smith (1968) 'the price they pay for their dependence is a loss of status and instead of the respect they command in traditional societies they tend to inspire pity in ours'.

The majority of people will be cared for within their family group. With the present mobility of population, this often presents a dilemma: to move to be with the younger relatives or to remain amongst familiar surroundings with comparative strangers. A variation on this theme concerns maintaining one's own home or moving in with other relatives. The outcome of such decisions can have far-reaching effects on individuals.

The health visitor needs to examine these problems in depth. She will then be in a position to help those faced with the situation to do likewise. It must be remembered that all the variations of human personality exist amongst the elderly in the same way as in other age groups.

The inactive retired person is in a *high-risk group* where health is concerned. The health visitor with her nursing background is in a good position to assess individual needs and mobilize resources which will be aimed at mitigating the effects of the four giants referred to in the opening paragraph.

It is perhaps worth considering, though, to what extent the problems which occur at this time are the result of unhealthy living in earlier years. There is room for considerable research into, for instance, the connection between arthritis and rheumatism and a sedentary way of life. Among her talents, the health visitor needs to develop an enquiring mind.

BEREAVEMENT

Of all the changes which can take place in the latter years of the family life cycle, the loss of a partner when death occurs can be the most disturbing and it is not unknown for the remaining spouse to die relatively soon afterwards. Disturbing though this event is, individuals in present-day society are unskilled when it comes to dealing with its effects. It is not now widely accepted that it is healthy to mourn. This involves showing emotion, talking about the dead person, reviving memories of shared events and so on. There may also be anger and distress at being left alone which may be hard to express. There may be a great need to talk to an understanding person, especially when society's general attitude is to prescribe a stiff upper lip and a change of scenery.

An understanding of the process of mourning is essential for the health visitor and will be needed in other situations, for instance following abortion or stillbirth, the death of a child or the birth of a handicapped child.

Special consideration is necessary when young children are in the immediate circle of mourners. For many years, adults have pretended that very young children do not notice the absence of a relative or are too young to understand. The social taboo surrounding death is nowhere more in evidence. However, child psychiatrists are concerned about this behaviour. They feel strongly that children must be allowed to be involved in the family mourning, to share the emotions expressed and to talk about life and death. In some areas, the Child Guidance Service makes special arrangements to see families as soon as possible after the death of a close member.

Health visitors are not immune to social taboos and they will need to think and talk through their own feelings about death. Here, their nursing background may be a disadvantage in that having dealt with the physical realities of death, they may feel they know about it. Unfortunately, the hospital setting does not always provide the necessary emotional support for staff and many trained nurses have unresolved anxieties arising out of their experiences with dying patients.

SECTION II   MINORITY GROUPS

In spite of the effects of inflation and unemployment in recent years, it remains true to say that living standards today remain considerably better for the majority of people when compared with those of previous generations. One effect of this, however, has been to isolate those individuals who, for a variety of reasons, continue to have a low income, for example the unemployed, those with disabilities of body or mind, chronic illness, poor educational opportunity and ability and those whose earning power is affected by social attitudes. Examples of the latter are women and recent immigrants. Legislation has attempted to improve matters for people within these groups, but such action can only be a partial solution and individuals in society must bear much of the responsibility for what occurs.

The health visitor needs to develop in depth her understanding of how social attitudes operate within society. She will also require considerable background knowledge of how society rewards success and behaves towards the less successful in this respect. There are two concepts which are particularly worth studying. The first is that society needs poor people as a baseline for measuring status and as a warning about the consequences of not working hard. The second is that society continues the Victorian approach and still attempts to help only the deserving poor.

As well as increased understanding about what makes people poor or compounds their difficulties, the health visitor should study the needs of particular groups. Even when financial resources are adequate, there are specific factors relating to special circumstances which vary according to the particular problem, the stage in development, when it occurred and the resources available for combating it. For this reason these groups will be considered individually.

THE HANDICAPPED

Although most people consider themselves sympathetic to the problems of others, there exists a kind of league table of conditions of the handicapped. Position on this table may relate to the extent to which the disability is apparent. The more normal in appearance, the easier is acceptance. For example, congenital heart defects and blindness are conditions which the public respond to well on flag days. Paradoxically, though, completely normal appearance is difficult to equate with handicap, hence emotional or educational handicap is less likely to arouse sympathy. Those suffering extreme physical and mental handicaps have been hidden by society, and currently much effort is being expended to re-educate society towards a more accepting role.

A further example of society's league table is available to those who consider the way finance is allocated to the handicapped person. Where blame can be attached to another person or group of people, a judge will decide the financial needs of the handicapped person. Benefit is higher if injury occurs at work or on active service. The needs of the excluded individual may be identical to those of the included but the difference in financial terms can amount to several thousand pounds. Knowledge of the historical basis for this state of affairs may help understanding of how the situation arose, but it does not justify its continuance. There is increasing pressure within society to alter this state of affairs.

Acceptance Acceptance of a handicapping condition needs to be studied from several angles: that of the individual, the family, the local social group and society as a whole. Professional workers involved with individuals and families need a depth of understanding and tolerance of human nature and behaviour. They should avoid simplistic approaches, interpretations and solutions. Acceptance itself is frequently seen in terms of where a handicapped child is cared for, instead of recognizing that rejection can appear in much more subtle ways. Some authorities prefer the term *realistic acceptance* which emphasizes the need to accept the facts and avoid the pretence that a situation does not exist.

Individual acceptance. The individual handicapped person is dependent, just like the rest of us, on a self-image. The infant who has not formed one will be dependent on those around him for help in this respect. Consequently, if the family has an image of helplessness, the individual is likely to mirror it. The adult, faced with sudden disablement, may be forced to rebuild his self-image. His ability to do so may be more dependent on his existing personality than on the actual disability, though, in some instances, the incapacity will affect thought processes and some individuals will escape this problem. However, it is not safe to assume that the mentally handicapped are altogether unaware of the difficulty. A teenage boy with *Down's syndrome* who appeared in a television programme for schools was asked about his hopes for the future. He expressed the wish that he might play with children who did not laugh at him.

Family acceptance. The family, faced with the imperfection of one of their group, have also to remake their image of that individual. For the parents of a newborn baby, their image of the expected baby will be destroyed and much of their emotional response can be likened to that of the bereaved. There is a need to mourn what is lost and accept what exists. Equally, for parents whose children become handicapped whilst young, there is still the hoped-for image to be mourned.

The extent to which families reject that which is imperfect is difficult to assess. It is possible that feelings vacillate from one extreme to the other. One must consider whether individuals are struggling to meet situations which society has already dealt with in a myriad of subtle ways. Extolling the virtues of individual success has implications for the less successful. When considering those about to enter the race with a handicap it is small wonder that many parents despair. Families then may have to attempt the difficult task of resolving conflicting social attitudes.

Neighbourhood acceptance. The acceptance of those who are disabled varies from place to place. The extent to which their needs have been ignored can be seen by studying such things as the inaccessibility of local government services such as schools, libraries and town halls. Architects are generally more likely to have the nimble in mind when designing public buildings.

Less obvious evidence of neighbourhood concern shows up when local organizations attempt to improve facilities. Premises suitable for playgroups for handicapped children may not be made available. Existing groups may pay lip service to the need for integrating the handicapped and then exclude them by insisting, for instance, that children are toilet-trained. This effectively prevents the more severely handicapped from involvement.

On the other hand the drive, energy and concern which are evident in some neighbourhoods on behalf of handicapped people are admirable. Increasingly though, handicapped people and their families want to play an active role in their own affairs and health visitors should be able to respond to this in a variety of ways.

Social acceptance. Western society with its emphasis on individual achievement and success may have to alter this view of life if it is to accept the less able in its midst. The opportunities which exist for some people are denied to others because of individual imperfections. For instance, it may be thought that the physically handicapped child has equal opportunity in the field of education. However, such a child may have to spend considerable amounts of physical and mental effort on the daily self-care tasks which the able-bodied perform without using much of either. Add to this time lost from school through illness, treatment and hospital attendance and one can appreciate the effect of disablement on a child. There may be little time or energy available for scholastic achievement and this may be more evident amongst average ability school children than the very bright. As yet, society has not felt it appropriate to accord further education facilities to the handicapped as an automatic right. At 16 they leave school unless they are sufficiently able to enter the field of further and higher education. Should they gain acceptance here through scholastic ability, they will be limited in their choice of establishment by the facilities of particular colleges. However, increasing attention is being paid to this by architects of educational institutions.

Opportunities in other spheres of training exist and continue to improve but are not necessarily matched by those in the labour market. The handicapped may find it more difficult to get a job, particularly when the general unemployment rate is high. Having got a job the onus is on the handicapped person to prove that he or she is as good as anyone else.

Society's apparent league table in relation to handicapping conditions has already been noted. Society's attitude towards mental handicap is changing as knowledge becomes more widespread. Hopefully this will continue to the extent to which people question why individuals who are different should be categorized at all or to a point where questions are more concerned with what constitutes a handicap. Depending on the criteria, it might be possible to argue that emotional and social handicaps which are less apparent and appear to be within individual jurisdiction are more serious than society admits at present.

The Congenitally Handicapped

Those born incomplete in some way have special problems which differ in many respects from those who acquire their handicaps later in life. Infants have certain needs, which if they are met, enable them to learn, develop and progress. These include interaction with other humans, opportunity to explore their surroundings and stimulation at appropriate times to encourage them further. For the child who lacks a special sense such as sight or hearing or whose mobility is restricted by an imperfect central nervous system, there is an increased dependency on those around to help fill the gaps.

Each handicapping condition known at present is the centre of an increasing body of specialist knowledge. It is doubtful if every health visitor can hope to learn all the relevant details concerning all handicapping conditions. When considering the average caseload and the incidence of handicapped children within it, there is some doubt about the need to undertake such a large amount of detailed study. It is essential, however, for the health visitor to have sufficient general background knowledge of handicapping conditions. When faced with individual babies the health visitor should be aware of the limits of her knowledge and where to go to extend it. Reference sources will include the medical personnel concerned with the child specialist centres, voluntary organizations, literature and consultant health visitors if the latter are available.

The Acquired Handicap

The further individual development has progressed, the less effect an acquired handicap will have on this aspect of a person's life. This does not minimize the total effect of such an event, however, because it may result in radical changes of occupation and therefore of life style. For the young man, doing well in his chosen work, with the expectations of even better things to come, disablement may mean a total readjustment of his concept of his life. This situation will be compounded if he has a dependent family. Here can be seen the effect of social attitudes referred to in the introduction to this section. His wife may return to work, but she will be fortunate indeed if her earning power equals her husband's. Even if it does there will be the extra expenses of child care, domestic help and labour-saving devices. The husband may no longer be able to do his own household maintenance and repairs. Here then, is a complex situation where an individual has to adjust to an incomplete image of himself both in physical and social terms. His needs will be varied and considerable.

Mental Health and Mental Illness

Many references have been made in other parts of this book (see Chapter 4) to the role of the health visitor in promoting mental health. Important aspects of this role lie in recognition of the early signs of breakdown in mental health and in giving support during periods of stress, anxiety or depression. The health visitor is well equipped to recognize these danger signals and call in appropriate expert help, where needed, and she is often required to give background support to a patient (or the family) undergoing a period of treatment, or returning to normal family life. The problems of acceptance which arise are very similar to those already discussed with the mentally handicapped, and similar adjustments are needed. In cases of long-term mental disorders, the health visitor may well be a frequent visitor to the family, particularly where the care of small children is concerned, and she may well be involved with the social worker in ensuring a continuity of care for the children during the absence of a parent, and always alert to the danger signals. In many areas, good counselling services now exist and it is important for the health visitor to have access to the local facilities, and the ability to recognize need and situations where families or individuals might benefit from such services.

The Chronic Sick

People who suffer from long-term illness are not always grouped amongst the disabled. The borderlines are hazy, but long-term illness may have the hope of improvement. Equally, avoidance of the word disabled may be employed as a manoeuvre for avoiding reality. Recent legislation has grouped them together for practical purposes and certainly many of the problems are identical. The criteria for registering people as disabled are more flexible than formerly. It is likely that more people meet the criteria than apply to be registered.

Apart from *chronic illness* being less easy to define, it must be remembered that individual response is not always a useful guide as to its disabling effect. Some people lead active and useful lives in spite of physical and mental illness; others less seriously affected find little to interest them except their own illness. Job satisfaction and individual personality may play a considerable part here and the flexibility or otherwise of working hours can have a bearing too. It must be recognized that the incentive to work part-time is often poor, because of the effect on Social Security Benefit.

Long-term illness probably means, in practical terms, more active treatment, contact with medical and nursing personnel and hospital admissions. Just as all these can apply to the disabled, so the contents of the preceding paragraphs may apply to the chronic sick.

LOW-WAGE EARNERS

There is a widely held view, presumably arising from the admiration accorded to the successful, that to be poor results largely from a lack of personal effort. Traditionally, certain jobs have been reserved for the less able: street sweepers and refuse collectors are good examples. Attempts to improve the lot of low-wage earners usually result in higher paid workers asking for more because the differentials are inadequate. Family Income Supplement is a benefit which has attempted to find an alternative method of improving the life of families in this predicament. Whilst it helps those who get it, health visitors must consider why eligible individuals do not apply and it is therefore necessary to study in depth the debate about selective and universal benefits and also the arguments for a national minimum wage. As well as the theoretical background, there is a need to understand social attitudes and one's own part in them.

The effect of low income on a family means in practical terms that they frequently live in poor accommodation, often lacking basic amenities. The rent may be high, although legislation has provided for rent allowances for those in private as well as local authority housing. There is often insecurity of tenure which is aggravated if the family falls behind with rent payments. Much of their expenditure is proportionately high because to make useful economies in heating or food requires suitable premises, equipment and capital. Care of children can be more difficult in overcrowded homes. For instance, to suggest controlling children by removing them to another room until they behave in the approved manner is impracticable if only one room is available, or if it is unsafe to leave a child alone in another room.

For the young parents with low income, it may not be possible to set up home away from the extended family. This was graphically portrayed in the television series *The Family*. The stresses and strains of child-rearing are increased in such situations and, similarly, marriages may not survive the effects of homelessness. Young couples in these situations need opportunities to discuss the avenues open to them with knowledgeable people. Health visitors should know what the local situation is where council housing is concerned and should also be informed about local housing associations, removals to new towns and, where applicable, the problems of tied housing. In areas where housing is a major concern, there may be useful resource centres which fulfil this role.

UNEMPLOYMENT

The relationship between employment and health and, conversely, unemployment and ill health, is a complex one and it would be dangerous to make simplistic statements about causal relationships. However, health visitors need to be aware of the possibility that a relationship could exist and to read the literature on the subject, particularly when the unemployment rate is high. According to Fagin (1981), prolonged unemployment can contribute to psychological and physical illness among all members of the family in a way similar to that of bereavement. Fagin describes a similar pattern of denial, followed by acceptance, when the individual feels undervalued, loses self-esteem which consequently affects the motivation to find work. Within the family there is likely to be stress, guilt, clinical depression and marital problems, leading to family breakdown in some instances. Problems such as these were found among the unemployed in the 1920s and, in the worst circumstances, complete apathy and despair were evident, from which a proportion of the population never recovered (Jahoda et al. 1966).

VIOLENCE IN FAMILIES

During the last 30 years, society has reluctantly recognized that some families resort to violence against their more vulnerable members. While children were the first to be recognized as victims, they have been followed by adults, usually women, then by the elderly and subsequently the handicapped. The causes of such violence are multiple and need to be studied in considerable depth by all those professional people who are likely to meet the problem. All the individuals involved require our understanding and sensitivity even in the face of the results of the violence. A major concern has to be the protection of vulnerable individuals, especially those who are unable to express themselves. In particular, the health visitor has to recognize the signs which may indicate that a family is reaching breaking point, or better still, help parents to explore their individual needs and resources and to involve other resources where this is seen to be appropriate.

FAMILIES WITH MULTIPLE SOCIAL PROBLEMS

For some families the difficulties of setting up and maintaining a home are insuperable. This is not necessarily only the result of a low income but may be more the result of inadequacies or immaturity of personality. Low income is increasingly a significant factor though, when there is only a limited amount of low-rent accommodation available. Failure to establish a home early in a relationship may be an important factor in the ultimate progress of a family. Homelessness and an immature inadequate personality may be precipitating factors which push families on to a situation where multiple social problems cause untold misery and shame. There appears to be a downward spiral which is very difficult to stop.

The multiple problems may involve any, or even all of the following: homelessness, overcrowding, child neglect and abuse, unhappiness, alcoholism, delinquency, truancy, criminality, illegitimacy, divorce and suicide. Psychologists have attempted to describe the condition. Bowlby (1965) calls it 'a social succession whereby an environmentally caused psychopathy or apathy traceable to maternal deprivation in infancy unfits a mother for parenthood and becomes the source of similar deprivations among her own children'. Howells (1963) maintains 'that the condition springs from individual psychopathology, i.e. dysfunction of the emotional substratum of the individual'. Resistance to help has been colourfully described as *gold-mines in reverse*, because of these families' ability to swallow up resources without any apparent benefit.

Family needs will therefore be multiple, particularly those of t children, whose individual needs are unlikely to be met. The health visitor should work out whose needs are most pressing and what kind of help will prove effective. An imaginative approach will be essential and little is likely to be achieved until some kind of rapport between the parties concerned has been established.

The health visitor will need to mobilize all available resources and resist attempting to fulfil all the necessary roles herself. Resources will include the active participation of the local authority social services department and possibly that of voluntary agencies such as Family Service Units. The local community may be able to play an active role. An example springs to mind of a couple with many children who were housed by the local authority amongst some well-established privately owned houses. The neighbourhood was relatively poor, but respectable and reacted strongly to ill-dressed, barefoot children in the street. The headmistress of the local primary school helped some of these neighbours to be a little more tolerant and meanwhile, with her staff, settled the children in school. In due course, a school journey was planned and two of the difficult family's children were included. The school helpers made clothes and provided suitcases and the exercise proved a success. The hardly legible letter of thanks which the mother wrote to the school was highly prized. The health visitor's role in all this was confined to helping the parents with decisions regarding future babies (the mother was sterilized) and coordinating with the various people involved. It would be unrealistic to pretend that all the problems disappeared. For the children, however, there was evidence of response to the caring attitude shown by the school staff.

This highlights the reasons for working with such families, which are firstly, the basic one of caring for those unable to care adequately for themselves and secondly, to mitigate the effects of such multiple problems on the children. For the infant and young child particularly, it may be necessary to draw into the family an adult who can meet some of their needs. A motherly daily minder can be an ally, but she needs to be involved intelligently to avoid frequent changes. At a later stage, a place in a playgroup or nursery class can supply some of a child's unmet needs. Again, the adults need to be involved and aware that special circumstances prevail.

Social services departments have a variety of ways to supplement parental care and this will vary from one area to another. A social worker may undertake intensive case work, or a family aide will become part of the family. Day or residential nurseries may also be used.

The health visitor, then, will be only one of several people concerned with such families and will need to liaise and communicate with the other workers. She will use all her skills in a variety of ways and will need to step back from time to time and make some assessment of her role.

FAMILIES WITH LESS OBVIOUS PROBLEMS

Since the health visitor is the only professional person to visit families with or without problems, she is in a unique position to recognize those families who have difficulties which are less obvious but where appropriate help may be beneficial. For example, Rutter et al. (1960), in a survey of the health and behaviour of a group of children aged between 9 and 12, found that for every child attending a psychiatric clinic another eight were experiencing undiagnosed psychological problems. The effects of these problems were apparent to either parents, or teachers, in some instances, but they were trying to help without the benefit of information or professional help. Like Caplan (1969), who discusses the possibility of preventing mental disorders by helping families in times of crisis, Rutter and his colleagues suggest that professional helpers already known to the family are the best source of help when they are supported and guided by a psychiatrist or a psychologist.

From the work of these and other authors, three conclusions may be drawn: firstly, that a proportion of families are unable to meet the needs of their children; secondly, that diagnosis and treatment which draw attention to the child can have undesirable effects; and thirdly, that help for these families should be provided by experts such as child psychiatrists through the medium of existing professional helpers.

While it is difficult to recognize those families experiencing difficulties, it is not impossible when one has sufficient knowledge and experience of normal child development. Some of the signs of emotional disturbance in a child may be a regression to an earlier, more infantile behaviour, or the continuance of a particular behaviour beyond the normal limits. Woolf (1973) describes two factors which are likely to require psychological assessment and skilled help for a child: firstly, a family crisis such as bereavement, severe illness or separation from parents; and secondly, persistent or severe behaviour disorders. For a more detailed description of such disorders see Lahiff (1981) *Hard-To-Help Families*, or the references already mentioned.

IMMIGRANT GROUPS AND RACE RELATIONS

Britain has always attracted settlers from other countries. They usually come because something is better than in their own country, either work opportunities, standards of living or greater religious or political freedom. Problems have arisen in more recent times for several reasons. There are greater numbers involved and immigrants have settled in more areas than formerly. Differences in skin colour make many groups more conspicuous than the indigenous population. The latter, however, have contributed to the difficulties, particularly in the post-war years when a paternalistic attitude prevailed. Membership of community relations committees, for example, originally consisted of local interested individuals not immigrants. This and other aspects of the problems are well documented by Hill and Issacharoff (1971) in their study of community relations committees in Britain. It is necessary to distinguish between problems arising from immigration and those arising from race relations.

For the health visitor there are two important areas to consider. Firstly, her own attitudes, prejudices and actual knowledge about immigrants. Secondly, the needs of the individuals and families who are trying to settle down here. It will also help to discriminate between problems which arise directly from the adjustment to a new way of life and those which stem from racial or colour prejudice.

The initial difficulties facing immigrant families on arrival include housing, getting jobs, settling children in school, providing an adequate familiar diet when prices of imported foods are particularly high, loss of the support of the extended family, communication difficulties, and a complex and unfamiliar social system. These factors can all contribute to a rising level of stress within a family with its consequent effect on personal relationships and also on individual health.

Just as the causes of difficulties are complex, help may be needed in a variety of ways. Contact with other families from a similar cultural background may provide some of the support previously provided by the extended family. Help with language may be supplied through attendance at classes or through a teacher visiting the home. Family dietary needs can be discussed so that a combination of acceptable cheaper foods can be mixed with the expensive imported familiar products. The Institute of Race Relations has published many useful books and leaflets on overcoming these and other practical problems facing recent immigrants, and health visitors may find them invaluable.

Problems arising in immigrant families who have lived here ten years or more may stem from earlier difficulties. There may also be fresh problems when, for instance, the second generation look for work. There are differences in school performance in immigrant children and also in job opportunities. The causes of these differences are complex and should not be dismissed simply as genetic endowment. Cultural differences in child-rearing patterns, expectations of parents and teachers, external factors concerned with racial prejudice may all contribute to this situation.

Studying such complex areas of human behaviour should not be confined to an information-getting exercise. As with all areas of study where personal attitudes and prejudices are involved, there should be group discussion and individual tutorial work as well. The sociological approach to this subject is discussed more fully in Chapter 5.

ONE-PARENT FAMILIES

Attention has been focused on alternately *fatherless* and *motherless* families. To spend time comparing their respective difficulties is fruitless. Their problems are basically the same: increase in expenditure probably combined with a decrease in income. This situation arises from a combination of factors which include inability to work, unsocial hours and overtime, immobility which results in loss of promotion, or for women, smaller pay packets and less job opportunity. Whilst working, alternative child care arrangements are required and can prove to be costly, difficult to arrange and often unsatisfactory. Less time and energy to shop and cook in the most economical way, make and repair clothes, do running repairs around the house, whichever partner is left with the children, can prove to be an overwhelming task.

For some parents in this position, providing a home at all may prove an insurmountable difficulty. This is particularly so for the unmarried mother and for the battered wife.

Focusing on the practical difficulties must not be allowed to obscure the emotional trauma within the family. To meet the emotional needs of young children is a demanding task for two adults. Indeed, some question the desirability of only two adults attempting to meet these needs. The extended family has an important role for the complete nuclear family. When one parent is coping alone with the children, isolation can become an overwhelming problem.

The health visitor will need to work at both the practical and the emotional levels. She will also need knowledge about the particular needs which arise in certain circumstances. These include fatherless families, motherless families, families broken up by discord, violence, bereavement. Each has some specific problems. Most share the ones already described.

OTHER MINORITY GROUPS

Reference must be made, albeit briefly, to other minority groups that health visitors may meet in the course of their work. Sometimes referred to as subgroups, they include gypsies, communes and others whose way of life is markedly different from the majority of society. Some may reject society's values, while others are rejected by society. Health visitors should be realistic in their evaluation of need in such groups. Their concern is for the total well-being of the individual. The child who looks scruffy may be emotionally more secure than his well-scrubbed peer in a semi-detached. The child in the commune may be exposed to less emotional trauma than one in a nuclear family. Assessment of need must therefore be based on available evidence in the family, not on the health visitor's feelings.

Some other minority groups are so small that it is not possible to do more than mention them here. They should not be overlooked. Townsend (1973) suggests the need for a more systematic study by sociologists of social minorities and of their relationships to social structures.

These minorities include gypsies, those living in communes, homosexuals and lesbians. Some of these are described by the de Berkers (1973) as 'misfits'—that is, someone who does not conform to the values and mores of society. They present a challenge to all in the caring professions. Health visitors who have faced up to their own attitudes towards those who choose different life styles may be prepared to meet them and help them in specific ways which do not underline the differences.

ETHICAL ASPECTS

In the course of her work with families, the health visitor will need to work closely with various other professional helpers. It is important, therefore, that she has an understanding of the following ethical issues: the nature of privacy, confidentiality, and the legal position of helper and client. In this context, some aspects of record keeping will need to be explored.

Privacy

Most people expect the right to be left alone to pursue their lives without interference from others. In our society, however, this right is exchanged for a variety of state services—education, health, employment, maintenance of law and order, to name but a few. To gain these services, individuals have to part with personal information. The idea of personal privacy then conflicts with the needs of the State. Membership of a group also requires the sharing of information, but as man is a social being he usually forgoes some of his desire to be left alone to enjoy the benefits of group membership. In this instance, the group will often claim privacy; concepts such as family and group loyalty have their origins in privacy. Personal information is shared, then, with officials of various kinds, but it is done willingly, consciously and in return for a service.

Confidentiality

Confidentiality is concerned with the protection of information entrusted to officials by individuals. Few problems appeared when professional relationships could be managed on a one-to-one basis, but this is no longer the case. Social problems are usually sufficiently complex to require the involvement of more than one kind of professional help. For example, the connection between health and social problems is widely recognized now. For the professional person involved with a family, the important questions are: what information needs to be shared, with whom and on what occasions? A subsidiary question is—what control can be maintained over where the information goes?

Various professional groups have published their own guidelines and comparison yields agreement on the following points. Firstly, information must be shared when a vulnerable individual, such as a child, is in danger. Secondly, the information given should be relevant to the situation. Thirdly, it should be ascertained that the receiving professional group shares a common confidentiality ethic. Finally, it is preferable that information is only passed on with the agreement of the client, although this has to be considered in the light of the first point.

The Legal Position

In law, a professional person can be prosecuted for the disclosure of information acquired in the context of a professional relationship, with the exception of evidence given in a court of law, or where information is shared in good faith with the intention of protecting a vulnerable person.

Record Keeping

Health visitors are responsible for both the quality of their record keeping and for the safety of their records, which should be stored in a suitably secure place which is only accessible to individuals who fully understand and accept the principles of confidentiality. The information recorded should be relevant to the objectives and underlying principles of health visiting, and should contribute to the selection of priorities and planning for health visiting for the individual or family concerned. Subsequent information, which necessitates reassessment of the situation, should be recorded as concisely as possible. Occasionally, confidential information is received which, in the opinion of this author, should not be recorded. Such a decision requires professional skill and confidence, but practising health visitors are likely to be the listening ear when a client pours out deep emotions, or past events, where the main value is the experience of sharing with another person.

SUMMARY

This chapter examines the health visitor's role in relation to the different groups with which she works. The first part of the chapter concentrates on life in the average family, considering the needs of the various age groups from the antenatal period to retirement, highlighting some aspects of need which the health visitor may expect to find. The chapter continues with a discussion on the specific needs of some minority groups, including the physically and mentally handicapped, and one-parent families, and looks at situations created by social problems, low earnings and unemployment, and race relations, concluding with a comment on ethical and legal issues. Throughout the chapter the student is guided to relate theoretical studies with real and practical issues and in a way that encourages the development of insight and understanding, along the lines of the search principle.

QUESTIONS FOR ESSAY OR DISCUSSION

1. What is meant by the 'Cycle of Deprivation'? Discuss the part the health visitor can play in breaking this cycle.
2. Discuss the value of parentcraft classes in the antenatal period. What evidence is there on the availability and quality of teaching during this period?
3. Discuss the emotional and psychological aspects of breast-feeding for the mother and baby. How would you attempt to promote breast-feeding in your work as a health visitor?
4. What factors might lead you to suspect child abuse, and what action would you take if this appeared to be a possibility?
5. Discuss the phases associated with bereavement. What is the role and contribution of the health visitor when visiting a bereaved family?
6. Discuss some of the problems of immigrant families in Britain today. Outline some of the ways in which the health visitor can be helpful in dealing with these.
7. Discuss the role of the health visitor when visiting a family where the young mother has multiple sclerosis.
8. Describe some of the problems which face a family when a young child is severely mentally handicapped. What services can the health visitor mobilize to be of assistance and how can she help the family to adjust to the situation?
9. What is meant by genetic counselling? Discuss the value of such counselling in relation to the prevention of congenital disease.
10. Outline some of the potential problems facing a one-parent family. Discuss some of the ways in which the health visitor can be of assistance in encouraging a stable home background for the children.
11. You are asked to participate in preparing a health education programme for a group of workers in industry, aged 45–55. Describe how you would go about this and the main subject areas you would deal with, giving reasons for your choice.

REFERENCES

Bowlby, J. (1965) *Child Care and the Growth of Love*, 2nd edn. Harmondsworth: Pelican.

Caplan, G. (1974) *An Approach to Community Mental Health*. London: Tavistock.

De Berker, P. & P. (1973) *Insights*. London: Pitman.

DHSS (1974) *Present-day Practice in Infant-Feeding*. Report on Health and Social Subjects, no. 9. London: HMSO.

Fagin, L. (1981) *Unemployment and Health in Families*. London: HMSO.

Fletcher, R. (1966) *The Family and Marriage in Britain*, Chapters 31 & 32. Harmondsworth: Pelican.

Frommer, E. (1973) Old problems handicap new mothers. *World Medicine*, 8 (2 May).

Hill, M.J. & Issacharoff, R.M. (1971) *Community Action and Race Relations*. Oxford: Oxford University Press.

Howells, J. (1963) *Family Psychiatry*. Edinburgh: Oliver & Boyd.

Jahoda, M., Lazarsfield, P.F. & Zeisal, H. (1966) Attitudes under conditions of unemployment. In: *Attitudes*, ed. M. Jahoda & N. Warren. Harmondsworth: Penguin.

Lahiff, M. (1981) *Hard-to-Help Families*. Aylesbury: HM & M Publishers.

National Council of Social Services (1954) *The Family*. London.

Rathbone, B. (1973) *Focus on New Mothers*. London: Royal College of Nursing.

Rice, R. & Seacombe, M. (1975) Attitudes of a group of mothers to breast-feeding. *Midwife, Health Visitor and Community News*, *II*, 6 (January).

Rutter, M., Tizard, J. & Whitmore, K. (1960) *Education, Health and Behaviour*. Harlow: Longman.

Smith, C.S. (1968) *Adolescence*. Harlow: Longman.

Townsend, P. (1973) *The Social Minority*. London: Allen Lane.

Wilkins, M. (1975) *A Family 'Affair'*. London: Michael Joseph.

Woolf, S. (1973) *Children Under Stress*. Harmondsworth: Pelican.

Wynn, M. (1970) *Family Policy*. London: Michael Joseph.

FURTHER READING

Baker, E. *et al*. (1976) *At Risk*. London: Routledge & Kegan Paul.

Brenner, M.H. (1979) Mortality and the national economy. *Lancet*, *ii*, 8142–7.

Butterworth, E. & Holman R. (1975) *Social Welfare in Modern Britain*. London: Fontana.

Butterworth, E. & Weir, D. (1972) *Social Problems in Modern Britain*. London: Fontana.

Carver, V. (ed.) (1978) *Child Abuse: A Study Text*. Milton Keynes: Open University Press.

Franklin, A.W. (ed.) (1977) *Child Abuse: Prediction*. Edinburgh: Churchill Livingstone.

Goldring, P. (1973) *Friend of the Family*. Newton Abbot: David & Charles.

Gravelle, H.S.E., Hutchinson, G. & Stern, J. (1981) Mortality and unemployment: a critique of Brenner's time-series analysis. *Lancet*, *iii*, 675–9.

Holman, R. *et al*. (1970) *Socially Deprived Families in Britain*. London: Bedford Square Press.

Jones M. (1974) *Privacy*. Newton Abbot: David & Charles.

Land, H. (1969) *Large Families in London*. Occasional Papers in Social Administration, no. 32. London: London School of Economics.

Madgwick, D. & Smythe, T. (1974) *The Invasion of Privacy*. London: Pitman.

Pincus, L. & Dare, C. (1978) *Secrets in the Family*. London: Faber & Faber.

Royal College of Nursing (1980) *Roles in Primary Health Care Nursing*. London.

Rutter, M. (1975) *Helping Troubled Children*. Harmondsworth: Penguin.

11. The Challenge of Health Education

SECTION I THE PHILOSOPHY AND ORGANIZATION OF HEALTH EDUCATION

Ann Burkitt

We all like to give other people advice and are flattered if they act on our information and unhappy if they ignore what we feel to be excellent advice. Health education in the sense of 'giving advice' appears to be such a natural function of human social intercourse that it is rarely considered and utilized seriously by the professional groups who claim expertise within this area. This is unfortunate because the normal impulse to advise is the origin and basis of health education.

Many of the laws of Moses related to health behaviour and prevention of the spread of disease, and subsequently the advice became embodied into a set of religious rules. Examples of this can be found in all cultures, such as ideas about being unclean after birth which had their origins in a form of birth control and spacing of children. Ancient Greek writers on medicine saw an *educational* role for a doctor as much as a scientific, curative one. In *Notes on Nursing* written in 1859, Florence Nightingale pointed out the folly of building yet more hospitals for sick children rather than teaching mothers in their homes how to care for their children, cook wholesome meals and keep a house clean. In her 1892 scheme for Lady Health Missioners in Claydon, Buckinghamshire, she saw their main role as *health educators* whose work should be personal, not lecturing people but working with them.

Not all advice giving is helpful or true, in fact some can be positively dangerous. In his book *The Anxiety Makers* Alex Comfort (1968) explores the frightening advice which has been given especially within the field of sex education. Masturbation, which has been shown to be a normal human activity, has been turned by many sex educators into an act of misery and guilt.

Misinformation is one problem area of health advice, and conflicting information is another. A common complaint of young mothers is that everyone tells a different story, especially in such areas as infant-feeding and crying.

A third problem area is concerned with the reasons why people do not act on advice which could help them to lead healthier and more comfortable lives.

A gradual recognition of these three problems has led to the slow development of a *specialist health education section*, normally located within the health service.

THE DEVELOPMENT OF THE HEALTH EDUCATION OFFICER

The second half of the nineteenth century was a period of increasing legislation within the areas of health, welfare and employment. Clean water, sewage, housing, regulation of hours of work, the Factory Acts and modification of the Poor Law leading to rapid expansion of public hospitals were some of the results. The increased legal framework of public health provision and the educational ideas of Florence Nightingale, are examples of two important aspects of health education, the first informing the public of their legal and social requirements to ensure the maintenance of public health (e.g. the use of vaccination services and antenatal clinics) and the second working with individuals or small groups to enable them to develop positive attitudes toward healthy behaviour and environments.

From 1900 there developed an increasing awareness of the personal aspects of the health services. Greater powers were given to the local authorities for the treatment of tuberculosis, venereal diseases, the maintenance of hospitals and the care and welfare of women and children.

The *infant mortality rate* of 154 per 1000 (see Chapter 7) caused public concern, and in 1908 the Notification of Births Act enabled medical officers of health to receive prompt information about all births in their area. The first infant welfare clinic opened in 1905, first on a voluntary basis, then taken over by the local authorities, who also started to appoint health visitors for the care of their children (see Chapter 1).

The Royal Commission on Physical Deterioration, set up when the Boer War revealed the appallingly low state of average physique of the nation, emphasized in its report of 1904 the importance of better food for the children of the poor. In 1906 an Act of Parliament authorized public money to be spent on the provision of school meals for children in need and in 1907 local authorities were given responsibility for the medical inspection of school children. This evolved into the school health service.

School has long been seen as a place to influence the new generation in habits more conducive to health than those of their parents. Before 1800, Sunday schools and the voluntary school movement included simple hygiene, needlework, cookery, laundry work and housewifery.

In his preface to *Unto the Last* (1862) Ruskin pleaded for the provision of schools by the government where a child could be

> imperatively taught with the best skill of teaching that the country can produce, the following three;
>   the laws of health, and the exercises enjoined by them;
>   habits of gentleness and justice;
>   the calling by which he is to live.

Hygiene became a prescribed subject in the syllabus for men and women in the examination for the Teacher's Certificate from 1894.

The growth of the public health and school health services has created a large number of people involved as health educators as part of their occupational role, including teachers, nurses and doctors. Some occupational groups who could enforce legal obligations, such as sanitary inspectors (who have evolved through public health inspectors to, from the 1 April 1974, environmental health officers) soon realized that in the long run it was better to educate people such as food handlers in the simple principles of food hygiene, rather than just resorting to the use of law. The law is now used as a last resort or as a warning to others.

As public health measures were introduced by law it became obvious that ways and money must be found to make the public aware of these measures. The Ministry of Health Act 1919 laid upon the Minister of Health the duty of securing the preparation, effective carrying out and the coordination of measures conducive to the health of the people. In addition, the first section of the National Health Act 1946 emphasized the importance of preventive medicine.

The Ministry of Health produced leaflets and posters on topics such as the maternity services and immunization and vaccination. This activity increased during the Second World War and included liaison with the mass media. Under Section 179 of the Public Health Act 1936 and in London under Section 298 of the Public Health (London) Act 1936, local authorities (counties, county boroughs, urban districts and rural districts) had power to arrange production of publications on health and disease, for the delivery of lectures, the display of posters and the showing of films. In the 1920s the London Borough of Southwark had a mobile van which toured the shopping areas as a travelling health education exhibition. Section 21 of the National Health Service Act 1946 specified that health education should be one of the facilities provided by the health centres that were to be built. In the event few health centres were built until the 1960s, due partly to the opposition of the medical profession. Counties and county boroughs had additional power under Section 28 of the National Health Service Act to undertake health education as one aspect of their powers to provide for the prevention of illness. A responsibility for health education was also implied in Sections 22 and 24 of the Act, which dealt with the care of mothers and young children and the role of the health visitor.

In 1954 WHO described the aims of health education as:

1. To make health a value asset;
2. To help individuals to become competent in and to carry out those activities they must undertake for themselves as individuals or in small groups, in order to realize fully the state of health defined in the constitution of W.H.O.;
3. To promote the development and proper use of the health services (World Health Organisation 1954).

In 1959 the Cohen Committee under the Chairmanship of Lord Cohen of Birkenhead was set up by the Conservative Government with the following terms of reference:

To consider whether, having regard to recent developments in medicine, there are fresh fields where health education might be expected to be of benefit to the public; how far it is possible to assess the results of health education in the past; and in the light of these considerations what methods are likely to be most effective in the future (Ministry of Health 1964).

The Committee's first meeting was in 1960 and reported in December 1963. The Report was published in 1964 and was accepted by the Labour Government. The Committee made 40 recommendations, 4 of which (19, 22, 27 and 28) are of particular importance to this chapter.

> *Paragraph 19*: The Government should establish a strong central board in England and Wales which would promote a climate of opinio' generally favourable to health education, develop 'blanket' programmes of education on selected priority subjects, securing support from all possible national sources, commercial and voluntary as well as medical, and assist local authorities and other agencies in the conduct of programmes locally.
>
> It would foster the training of specialist Health Educators; promote the training in health education of doctors, nurses, teachers and dentists; and evaluate the results achieved by health education.
>
> *Paragraph 22*: Local authorities should appoint Health Educators as these become available.
>
> *Paragraph 27*: There is scope for a new profession of Health Educators and the new national boards should consider how suitable training courses for them could best be provided. Training should include instruction in journalism, publicity, the behavioural sciences and teaching methods.
>
> *Paragraph 28*: The Medical Officer of Health must be much more concerned with health education and should assist his Health Educator in securing the support of medical and community leaders.

The recommendation of Paragraph 19 was accepted and in 1968 The Health Education Council was created which took over the functions of the Central Council for Health Education. This Council had been formed in 1927 to supplement central government efforts in producing publicity material. After the war it had become increasingly involved in providing in-service training for health service staff and teachers. It had a very small budget but it had become the central body for discussion about the development of health education.

In 1957 the Institute of Education, London University, started the Diploma in Health Education. Although this course no longer exists it was superseded in the early 1970s by two diploma courses, one at Leeds University and one at the Polytechnic of the South Bank.

The 1936 Public Health Act gave local authority public health departments powers to become involved in public education, but did not specify the need to appoint specialist staff. As far as it is possible to ascertain, between 1936 and 1940 only 1 health education officer was appointed. Between 1940 and 1960, 10 were appointed and between 1961 and 1970, 79 chief health education officers were appointed, some having assistants. In 1965, the year after the publication of the Cohen Report, 27 appointments were made.

On the 1 April 1974, under the provisions of the National Health Service Reorganisation Act 1973, health education officers were transferred from the employment of the local authority to the National Health Service. The arrangements for health education were changed again in 1981 in the creation of district authorities.

THE ORGANIZATIONAL STRUCTURE

Health Education Since April 1974

The reorganization of the health service provided a definite place for a health education service at area level with a national salary structure.

The local education authority retained its responsibility for health education within the educational service while at local government district level the Environmental Health Service had responsibility for environmental health education and home safety. The joint liaison committees between the area health authority and the local authority provided a formal system to decide a common policy.

At a national level the Health Education Council (funded by the Department of Health and Social Security) provides national campaigns and posters and leaflets for use at local level plus an information library and resource centre. The Education and Training Division provides a service for teachers' initiation and support for health education courses, conferences and seminars.

The Department of Health and Social Security and the Department of Education and Science have responsibility for policy within the health and education services, while the Home Office is in charge of home safety. Numerous voluntary bodies have clear educational roles within the area of specialized interests, for example The Royal Society for the Prevention of Accidents, The Family Planning Association and The Marriage Guidance Council.

While the 1981 reorganization broke up the teams based at area health authority level, the basic work covered by a health education unit is maintained as far as possible in the new district health authorities.

If the aims of WHO are to be achieved it requires, however, a joint effort of everyone involved in the health service, although some, such as the health education officer and the health visitor, have larger roles than others.

The Functions of a Health Education Unit

Most health education officers have nursing/health visiting, teaching or administrative backgrounds and frequently now hold a Diploma in Health Education.

The four main functions of a unit are as follows.

1. *Administration and management*
   Management of manpower in the education section
   Planning of short- and long-term health education projects
   Execution of health education projects
   Budgeting
   Provision of and control and lending of educational technology and visual aids
2. *Involvement in the provision of in-service training of other staff*
3. *Collection of data relevant to health education which includes*
   liaison with the epidemiologist
   evaluation of health education projects
4. *Cooperation with and coordination of the health education*
   Activities of staff in the health service, education service, environmental health, community and voluntary organizations.

Except for the staff of the health education unit, the health education officer has no executive power over any of the other professions which have a health education function. Indeed, the health education officer has little influence on the most active educators who are the clients' friends and relatives.

THE HEALTH EDUCATION OFFICER AND THE HEALTH VISITOR

The relationship between the health education officer and the health visitor is an important one and therefore needs further examination. Decisions on the health education role and functions of health visitors within a district are the responsibility of the nursing managers and the individual health visitors. In her study *Aptitude or Environment* Hobbs (1973) showed that the more support a health visitor had, the more likely she was to be involved in health education. With the cooperation of the nursing officer, the health education officer can give that support by providing up-dated information, a forum for discussion to decide a common approach and by providing some evaluation to see whether or not the clients have understood and accepted the health education provided.

The health visitor has many opportunities for health education but the extent to which she can exploit these will depend on how interested she, as an individual, is in health education, and the amount of support given in terms of time allowance, in-service training and the provision of teaching aids. Techniques of health education are covered in a later section but it is worthwhile to consider what those *opportunities* are.

1. *Face-to-face*. All interview situations are potentially educational opportunities (see Chapter 8). Unfortunately, for far too many people the word education means students sitting at desks being lectured at, but if Florence Nightingale's idea of not lecturing but working with people is accepted, it is clear that all contacts with clients can be used either consciously or unconsciously for positive education, reinforcing information and knowledge and increasing the client's confidence in his or her own ability to cope. This is the second aim of WHO in health education.

2. *Small groups* formed on the basis of people who attend a clinic or doctor's surgery present ideal opportunities for education. The group may be formed of people with a common need, as for example with antenatal groups, elderly people with diabetes mellitus or overweight middle-aged men, or it may be more general like a mothers' club or old-age pensioners' group. The health visitor may have both an organizational role and an educative one or she may share these with the health education officer or other nursing staff such as the midwife and district nurse.

3. *As a specialist speaker* there are opportunities with voluntary organizations, schools, colleges and other statutory services. Subjects of such talks are frequently the local services or the action needed to avoid a health hazard. These are the first and third aims of health education.

4. *As a part-time teacher or advisor to the education service*, the health visitor's involvement with the statutory education service varies greatly from area to area depending on the particular arrangements made for the school health service, school health education and staffing ratios.

Many areas do use health visitors as part-time teachers while others see her role as a specialist speaker and advisor. Whatever the arrangements, to be successful, the health visitor must feel confident and supported in that role. The function of the health education officer is to provide that support and any necessary in-service training once the overall policy has been decided upon by the management team.

ETHICS AND HEALTH EDUCATION

Health education is not just about encouraging people to live healthier lives but also encouraging people to take decisions which may be moral ones. This is particularly true in the area of sex education, the prevention of venereal disease and birth control. We each have personal views on the kind of behaviour that is desirable, also on what is good and bad. These are called value judgements. There are also facts which are derived from information which has been scientifically tested and found to be true within the limits of present knowledge. In a rational world the presentation of facts (for example the strong statistical connection between people smoking and the subsequent development of lung cancer) should be enough to modify people's behaviour. But we do not live in a rational world, and people, including health educators, have strong views and opinions which influence the way they both present and perceive facts.

The presentation of unpleasant facts about what some people consider to be a pleasant occupation (e.g. smoking) can cause anxiety levels in those who, while accepting the facts, do not believe they can give up the habit and this poses a moral dilemma. We have a duty to present people with information about danger but because of our own beliefs we may choose to put values on the presentation, so that the individual is also led to see himself as 'bad' or 'wicked'.

The health educator's views of a healthy life may well conflict with those of the individual or group concerned. To take an extreme example, someone who believes that free expression of sexual drive is the basis of mental health is not likely to find much sympathy at a Mother's Union meeting.

It is the conflict in opinions as to which facts are the most important which leads to the moral dilemmas in health education. Even in well-established areas of public health such as immunization there is the problem of children harmed by vaccines. The question is whether to tell parents about the relatively minimal risks, with the result that immunization levels fall and there is a recurrence of whooping cough or diphtheria, or to say nothing about the risks involved and maintain a high level of immunity.

There are no general answers to these questions, but as health education becomes more formalized it should be possible for all groups of health educators to decide on a common policy.

Students may well feel reading this section that health education presents too many complexities, but it is this that makes it an exciting challenge. Research has shown that friends and relatives are the main health educators and we have no control over their advice, but as professionals, health visitors do have access to up-to-date information and professional standards and are also in a position to meet the friends and relatives.

Ignorance is not bliss and health education is the way by which the health service can give back to people the right to make sensible decisions about their own health, based on knowledge. The DHSS publication *Prevention and Health: Everybody's Business* (1976) is a step in this direction.

SECTION II HEALTH EDUCATION AND THE HEALTH VISITOR

Grace M. Owen

Discussion of the general philosophy of health education in the current cultural and administrative setting in the United Kingdom has set the background for the examination of some principles underlying the process of health education for the health visitor. This, however, needs to be done in the context of the current interpretation of her role and function, which has been fully discussed in Chapter 2, but it may help to recapitulate here in terms of her role as a health educator.

Health education has been an integral part of a health visitor's work since the early days of the Ladies' Sanitary Reform Association in Manchester (Hale *et al.* 1968). One of the problems, however, has been the difficulty in defining exactly the *nature* of her role in health education. For some health visitors health education is so much an essential and integral part of health visiting that it is not specifically spelt out, on the assumption that it always takes place, particularly in the face-to-face situation of home visiting. For others, however, any reference to health education is interpreted in terms of *group teaching* and is seen as a specific area of work which is either to be undertaken with enthusiasm, or to be avoided at all costs as a time-consuming and demanding occupation. This ambivalent approach has existed for many years and does present difficulties in interpretation of role. Clarification is essential if principles are to be selected for application to practice.

By definition, the primary function of the health visitor in the Report *An Inquiry into Health Visiting*, is *health education and social advice* (Ministry of Health 1956). The Report interpreted health education as *practical advice* given to families in their own homes or elsewhere on personal health, and also (for those with special aptitude) the *teaching of groups*.

In 1972 the Report of the Committee on Nursing (HMSO 1972) envisaged the responsibility for health education, extending to all midwives and nurses. In 1979 the Health Education Council organized its second workshop on Health Education in Nursing (Perkins 1980), the aim being 'to explore health education as a function of the role of the nurse as developed in the basic preparation for general nursing'. Thus there has been a growing awareness of the need for all nurses to be involved to some extent in health education. In time, this approach could ultimately affect the perspective of nurses entering health visiting courses.

The leaflet produced by the Council for the Education and Training of Health Visitors in 1967 included *health teaching* as one of the five main aspects of the health visitor's work. The 1973 version of this leaflet expanded this more fully, saying:

> Maintenance of health depends upon adequate knowledge being both available and acceptable and in this connection the health visitor has a key role. . . . Individual teaching is undertaken by all health visitors, and those who discover they have an aptitude for group teaching have opportunities of developing from the knowledge and skills . . . the health visitor can be concerned with professional and lay audiences, her sessions take place in health centres, clinics, the school classroom or group practice premises. Her approach and methods vary. . . .

Hobbs comments on this tendency (as expressed in the Jameson Report and reiterated in the Council's leaflet) to assume that not all health visitors may have the aptitude for group teaching.

However, at the same time, the Council's syllabus as set out in 1965 includes health education in these terms:

> Present-day aims and scope of health education.
> Elementary principles of educational psychology and their application to group teaching.
> Methods of teaching—including group techniques.

In addition, the Council's 1972 *Guide to the Syllabus of Training*, points out that:

> The technique involved in presentation should be practised and part of the tutor's responsibility is to ensure contact with appropriate groups in the community.

Hobbs (1973) demonstrates the wide variation in the amount of emphasis given to health education in the student's training, and also the extent to which practising health visitors carry out group teaching, varying with personal inclination, and the attitudes of the local health authority.

The Royal College of Nursing's *Report of the Working Party on the Role of the Health Visitor* (1971) identifies four areas of *core* skills in health visiting, one being 'skills in communication', and another 'technical expertise in the promotion of health . . .'. The Report states categorically that the health visitor has a primary role in health education, individual health education being an integral part of her contact with people—she 'will be involved with group health educa-tion' and may also have a role as 'consultant and advisor in the planning of courses and campaigns'.

This slight ambiguity in defining the health visitor's role is appar-ent in *The Report of the Work of Health Visitors in London* (Marris 1972), where there was an obvious omission in classification of activities carried out by health visitors. Health education was left off the main list compiled as a result of the pilot survey and a separate class for it had to be created in the general questionnaire. This omission could well have been a reflection on the perspective of the health visitors involved in the pilot survey, who classified the valuable health educational content of their routine home visiting in some other category such as *'advice'* or *'information on services'*, rather than *health education* or even *interviewing*.

From this brief resumé of the attempt to clarify the health visitor's role in health education, it appears that there is definite general agreement on the fact that health education is an integral part of all the health visitor's work and all health visitors appear to be involved in general health education, particularly in the individual situation in home visiting and at clinic sessions. There is, however, a some-what less clearly defined role in terms of group teaching. The Council for the Education and Training of Health Visitors obviously includes it in a positive way in their syllabus, and literature and training centres include a varying amount of preparation for group teaching in their courses. There does appear, however, to be some acceptance of the fact that not all health visitors will want to be involved in group health education.

It is thus evident that the health visitor needs to be equipped with a wide range of skills to enable her to fulfil this role satisfactorily. Also that the principles underlying the development of these particular skills can obviously be applied in other aspects of her work, such as assessing need, interviewing, counselling, communication, education and group leadership.

Inevitably some of the principles of educational psychology will have been discussed previously in a different context (Chapter 4) leaving only certain areas to be developed in this section, concerning groups and group leadership, communication principles and their application to health education.

A general appreciation of the factors influencing the learning processes helps in understanding any teaching situation, whether in individual or group discussion, and a brief recapitulation of the relevant educational principles will lead into the present discussion.

Motivation is a vital factor—people learn what they want to learn and when they want. They want to learn things that interest them and are meaningful, and therefore anything relating to individual or basic need is welcomed. Factors relating to fulfilment, *satisfaction* or *security* are important, therefore anything that increases *confidence* aids learning. *Pain* or *fear* are *inhibiting factors*, and hunger, tiredness or unhappiness can prevent the learning processes. A strong *goal* or purpose facilitates learning and any methods stimulating *attention* or provoking *curiosity* are useful. *Readiness* to learn is governed by previous *experience*, pleasant or otherwise, and existing *knowledge* of the subject. Active *participation* encourages concentration and involvement and absorption in the task, action helping to *reinforce* a concept that has recently been learned. Action also reveals any lack of knowledge and gives some *feedback* on progress.

All these factors are important to remember in any health education situation. Much of the health visitor's most valuable teaching is done in the individual situation as she visits in the home, or interviews clients in the health centre, giving guidance on a variety of topics relating to health care. Anticipatory guidance, counselling skills, and the principles of interviewing are inseparable from any techniques used in health education in these situations. One major advantage of carrying out health education in the individual setting is that it is often given in response to an expression of immediate need, or directly linked with the interests of the recipient, and this facilitates the learning processes. Frequent reinforcement and encouragement are essential, however, as this kind of learning lacks the advantages of the strength of group decisions, as seen later in this chapter.

One other point of significance to bear in mind is that there are *individual differences* between learners, including factors such as intelligence, culture and group pressures in addition to those already noted above, and these can affect the rate of progress or the individual's attitudes and receptivity.

GROUPS AND GROUP LEADERSHIP

Groups are basic to the structure of our society and everyday life, each individual living out his life in the context of many different groups, with different constraints and influences. Whenever a group is formed, certain members are likely to assume a more active role than others, to be preferred or listened to more often or to dominate the group. As the group becomes established so the leaders' role becomes more important. Some groups are more effective than others and groups of all kinds affect their members in different ways (Krech *et al.* 1962, Chapter 1).

It is helpful for the health visitor to understand the principles of *group dynamics* and *leadership* for application to many situations in which she works, but most particularly in relation to health education. She is concerned with gaining insights into a variety of different kinds of groups, how the members react and respond to change, also the factors influencing change of behaviour and the processes of *attitude change* and *decision making*.

Insights thus acquired may be useful in a variety of situations, such as organizing a mothers club or weight watchers group, leading a team, in a health centre or general practice unit, chairing a committee or leading a discussion group. They also assist in understanding the influences of *reference groups* and taking them into account when planning the approach to health education. Obviously many of these skills are only acquired with practice over a period of time and newly qualified health visitors will not find themselves engaged in all these activities at first, but an awareness of the principles involved gives a good basis upon which to develop skills ranging across a wide variety of group activities with a potential for health education opportunities.

It is possible to select only a few studies for consideration here, from the extensive literature available, but this discussion may demonstrate their relevance for the health visitor in group work and stimulate further interest in an intriguing field of study full of potential for application in health education.

Sprott (1958) defines a group as 'a plurality of persons who interact with one another in a given context more than they interact with anyone else'. This relates mostly to small groups, often referred to as *primary groups*, which are characterized by face-to-face contact of their members, who often come together for a specific purpose. *Secondary groups* are indirectly related groups, such as nations, or professional associations, with some unity of administration but whose members are not in face-to-face interaction.

Homans (1950) suggests that for those of us concerned with the application of group theory to everyday activities, there are three kinds of aim:

1. the easing of human relationships
2. the enrichment of human personality
3. getting people to do things they would not otherwise do.

The first point involves understanding human behaviour in terms of enabling the establishment and maintenance of satisfactory relationships. A relaxed and friendly atmosphere is valuable if learning is to take place effectively.

The second point relates to the satisfaction of belonging to a group. Homans (1950) gives useful chapters on the ways in which group activities meet human needs, stressing the value of approval, security and a sense of belonging gained through group interaction. This indicates the therapeutic value of a well-integrated group which all adds to creating a favourable climate for successful health education.

Thirdly, people tend to conform to group norms and standards of behaviour and therefore clear aims and objectives are helpful. There is a considerable amount of evidence indicating that decisions made collectively tend to be acted upon, and are more effectively carried through, than those made by individuals, or through pressure from without (Cartwright & Zander 1968, Chapter 1). This is a very important factor underlying the value of using discussion groups in health teaching. An appreciation of theories of communication and attitude change is also helpful in understanding the decision-making process.

The effectiveness and therefore success of groups depend upon a number of variables. Cartwright and Zander (1968) include size, composition, status, hierarchy, communication channels, leadership styles, task motivation and friendly relationships as being important features. A well-integrated group provides goals, norms and satisfaction for its members, and functions well. Such groups attract new members and keep them. A less well-integrated group lacking in positive aims and goals functions poorly, breeds dissatisfaction and discontent and ultimately fails to thrive.

A careful study of these principles and their application to a specific situation in establishing group teaching will go a long way towards ensuring success. A mothers' club established in congenial surroundings, efficiently led by members of the community acceptable to the group, with clearly defined objectives and a stimulating programme, is likely to attract members and provide excellent opportunities for a continuing programme of health teaching, where members learn and enjoy the therapeutic benefits of belonging to a group. Where a group does not thrive it is probable that some of these basic principles have been overlooked, and no teaching programme in itself, however well planned, is likely to succeed if they are ignored.

Group pressures to conform to group norms are strong and can have undesirable effects, as well as influencing members for their good. A study of the work on reference group theory (Hollander & Hunt 1971) will give some indication of the kind of influences which need to be taken into account in planning any approach in health education. The reference group can provide strong adverse prejudices or attitudes or it may provide a useful starting point for a successful campaign in promoting health. An example of this was seen in the successful establishment of 'non-smokers clubs' in the senior forms of some secondary schools in London.

Group Leadership

Group effectiveness is particularly closely related to one of the variables outlined by Cartwright, and leadership has been an absorbing subject of interest for social psychologists for many years. Some kind of leadership exists in all groups but the problem of identifying the leader and defining the style of leadership is a complex one. We all live in the context of groups and therefore under the influence of leaders, and most of us find ourselves exercising the skills of leadership at some time in a variety of situations.

For the health visitor these skills are particularly pertinent in the field of health education.

Research on leadership has shown the futility of attempting to identify the qualities that make a 'good leader' or to establish a set of 'rules for leadership' (Cartwright & Zander 1968, Chapter 1). The only generalization that can be made is that leaders tend to be mostly responsible and dependable people, generally slightly more intelligent than their group; they tend to be dominant and to interact most frequently with group members. It is also recognized now that the leadership of a group is determined by the structure of the group, the situation and the task in hand (Cartwright & Zander 1968). In this context interaction theory makes an interesting contribution to the understanding of effective group leadership (Gibb 1969).

Leaders may be the formal type of 'office holders' with recognized and designated authority (as for example, a senior nursing officer working for the area health authority). They may also be informal leaders who tend to emerge in response to a particular group need in a situation. Two other types of leadership as described by Bales (see Krech *et al.* 1962) are often seen in group work. They are the 'task specialist' who has skills specific to a particular situation, or the 'socio-emotional' leader who helps to resolve conflicts and maintain good relationships within a group.

Some of the earliest investigations on leadership by Lewin, followed by Lippett and White, have observed different styles of leadership which are of particular value for those engaged in group discussion activities (Cartwright & Zander 1968, Chapters 25 & 28).

1. *The 'authoritarian type'* of leader who gives orders, expects obedience and lets the group get on with the work. This tends to get a lot of work done, but the quality of performance is poor, there is much aggression and the members demand attention.

2. *The 'democratic leader'* is one who frequently consults the group, leads and guides imperceptibly and encourages the group to make its own decisions. At the same time the leader works alongside the group members. The group integrates well and continues to function well in the leader's absence, performance is good and morale high.

3. *The 'laissez-faire type'* of leader tends to be a happy-go-lucky type—often popular but tends to leave the group to fend for itself and there is low performance and much frustration,

particularly on the part of more able members. Strictly speaking this cannot be called leadership as the group often disintegrates.

Authoritarian style of leadership is best suited to crisis situations and people often feel more secure with this approach. Democratic leadership is more useful for routine team work and gains a good response in long-term achievement and integration and with more intelligent groups. These classifications are used for descriptive purposes but in practice it is often found that a combination of leadership styles exists, in order to meet the needs of a particular situation. The experienced leader will vary the approach to suit the needs of the group, or change the situation to suit the kind of leadership available. Leadership can be learned and people often acquire leadership skills as a result of holding 'office'.

Fiedler (see Cartwright & Zander 1968) has shown that individuals who have strong personality tendencies in either direction can adjust according to the needs of the group, and the task in hand, or they can restructure the situation

All these basic principles are very applicable to discussion in group work, where it is often found that the more 'democratic' kind of approach creates a favourable atmosphere for dealing with controversial issues, especially where attitude change is involved. An experienced group leader or teacher will vary the approach according to the kind of group, and the topic under consideration and the extent to which behaviour modifications are required.

Communication

Cartwright included *communication* as another variable important in establishing a well-functioning group (Cartwright & Zander 1968). Communication consists of a much more complex process than simply 'telling' people what to do, or passing on information. It is a two-way process and to be effective there must be a *response* on the part of the recipient. It is very easy in group teaching to assume that information passed on means that the recipient has absorbed the information and will act accordingly, only too often to discover a subsequent failure of communication.

Communication can be considered conveniently under these headings.

1. The 'communicator'
2. The 'message' or information to be communicated
3. The 'recipient' of the message.

For effective communication the recipient must understand the message as intended—one of the best ways of assessing the accuracy of interpretation is through 'feedback' or the response of the recipient.

The *communicator* initiates the process and needs to have the aims and purposes of the communication clear. Speech, language and writing are important media, and understanding involves more than just speaking the same language. People communicate most effectively if they have comparable experiences in life and have faced similar situations. Childbirth may have been a harrowing and traumatic experience to one mother, while another may have had quite a satisfying experience, and these two mothers can place quite a different interpretation on a particular communication. The communicator's attitudes and perceptions can also influence the manner of presentation. A prestigious personality has considerable influence, and information from such a source is shown to be more readily acceptable.

The *message* needs to be presented in a way which can be understood, and the *order* of presentation of facts is important. It is more effective to put the acceptable and desirable facts first and then go on to deal with unpleasant issues. Where fear is aroused early in the process, recipients build up a resistance and can then miss the positive aspects of the teaching. People tend to listen most readily to facts they already agree with; it is, however, more effective to place two sides of an argument to a highly intelligent group likely to draw their own conclusions.

To secure maximum effectiveness the contents of discussion should be arranged to awaken an awareness of need which can be followed by the appropriate factual teaching. Any process of attitude change may well be accompanied by some expression of aggression as the faulty attitudes disintegrate, but this soon disappears as new information builds up a sense of security and solution, which is then reinforced by the leader's encouragement as new attitudes are established. The leader must be fully aware of the process of attitude change which is fully discussed by Krech *et al* (1962, Chapters 7 & 8).

The *recipient*, like the communicator, is influenced by his own attitudes and previous knowledge in interpreting the information. Individual differences are important here and the recipient must be seen in the context of his own reference groups. Public commitment ensures that the recipient is less likely to change his mind later, which is why it is quite a good idea to help a group to reach a decision and express a possible course of action towards the end of a discussion. This is a principle which has been applied and shown to be of value in the success of 'weightwatchers' groups, and is one reason why they achieve considerable success.

The *non-directive approach* in group work, as described by Batten (1967), is one which makes full use of many of the principles outlined above. This is a technique which is currently in frequent use in community work and health education, particularly with groups which fail to respond to a more directive approach. It is used in an attempt to encourage a group or individuals to identify their own needs and to formulate a plan to meet them. Here the role of the leader is one of helping in the identification of need, provision of information required, suggesting sources of help and assisting in interpersonal relationships within the group.

The leader's function in any group situation may thus be summarized briefly.

1. To represent the group, establishing good communications within the group and with other groups.
2. To represent the group norms.
3. To make contact with group members, establishing and maintaining satisfactory relationships.
4. To help the group to define its aims and objectives and work towards them.
5. To establish an atmosphere of friendliness and cooperation.
6. To ensure that all members participate in activity, contributing individual skills, developing potential and gaining satisfaction.
7. To assist in resolution of conflict, changing attitudes, solving problems and completing tasks.
8. To coordinate activity, thinking and planning ahead.
9. To assist in the decision-making process.

All of these principles are basic to any group work and can be particularly important in group discussion in health education. It has been suggested that some health visitors who find difficulty in group work, do so because too much emphasis in training is placed on methods, techniques and content of teaching rather than the understanding of groups and group leadership in general. Health visitors have considerable understanding of human behaviour in other contexts, and considerable prestige in the community, as well as the knowledge and expertise in the subject matter required.

These assets, with an understanding of the foregoing principles, are excellent equipment for group work and when put into practice with the appropriate methods and techniques described in the next section, should ensure successful health education in any situation, and lead to the satisfaction and rewards of developing new skills.

SECTION III HEALTH EDUCATION: METHODS AND TECHNIQUES FOR HEALTH VISITORS

Paula Crouch

Health education is concerned with choices an individual makes in relationship to his health behaviour. One of the most potent sources of influence on this is the family. The health visitor's unique role with the family is one of potential influence on its health behaviour, and much of her work is, of course, carried out on a one-to-one basis, relating health education to individual needs. However, as discussed earlier, health education carried out in groups can be extremely effective, as the group itself provides an added dynamism regarding any decisions made, the achievement of the group often being greater than the sum total of individual achievements. The success of numerous slimming groups and clubs is an example of the total group effort.

The health visitor is one of many possible health educators who may contribute towards the provision of health education within the community. In order to discuss how the health visitor might be able to make the best use of her skills as a health educator, it will be necessary to consider some of the principles, processes and techniques involved.

The material presented here aims to give an introduction to the practice of health education and should not be regarded as an exhaustive exposition on the subject.

ASSESSMENT OF NEED

Various attempts are made to *assess the health needs* of the community and to highlight areas where health education may best meet these needs. The mortality and morbidity rates relating to a particular

health authority have long been used for this purpose and the health
visitor would be well advised to study the current statistics. These
statistics may give a broad indication of some of the needs within the
community and will be of considerable value if related to the particular population with which the health visitor is working. The
increasing use of age/sex registers may also be helpful in highlighting potentially vulnerable groups (see Chapter 7).

One of the aspects of assessment of need in relation to health
education which is only recently receiving the attention from planners of large-scale health education campaigns it deserves, is
ascertaining what the *consumer* himself wants in terms of health
education. The very nature of the health visitor's work, primarily in
the homes of families, has meant that she has always carried out this
function of assessment of need before she can attempt to introduce
effective health education to the individual. Where health visitors
can share their knowledge of the needs of the community with other
primary health care and community workers, a comprehensive
picture of the needs of the community may emerge.

It must always be remembered that needs are not static, that
constant reassessment is necessary and should be matched by a
flexibility in the provision and approach of health education. Health
educators themselves should be aware of their own influence on
need. Their own expectations or particular bias may be reflected in
the criteria used for assessment of need. The choice of health education programmes may reflect various interests within the
community, as well as local or national policy and availability of
resources.

PLANNING AND PREPARATION

Having ascertained need within the community for health education, the health educator must then decide how the available
resources in terms of personnel, skills, time, equipment and space can
be used most effectively. If the need is shared by a number of people
in similar circumstances, a group might be the most effective way of
attempting to meet the need. Alternatively the formation of a group
may be requested by potential members. This may be particularly
appropriate for lonely young mothers who may find that a group
will meet some of their social needs as well as a need for sharing
experiences and anxieties, for reassurance and possible advice on
child development and child care.

The health visitor's involvement in various group activities may vary a great deal, both in terms of initial involvement and continuing responsibilities. The involvement may range from a total planning and teaching commitment, for example in an antenatal series, to being an instigator of a group such as a mothers club, aiming to encourage the group to become self-supporting administratively whilst the health visitor acts primarily in an advisory capacity. Continuity of involvement, regardless of degree, is important in order to assess the continuing and changing needs of the group and its members and to meet their needs, in the group situation or with a home visit, as the occasion demands. Continuity of leadership is particularly important in groups where a specific need is to be dealt with in a relatively short time span, for example in an antenatal parentcraft class or slimming group. It is also important when working with groups of elderly people, who may not like frequent changes.

If involved in planning a health education series, the health visitor may consider it necessary or desirable to involve others in the running of the group, for example a midwife or physiotherapist to participate in antenatal teaching, or a number and variety of speakers invited to talk with a mothers club. Alternatively, the health visitor may be invited to participate in a series of health education. In any of these circumstances it is most important that all those participating in the planning of a group meet together to work out their objectives and how these are to be most effectively met. If 'guest' speakers are invited, the group leader should ensure that the speaker is adequately briefed about the group and its purposes.

The health visitor may be invited to participate in health education in a *school*. Here again, the health visitor will need to consider how she can make the most effective use of her time and skills— either in actual teaching or by working with the school teaching staff, stimulating and encouraging the staffs' own involvement. In this situation, the health visitor may be a catalyst and resource person, perhaps occasionally participating in teaching where her specialist knowledge and skills are appropriate.

In some working situations, lack of appropriate facilities, including space, may discourage the health visitor from participating in group health education. Fortunately, many of the new health centres now being built have incorporated within them facilities for group health education. A cheerful, relaxed atmosphere, with facilities for refreshments and demonstrations, and wherever possible and appropriate, staffed creche facilities, all contribute towards the success of health education. However, not all health visitors will be working in ideal facilities, so ingenuity and occasionally persistence will often overcome some of the most difficult circumstances. Some very successful mothers groups meet in the mothers' own homes, turning initial necessity into a virtue, by attracting people who may otherwise be put off by the more formal surroundings of a clinic or health centre.

TEACHING OBJECTIVES

Once a need for health education has been established, the parallel task for the health educator is to establish the teaching *objectives*. These objectives can then be used as a guide both to the content of the teaching and the most appropriate teaching methods to be used. The objective of a particular parentcraft session may be to encourage parents to provide suitable play opportunities for their children. Once this main objective has been established, subsidiary objectives become apparent, i.e. to discuss the relevant stages of child development, to promote an awareness of the child's capabilities and potential and link these to the need for appropriate experiences; to encourage the parents' awareness of the importance of the need for appropriate learning experiences.

The above example illustrates an instance where the main objective is concerned with promoting positive health behaviour; for some it may involve an actual change in behaviour. These basic objectives relating to the encouragement of positive health behaviour are the basis of most health education. Information needs to be provided in order for individuals to make informed decisions, but the provision of knowledge by itself is not usually enough to change behaviour: many people continue to pursue habits they know to be injurious to their health and safety. Previous experiences, the influence of family and friends as well as individual motivation, all influence health behaviour and the potential for change. Chapter 4 on psychological insights discusses more fully these and other factors which will hinder or enhance learning as a prerequisite for behavioural change and could beneficially be referred to at this point.

Education research (Bligh 1972) indicates that teaching methods which involve the groups in active participation in discussion are more likely to be successful in achieving attitude and behaviour change than the straight lecture. Consequently, the group discussion method is often preferred to the more formal lecture. A combination of a short talk followed by discussion may be appropriate on occasions where the group is well motivated and needs to have some information upon which to base a discussion. Factors involved in leadership of discussion groups have been discussed earlier in this chapter.

PREPARATION FOR TEACHING

Whichever teaching method or groups of methods are employed, it cannot be stressed too strongly that adequate *preparation* of the teaching is absolutely essential. A knowledge of the size of the group, age range, sex, intelligence, cultural and social background and previous experiences and knowledge of the members of the group and the time available will all help the health visitor to plan her teaching. It will be helpful to incorporate a note of these factors into the teaching notes, so that if the teaching session is to be repeated at a later date, the appropriate adjustments can be made if the composition of the group differs from the original one for which the notes were initially prepared. Teaching notes should also incorporate a *plan* of the sequence of the session with reference to appropriate *content* and methods to be used, including any audiovisual aids. It is often helpful to write out carefully phrased *key* questions, used to aid the development of a teaching session, in full in the teaching notes. Skill and time are needed in order to phrase productive questions. The use of questions has been discussed at length in Chapter 8, and the same principles can be applied when considering the use of questions in the teaching context.

A logical sequence of presentation should always be aimed for. It is advisable to start from that which is *known* by the group, moving on to the *unknown*, hence the importance of knowledge of the previous experience and education of the group members. Similarly, moving from the *simple* to the *complex* and the *whole* to the *part* will also aid the learning sequence.

The *timing* of a teaching session should be planned as carefully as possible. As with other skills, this should develop with experience. Initially there is usually a tendency to prepare too much teaching material for one session.

It is often helpful to make very full teaching notes initially, condensing them to main headings, key questions and a note of methods, when one has become familiar with the content and outline of approach. Many group leaders find that for teaching notes, small cards secured in sequence are easier to handle and less distracting to a group than sheaves of file paper.

TEACHING TECHNIQUES

Having discussed the importance of adequate preparation, it is now appropriate to consider some of the teaching *techniques* which may be employed to make the most effective use of that preparation.

The most important initial task for the health visitor is to establish *contact* with her group. Non-verbal signals may be picked up before any words are used. The health visitor should be aware of the importance of eye contact and signals (Powell 1973). If possible the whole group should be acknowledged, but the glance should not be so long as to cause embarrassment to any individual so that, although the leader is addressing a group, the individual feels that it is he who is being addressed. Eye signals can be useful in maintaining contact and estimating responses of the group members. Other non-verbal signals such as facial expression and hand gestures can communicate a wealth of meaning. It is often very revealing and somewhat disconcerting to be made aware of one's own particular mannerisms and gestures, but if one is aware of them, attempts can be made to modify or eliminate those which hinder communication whilst retaining those which enhance it.

It may be necessary to attract the *attention* of the group at the outset of the session. This does not have to be done abruptly by calling people to order, but can be achieved more subtly by such techniques as asking if people are comfortable, if they would like a window open, or whether everyone can hear. At an initial meeting of a group it will be appropriate for the group leader to introduce herself, and if it is a small informal group, invite members to introduce themselves.

The introduction to a subject topic should give an idea of what is to be discussed and should aim to stimulate and motivate the group. Remembering the principle of moving from the known to the unknown, the session should start with a point familiar to the group. As there may be differences within the group on this aspect, it may be appropriate for the group to be invited to share its knowledge and experience.

One can then move on to presenting new material, followed by the introduction of any provocative or new ideas to stimulate further thought. When deciding how best to deal with a particular topic content, it is helpful to look at the nature of the material. The material may be *factual*, some may be based on *opinion* and much may have *emotive connotations*. There are few *facts* today which remain undisputed. The rapid increase in the volume of research undertaken relating to many aspects of our daily lives, lays open to question many previously held ideas. Whenever possible the health visitor should ensure that she has access to up-to-date information and research. The aim should be to present a balanced view, based on the basic principles the health visitor has learnt during her professional training. Those facts which remain undisputed can be presented in a straightforward manner, whilst concepts need to be put forward more tentatively. Much of health education is threatening, it may threaten lifelong habits and firmly held beliefs and prejudices. Threats, if harsh, can make people antagonistic. One is more likely to evoke a desirable response by adopting a democratic approach, inviting people to take up a suggestion and giving the necessary support for that action.

Research (Bligh 1972) into the effects of *memory* on learning indicates that one remembers more of the beginning and of the end of the learning session than one remembers of the middle. Hence, the importance of both the introduction and the conclusion. Adequate time should be allowed at the end of any teaching session for a summary of the main points discussed.

One of the ways in which a knowledge of the previous education of the group can be useful to the health educator is to indicate the most appropriate use of *language*. Bernstein's (1970) work on language use indicates that people who have been exposed to the use of explicit forms of meaning from an early age may be able to interpret complex verbal messages without too much difficulty. On the other hand, people who have been exposed primarily to context-bound language may find abstract concepts and generalizations more difficult to cope with.

Some people, particularly children, find it difficult to concentrate for long time spans. Knowing this, the health visitor can plan a teaching session accordingly, making good use of audiovisual aids and introducing various activities in which the group can participate. Where appropriate, practical skills can be demonstrated and then practised by the group members. Alternatively a large group may be reformed into smaller *buzz* groups to discuss a particular topic and then report back to the main group. Active participation, by both adults and children, can be encouraged by project work. A topic may be dealt with in some depth, each individual undertaking appropriate research, culminating in presenting the findings to the rest of the group by various means such as an exhibition.

ROLE PLAY

Another teaching method which can be used to encourage active participation is *role play* and this is particularly appropriate where feelings are being considered. In role play several volunteer members of the group act out a situation, having conferred for a few minutes to allocate roles and decide upon the approach to be adopted. The situation to be acted out is usually prepared beforehand by the group leader, but a suggestion from the group might be acted upon. Role play compels the participants to address themselves to a particular social situation. Feelings which have previously been masked may be expressed and the situation may be used to encourage participants to consider a different point of view or situation than their own. The leader may interrupt the role play when she feels that several useful points have emerged which can then be discussed by the group. It is sometimes appropriate for another group to act out the same situation, presenting alternative approaches. If used in appropriate situations with adequate preparation, the technique can be used with a number of different age and interest groups—and groups whose members are not all of the same age range or background. Role play has been used extensively with young people dealing with such topics as responsibility and authority. However, it has been used equally successfully with a group of parents, the parents taking on the roles of children, leading to a greater understanding of their children's feelings, fears and frustrations.

AUDIOVISUAL AIDS

In addition to a wide range of teaching methods and techniques available to the health visitor, education technology can be employed to help put across a particular message and aid learning. The principle which governs the choice of suitable teaching methods can also be applied to the use of appropriate audiovisual aids, i.e. the method or aid used should be the most appropriate for the achievement of the teaching objectives. Any aid used should *assist learning*; it may supplement verbal information or may be used to illustrate relationships between various factors. Audiovisual aids can be used to focus attention on a particular point, as well as helping to put over a point. They are a *means* to an end—*never* an end in themselves. All of these factors add up to effective communication, the basis for effective teaching and learning. The source of the message needs to be effective, be it a film projector which is properly maintained and operated or a poster which is displayed in a suitable position with adequate lighting. The message (Cartwright & Zander 1968, Chapters 25 & 28) itself needs to be clear and relevant to the recipient, who should be able to understand it, appreciate its significance and store the main essentials.

Space being limited, it is not possible to go into any great detail concerning the main types of audiovisual aids available and their particular uses. More detailed reading is recommended at the end of the chapter. It is only possible here to focus on some of the factors the health visitor may find relevant when considering the use of more readily available aids.

One of the most readily available, but often overlooked, aids is of course the real thing. This is particularly appropriate when dealing with practical skills. However life-like a doll is, there is nothing to equal a real baby, slippery and wriggling, when it comes to demonstrating bathing the baby.

The Chalkboard
The humble blackboard, or *chalkboard* as it is now more commonly called (many are no longer black), should not be overlooked by the teacher. It can be useful for making a summary, quick diagrams and technical words. If using the chalkboard, several points should be kept in mind. Always start with a clean board, both for legibility and avoiding distraction. It is helpful to start with a subject heading as a focus of attention (Fig. 16). Legibility can be enhanced by: adequate lighting and avoidance of glare; chalk colour, yellow and white being the most clear on a dark board; firm script, made by standing squarely in front of the board with the elbow of the writing arm well up; and lettering large enough for everyone to see. One should avoid addressing the group whilst facing the board with one's back to the group.

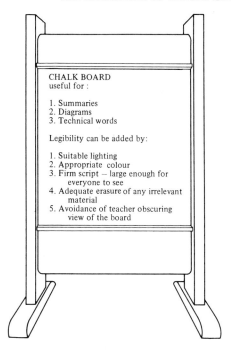

CHALK BOARD
useful for :

1. Summaries
2. Diagrams
3. Technical words

Legibility can be added by:

1. Suitable lighting
2. Appropriate colour
3. Firm script — large enough for
    everyone to see
4. Adequate erasure of any irrelevant
    material
5. Avoidance of teacher obscuring
    view of the board

Fig. 16. The use of the chalkboard.

Overhead Projectors

The streamlining of the design of many overhead projectors now means that they are easier to transport and use in many teaching situations. Originally the overhead projector was designed to be used as a substitute for the chalkboard. It can be used as such, but has a variety of other uses which can make it a valuable teaching aid. The only other equipment needed for use with the overhead projector is some acetate sheet and felt-tip pens for making the transparency, a screen which can be raked at an angle to avoid a keyhole effect of projections, and a handy electrical socket. No blackout is necessary. The acetate transparencies can be prepared before the teaching session, if appropriate, either by hand or else various photographic and heat processes can be used to reproduce printed script or diagrams and the like. Overlays can be used to gradually build up a transparency, enabling one to deal in stages with particular factors being considered. Many commercial firms now produce some excellent material for this medium, which may be particularly useful for dealing with such technical subjects as anatomy and physiology.

Other Projectors, Slides and Films

Ciné and still projections have for some time been used by the health educator and there is a variety of good health education material available for use with these media. It should be remembered that a ciné film is still an *aid* and should be used as such with adequate preparation, including the essential preview by the health visitor using the film. The choice of film is most important, as whilst it is showing, the health visitor hands over her role of teacher to the film. The film itself should of course be suitably introduced and followed up by discussion.

Slide transparencies and film strips can also play a valuable part in teaching. They have an advantage over the ciné film in that it is easier to stop and discuss a particular point as it arises rather than wait until the end of the 'show'. The use of slide transparencies tends to be more flexible than that of a film strip in that they can be rearranged in order to suit different needs; those which are considered inappropriate for a particular group can be omitted. Some slides and strips are produced with an accompanying tape-recorded commentary. This may be helpful, but ties one to a given sequence and unfortunately many seem to use a rather monotonous voice tone. It is often more effective and stimulating for the health visitor to give any commentary or explanation herself as she can respond immediately to the particular needs of the group. Slides and continuous film loops can also be used in conjunction with back projection equipment (which requires no background) to give continuous displays in such places as waiting areas in a clinic or health centre. These might be used in conjunction with a tape recording. Short tape recordings may be also used to stimulate discussion or illustrate a particular point to a group. A number of tapes have been produced commercially to be used as *triggers* for discussions with young people on such subjects as alcoholism and personal behaviour and responsibility.

Flannelgraph

The flannelgraph has been firmly established as a teaching aid in health education for some considerable time. Unfortunately it has, on occasion, been rejected mainly on the grounds of being unsophisticated. However, if a flannelgraph is prepared with thought and imagination, it can be a very useful teaching aid with a wide variety of groups.

Posters
The opportunities which clinic and health centre premises offer for static displays of health education should not be overlooked. The long established favourite for this purpose remains the poster. The poster must be able to attract attention and communicate its message. It is often helpful to have a particular theme in the clinic or health centre with posters and other display material relating to the theme. Posters need to be changed at frequent intervals in order to maintain interest, and those responsible for choosing posters should consider that the poster's main aim is to communicate a message which will promote positive health behaviour. Shock tactics, especially when presented visually, can be very threatening, and as discussed earlier, threats can produce antagonism—which in turn blocks the message, so defeating the object of the exercise.

Leaflets and Literature
Another aid which is often easily available is the leaflet, booklet or handout, a large number having been produced commercially. The importance of this medium should not be underestimated. It is the leaflet which is taken home and can be referred to at a later date. Hence, the importance of ensuring that the printed material transmits the message intended by the health visitor. Leaflets can be useful for a variety of groups and purposes, but may be particularly helpful where language barriers hinder communication. Many leaflets are now produced in various languages on a variety of health education topics. The Health Education Council has prepared some excellent material on a wide range of topics which has the advantages of aiming at the positive promotion of health and is not influenced by the need for commercial advertising of products.

Mass Media
Finally, one should not forget the potential use of radio and television in a continual health education series. These media are used primarily in school health education programmes and could form a useful basis for health education with other groups—given that the

screening times are convenient, such programmes may be useful in providing information and a stimulus to discussion.

The health visitor should be aware of the teaching aids which are at her disposal through the local health education department of the authority in which she works. When using any aid the health visitor should make herself familiar with the material and ensure that it is suitably prepared. Adequate notice should be given when ordering specific equipment. Any equipment should be adequately maintained and, where appropriate, manufacturers' instructions followed. It is advisable to keep suitable *spares* at hand for electrical equipment—particularly bulbs for projectors. The health visitor should ensure that she is competent to use the equipment or has the services of one who is qualified to do so.

The total learning and teaching environment, the content and methods of teaching and aids used all contribute towards the effectiveness of health education. Thorough preparation of these factors is vital in order to make the best use of resources available. Having prepared thoroughly for the teaching session, one must always be alive to the needs of the group and be flexible enough in approach to deal with any circumstance as it arises. The techniques and skills which the health visitor uses in her teaching will contribute to its success. Nevertheless, one of the most important contributions towards successful teaching is an attractive, sensitive personality. Teaching and learning should be enjoyable experiences and the teacher who is able to put people at their ease has a valuable asset.

EVALUATION OF TEACHING

In industry it is common practice to evaluate the effectiveness of a process after it has been introduced. However, health visiting and health education are fields where immediate effectiveness is not always evident. Often the influence of health education cannot be isolated as a factor contributing towards behaviour change. Nevertheless, some attempt at evaluation needs to be made in order to try to assess whether the client is receiving the best *service* and to promote job satisfaction for the health educator.

During her training the student health visitor will probably have any teaching she does assessed by her fieldwork teacher or tutor. Guidance can be given as to overall presentation, use of techniques and aids and the achievement of objectives. These comments can be used to help the student to continue to develop her teaching skills. However, in addition to this she should also get into the habit of making her own evaluation of the teaching session. Once qualified, the 'expert' opinion will often no longer be at hand and the development of the ability to make a critical self-assessment will continue to be a guide to teaching effectiveness. Immediately after the teaching session, the health visitor should make a note of any comments she considers relevant to the session, including a note of any changes in content, presentation or approach she thinks would be advisable if repeating the session at a later date.

The opinion of the members of the group will also be a useful form of evaluation of the teaching session. However, one must be aware of the limitations of this assessment as long-term effects will not be evident and the assessment itself will be limited by the type and scope of quesions asked.

As with other aspects of the health visitor's work, the effects of health education may not be seen for a very long time. Prevention is a difficult if not impossible factor to measure. Nevertheless, health education as carried out by the health visitor on a one-to-one basis or in groups is an integral part of her work. In trying to make an assessment of her contribution to health education both with the individual and the group, the health visitor needs to be aware of the influence which her own behaviour, by example, may make to the total effect. The way she communicates with a child can provide a behaviour model.

Any theoretical consideration of the health visitor's involvement in health education needs to be supplemented by discussion with practising health educators as well as opportunities to put theory into practice. As pointed out by the Council for the Education and Training of Health Visitors (1974), the health visitor student period 'is the time to use imagination and to experiment with new ways of teaching'. As highlighted in Hobbs' study (1973), local situations and philosophies will often influence the health visitor's involvement in group health education activities.

Health education continues to develop in the light of new knowledge, methods and technology. Those involved should be aware of current developments, for example the potential of video cassettes and simulation games. Professional organizations and journals are often useful forums for reviewing and exchanging new ideas, whilst further training courses may provide opportunities for a study of the subject in greater depth.

SECTION IV EVALUATION AND HEALTH EDUCATION

Ann Burkitt

It would not be fitting to complete a chapter on health education without some further reference to evaluation. This has been discussed with reference to teaching, but needs further thought in the wider and more general context.

Although there is general agreement among health professionals and school teachers that health education is a 'good thing', there is still little money or other resources devoted to it. One of the reasons for this is that it is so difficult to prove that health education has achieved anything. Even if a mother does modify her behaviour to a more positive one towards the handling of her child, how can the health visitor prove it was because of her health education rather than the advice of friends, relatives, books or television? It is relatively easy to make a case for money and staff for kidney units, but if a home safety campaign is organized and the next year the number of home accidents is slightly decreased, it is not easy to decide whether this is due to the campaign or other factors such as rising living standards or a better home help service that contributes to the result. Most evaluation of health education is of a simple kind, for example calculating the number of leaflets distributed, the number of organizations requesting talks or the number of people that come forward for screening after a publicity drive.

Long-term studies on growth and development such as the Douglas (1962) cohort study or the 1957 cohort (National Children's Bureau 1967), have never as yet been attempted with health education. Even so there is a growing interest in research into many areas of health education. Medical sociology, educational and social psychology and epidemiological studies are contributing to our understanding of how people value health and the factors that motivate individuals and groups to alter their behaviour to improve their health.

Two American social scientists, Rosenstock and Hochbaum (Rosenstock 1960; Rosenstock et al. 1960), have written articles examining the steps through which people modify their behaviour. The following steps are based on their work, and possible forms of evaluation and research are indicated for each step.

1. Motivation towards health behaviour can be in conflict with other aspirations, for example to be wealthy, to be seen to be adult or to prove one's sexuality by becoming pregnant.

People with strong drives to be successful and powerful may ignore their bodily needs and yet if they can be shown that fitness is an asset in their quest, they may listen to the health educator. It is important to establish the main aspirations of a client or group and use that desire as a positive force in the health education programme. This is an area for social science research but the health visitor, by sympathetic listening and asking questions before launching into a programme or an advice session, will come to some considerable degree of understanding. A young mother's main desire may be to differ from her own perception of her mother. Therefore to build up her confidence in her *own* decisions may well help her to accept the professional's advice which might, in fact, sound very much like her mother's.

2. The individual or group must recognize that they are susceptible to health hazards or pregnancies, for example. One of the problems in contraceptive education is the number of girls with unplanned pregnancies who say, 'but I didn't think it could happen to me'. In addition, although the doctor, health visitor and social worker may consider that it would not be right for social or medical reasons for a woman to start a pregnancy, the girl herself may reject the danger.

Belief in susceptibility and seriousness is an obvious problem in smoking education. To a 15-year-old, 55 seems years away and of no consequence. Other individuals may respond with an exaggerated sense of susceptibility and seriousness. We all have a tendency to diagnose obscure diseases in ourselves that are described on the television. The more a health visitor knows her group the more able she is to evaluate the response.

3. Individuals and groups, if they accept the second point, will have varying perceptions of the intensity of the threat, for example during epidemics it is easy to get people vaccinated but when there is no obvious danger it becomes more difficult to maintain a high level of immunized people.

If the intensity of the *threat* creates too high a level of *anxiety*, it may cause 'switching off' and the message is rejected. Research has shown that the horror approach to smoking or road accidents succeeds at first but then causes rejection as the target group cannot cope with the anxiety aroused, and indeed the amount smoked or the speed of driving may increase. The art in health education is to show people they are in danger so that they wish to change their behaviour, but not to frighten them. This is in line with the earlier discussion on communications.

4. The *time* between acceptance of the above points and the availability of *action* is a crucial factor. This is an essential aspect of health education for the health visitor to remember. It is no use convincing a pregnant mother she should stop smoking and that the smoking advisory clinic will help her, if the next session does not start for another three months. Any type of health education that requires supportive services must be planned in conjunction with those services.

5. There must be a belief in the advantages of action. Many people claim to put on weight if they give up smoking and they see weight gain as a bigger problem than lung cancer. Or their friends may have told them that having a cyto-test in painful, so although they have accepted the need for action, the action can be seen to have a negative effect when set against the advantages. Health visitors should be prepared with reassuring examples and even introductions to people who have had positive experiences.

6. Cues for action often come through general health education programmes. An individual may have gone through the first five stages but still needs that added push. It could be a poster or leaflet, a group discussion or counselling that finally makes the person act. A valuable form of evaluation in screening services is asking people on their initial visit what made them come. This can provide a useful guide as to what form of health education is having the most effect on that group which comes forward.

7. Good experiences when action is taken are likely to lead to repeated action or maintenance of positive health behaviour, whereas bad experiences are likely to lead to rejection of the action and the health message.

For example, a mother of four has been convinced she needs family planning advice and has accepted an appointment, but at the clinic is greeted by an offhand receptionist and a doctor who treats her as yet another sausage on a conveyor belt. It would not be surprising if she did not go back. Therefore evaluation of the way in which our services approach clients is an important aspect of health education. Good and bad experiences have a ripple effect, remembering that friends and relatives are the main health educators.

8. Public pressure either provides positive or negative reinforce-

ment of the health education campaign. The more your health education is topical and in line with public opinion, the more successful you are likely to be. That is not to say that health education should not be ahead of public opinion, but if it is wildly out of tune it has little chance of success or acceptance in the long term and then only if it is based on fact. Health education led the campaign against smoking and there is a gradual development of public opinion against smoking providing positive reinforcement of the health message. The growth of no-smoking areas is accelerating. When you remember that spitting was a widespread practice at the turn of the century you can see the extent to which public opinion and health education can act together.

New ways of evaluating health education programmes and research projects into fundamental areas of human motivation are growing. These are published in a wide variety of professional and academic journals. Specific information can be obtained from the library service of the Health Education Council.

The health visitor has only time for the simplest forms of evaluation but hopefully as health education units grow and develop, a useful partnership will evolve and a better form of fieldwork evaluation emerge.

SUMMARY

This chapter looks first at the philosophy and organization of health education, noting the current uncertainties created by new administrative structures. The next section concentrates on the role of the health visitor in the individual and group settings and attempts to relate some communication and group theory with practice. The third section describes some of the techniques in use and the methods suitable for health visitors. The chapter concludes with some discussion on the difficulties of evaluation.

QUESTIONS FOR ESSAY OR DISCUSSION

1. Discuss the view that the prevention of disease today depends more on education and personal conduct than on environmental controls.
2. Discuss the main problems facing the health educator in relation to: *either* (a) International health needs; *or* (b) Sociomedical problems in Britain today. How are these challenges being met and to what extent can achievement be assessed?
3. Discuss the usefulness of local statistics (indicating their source) in

planning a health education campaign against either accidents in the home or drug dependency.

4. What educational principles would you take into consideration when planning a series of lectures for 16-year-olds on sexually transmitted disease?

5. Discuss the value of mothers clubs. How would you plan a programme for a winter session for a group of young mothers in an urban area of an industrial town?

6. To what extent can the skills of leadership be learned? Discuss the importance of this in the context of group leadership in health education.

7. What is the significance for the health educator of the evidence on effective communication?

8. Discuss the role of the health visitor in carrying out health education in schools.

9. What are the prerequisites for a cohesive group? Show how you would apply this evidence to your work when establishing a new mothers club.

10. Discuss the value of teaching aids in group health education. What are some of the main principles to consider when preparing to use visual aids?

REFERENCES

Batten, T.R. (1967) *The Non-Directive Approach in Group and Community Work*. Oxford: Oxford University Press.

Bernstein, B. (1970) Education cannot compensate for society. *New Society*, *387*, 344 (26 February).

Bligh, D. (1972) *What's the Use of Lectures?* Harmondsworth: Penguin.

Cartwright, D. & Zander, A.Z. (1968) *Group Dynamics*. London: Tavistock.

Comfort, A. (1968) *The Anxiety Makers*. St Albans: Panther.

Council for the Education and Training of Health Visitors (CETHV) (1965) *The Syllabus*. London.

CETHV (1967) *The Function of the Health Visitor*. London.

CETHV (1972) *Guide to the Syllabus of Training*. London.

CETHV (1973) *The Health Visitor, Functions and Implications for Training*. London.

CETHV (1974) *Bulletin* (March). London.

DHSS (1976) *Prevention and Health: Everybody's Business. A Consultative Document*. London: HMSO.

Douglas, J. (1962) *Home and School*. St. Albans: Panther.

Gibb, C.A. (ed.) (1969) *Leadership*, Part IV. Harmondworth: Penguin.

Hale, R., Loveland, M.K. & Owen, G.M. (1968) *Principles and Practice of Health Visiting*, Chapter 1. Oxford: Pergamon.

HMSO (1972) *Report of the Committee on Nursing*, para. 27. Cmnd. 5115. London.

Hobbs, P. (1973) *Aptitude or Environment*. London: Royal College of Nursing.

Hollander, E.P. & Hunt, R.G. (eds.) (1971) *Current Perspectives in Social Psychology*, Chapter 8. Oxford: Oxford University Press.

Homans, G.C. (1950) *The Human Group*. New York: Harcourt Brace.

Krech, D., Crutchfield, R.S. & Ballachey, E.I. (1962) *The Individual in Society*, Chapter 1. New York: McGraw-Hill.

Marris, T. (1972) *The Work of the Health Visitors in London*. Research Report no. 12. London: GLC Department of Planning and Transportation.

Ministry of Health, Central Health Services Council and Scottish Health Services Council (1964) *Health Education. Report of a Joint Committee of the Central and Scottish Health Services Councils*. London: HMSO.

Ministry of Health, Department of Health for Scotland and Ministry of Education (1956) *An Enquiry into Health Visiting. A Report of a Working Party on the Field of Work, Training and Recruitment of Health Visitors*, para. 25. London: HMSO.

National Children's Bureau (1967) *National Child Development Study*. London.

Perkins, E. (1980) *What is Health Education in Nursing Practice?* Report of a developmental workshop. London: Health Education Council.

Powell, L. (1973) *Lecturing*. London: Pitman.

Rosenstock, I.M. (1960) What research in motivation suggests for public health. *American Journal of Health, 50* (3 March).

Rosenstock, I.M., Hochbaum, G.M. & Skegeles, S.S. (1960) *Determinants of Health Behaviour. Golden Anniversary White House Conference on Children and Youth*. Washington DC.

Royal College of Nursing (1971) *The Role of the Health Visitor*, p. 11. London.

Ruskin, J. (1862) *Unto the Last*. London: Doves Press.

Sprott, W.L.H. (1958) *Human Groups*, Chapter 1. Harmondsworth: Pelican.

World Health Organisation (1954) *Health Education of the Public*. Technical Report no. 89. Geneva.

FURTHER READING

Anderson, D. (ed.) (1979) *Health Education in Practice*. London: Croom Helm.

Bell, J. & Billington, R. (1980) *Annotated Bibliography of Health Education Research Completed in Britain from 1948–1978*. London: SHEU.

Caprio, B. (1974) *Poster Ideas for Personalised Learning*. Harlow: Argus Communications.

Dalzell-Ward, A.J. (1976) *Textbook of Health Education*. London: Tavistock.

DHSS (1976) *Prevention and Health: Everybody's Business*. London: HMSO.

Douglas, T. (1978) *Basic Groupwork*. London: Tavistock.

Galli, N. (1978) *Foundations and Principles of Health Education*. Chichester: Wiley.

McQuail, Denis (1975) *Communication. Aspects of Modern Sociology*. Harlow: Longman.

Parker, E. (1975) *Introduction to Health Education*. London: Macmillan.

Perkins, E. (1980) *Education for Childbirth and Parenthood*. London: Croom Helm.

Read, D. (1971) *New Directions in Health Education*. London: Collier-Macmillan.

Redman, B.K. (1976) *The Process of Patient Teaching in Nursing*. St Louis: C.V. Mosby.

Sutherland, I. (ed.) (1979) *Health Education*. London: Allen & Unwin.

Wilson, M. (1975) *Health is for the People*. London: Darton, Longman & Todd.

Journals:
Health Education Journal
International Health Education Journal
International Health Services Journal.

IV. Looking Ahead

12. Integration and the Future of Health Visiting

Grace M. Owen

> The fabric of the day after is woven from the fibers of the day before, and the fibers of the day before were grown from the seeds and seedlings of the day before that. A tapestry of the day after that can only be woven from the skeins of the present—the colours of which may seldom seem to match. Yet elements of time assure us that events will and do occur and take their shape from the now, the yesterday, and the day before that. Events we once thought impossible are even now so well accepted that the resistance and drama which accompanied their arrival are already forgotten; for the social anxieties and fears of today are but the heralders of the changes awaiting the new tomorrow, the day after, and the day after that . . . (Reinhardt & Quinn 1973).

This quotation comes from the introductory paragraph of a paper given in 1958 in which the speaker was visualizing the shape of things to come in the nursing profession at approximately the end of the twentieth century. She foresaw a change in the image of the professional nurse from that of the 'floor nurse' (p. 21). She suggested the use of the term 'nurse' will have returned 'to the hearth'—and 'health services will be largely dominated by health visitors'. She saw them as holding degrees and known as 'health service workers' with a preparation of five to six years' education. Four of these years would be concentrated on the humanities and social sciences. This is a very interesting speculation when viewed from the perspective of even 24 years later on, and one worth returning to later in this chapter.

Any attempt to speculate about future developments inevitably rests on the threads which are identifiable in the relevant history and are apparent in the present order of things. Such attempts must also make certain assumptions about the way the future will unfold and this is where difficulties arise. Certain things, however, are reasonably predictable, such as the fact that we have to begin with the present structure and situation and assume future developments will have their roots here. Also, it is now increasingly obvious that it is no longer possible to assume unlimited expansion of resources or technological growth and change. It is much more likely that quite drastic reconsideration of priorities will have to be undertaken, with a reassessment of the areas of greatest need. Another reasonably predictable factor is that we are likely to be living in a situation of rapid social change, with corresponding shifting values and changes in medical and technical knowledge and environmental conditions (Toffler 1970).

As the history of the development of health visiting unfolded in Chapter 1, it was possible to trace how the 'fabric of today' was in fact woven from the 'fibers of the day before', and at this point we may well be curious to speculate about the tapestry of the future, and indeed wise to do so to some extent, so that we may be prepared to anticipate any changes that are reasonably predictable. Several threads emerge with some clarity, the first being that although some of the basic objectives of health visiting have changed very little, the skills and knowledge required have changed considerably, becoming more complex and specific. Health visiting practice too has changed according to the new needs facing the present-day health services. The provision of a professional education and training equips the student with basic knowledge and skills which may readily be modified and extended according to the changing needs of the individuals in the community served.

The discussion in Chapter 1 commented on the period of uncertainty and the 'dilemma of identity' which appeared to undermine health visiting for a while and from which 'the new breed' of health visitor emerged in the 1970s, with a much more clearly defined role and status, and a function in the primary health care team. She also had a recognized set of specific skills unique to health visiting and acquired in addition to basic nursing education (p. 36). Chapter 1 concluded with a full quotation from paragraph 548 of the Report of the Committee on Nursing (HMSO 1972), and it is from that point, on the basis of that statement and in the knowledge that the new statutory bodies have been established and have begun their deliberations, that any future speculations emerge. Such philosophizing must also be set in the context of changing individual and community need, the function of different professionals in meeting such need, the skills required and possible implications for future preparation, and, not least, the resources available to provide the service.

CHANGING INDIVIDUAL AND COMMUNITY NEEDS

A wide range of different kinds of speculation can be found among the many forecasters of changing needs in the community. Those whose work is particularly relevant to this discussion—such as Nuttal (1976), Mussallem (1970) and Parker (1970)—all stress the importance of demographic changes which affect the possible patterns of need in terms of vulnerable and dependent groups. Other factors frequently noted include the changing character of disease as medical and scientific knowledge advances, with the emphasis shifting from mortality to morbidity.

Attention has been focused by the DHSS (1976) on the effects of possible demographic changes (including the effects of migration) and emphasizing the probability of an increasingly ageing population. The same document emphasizes the possible effects of changing patterns of health behaviour, such as increasing alcoholism, and the effects of smoking or air pollution, also the relationship between affluence, leisure, the environment and health. The beginning of the second half of this century saw an emphasis on ensuring that provision of specialities in hospital and medical care was available to everyone, but now emphasis must be placed on the role of the primary health care services, and the responsibility of each individual in maintaining personal health.

In the Report of the Committee on Nursing (HMSO 1972), an assessment of community need as seen in 1972 was outlined in para. 547. It was noted that the community health services must be considered a main element in an integrated National Health Service, and would have needs related to the positive promotion of health, and provision of health care (apart from hospital admission) and would include the following.

1. A preventive health care service.
2. Health supervision of children under school age and school children.
3. Developmental paediatrics and early assessment of physical and mental handicap.
4. Ascertainment and provision of health care for families at risk.
5. Care for the chronically sick, handicapped and disabled.

6. Treatment and care of the mentally ill and frail elderly.
7. The development of public understanding and support of community health measures, to include health education.
8. Cooperation in domiciliary family planning services.

The following paragraph (548), as already noted, outlines the role of the health visitor in meeting these areas of need, and paragraph 553 sees this placed firmly in the context of an integrated health service, with emphasis on integration at area and district levels (HMSO 1972).

Another consultative document issued in 1976 (HMSO 1976a) set out some of the priorities in the health and social services in an economic situation, where difficult choices had to be made. Special emphasis was given to the expansion of the family practitioner services, maintaining health centre programmes and vital supporting services, such as health visitors and home nurses, with a 6 per cent increase during the year. These two consultative documents taken together indicated a noticeable trend towards the recognition of the need for priority to be given to preventive services and the promotion of health. This trend, seen together with the statement on community needs and the description of the health visitor (HMSO 1972) and recognition of the need for no services, leaves no room for any gloomy forecasts about the continued need for the services of the health visitor. This was followed in 1977 by a further discussion document, *The Way Forward* (HMSO 1977), setting out priorities in the use of resources. The emphasis was again on prevention and primary care. In addition, the report *Fit for the Future* (HMSO 1976b) recognized the value of the health visitor's skills in the field of child health and care, especially if prepared along the lines of the proposals of the Report of the Committee on Nursing, with special modules on paediatrics, community nursing, followed by health visiting. Obviously the possibility of this kind of health visitor specialist becoming a reality is dependent on the future pattern of basic nursing education, and the discussions are as yet only in embryonic stages. The Report, however, opened up interesting possibilities and pointed out that the number of practising health visitors needs to be doubled to reach even the proposals of the *Inquiry into Health Visiting Report* of 1956 (Ministry of Health 1956).

The key role of the health visitor in health education is also widely recognized by such organizations as the Health Education Council and the General Dental Council.

The important thread emerging here is the recognition of the need for a professionally trained person with skills such as those possessed by the health visitor and the increasing recognition being given to the value of her services, particularly with vulnerable groups and in health education, and the primary health care team.

NEEDS—RESOURCES AND MANPOWER

Nuttal (1976) draws attention to the fact that approximately 95 per cent of people who are sick in the UK are cared for in their own homes, by friends or relatives—or by no one at all! Also about 92 per cent of actual nursing care is given by totally untrained people. The delivery of health care is a 'labour intensive business' and with the question of priorities dominating the political scene, health care must now compete with social services, education and other necessities for resources. In order to survive as a profession, nurses will need to pay more attention to the kind of nursing that is carried on *outside* of the hospital.

McFarlane (1976), in 'Charter for Caring', notes that in this country our orientation in nursing practice has been dominated traditionally by the aspects of 'doing', and we know very little about the aspects of the principles which guide in 'supporting and teaching' others in maintaining health, although these skills have in fact been developed in the speciality of health visiting.

Mussallem (1970), exploring possible future developments as seen in Canada, sees also a move towards general integration of hospital and home or community care, but, however, adds:

> *Homo sapiens* will be much as he is now, a creature of reason who is born once, dies once, and in the interval between birth and death will be subject to most, if not all, the conditions and motivations that have applied to man since he first walked this earth. He will be happy and depressed. He will be lonely, fearful, gregarious and brave. He will feel pain when injured, anger when abused and pleasure when pleased. He will in fact, be the same human being . . . and will respond then (circa 2020) as now to tender care and skilled competence the professional nurse contributes to the world of health.

Human nature itself is unlikely to change—and human need therefore will continue, but Mussallem goes on to ask the important question '*where*' will the care be given, and predicts a much freer movement of nurses between hospital and home. Nursing, she stresses, is a dynamic component of any health service—but nurses of the future will be much more concerned with total health care.

Before leaving the 'forecasters' we should return to Bartholomew, who envisaged the health visitor at about the year 2000 as a composite mixture of the 'good old nurse', a disciplined social worker and an educator—a product of merging three disciplines—not so very different, in fact, from the health visitor of today! Nurse educators are challenged to come to grips with these trends. For too long they have been overconcerned with biological sciences; they must now learn to train professional health workers to meet the needs of a changing society (Reinhardt & Quinn 1973).

These few glimpses of current thought may well stimulate us to ask what they have to say for the future of health visiting.

THE HEALTH VISITOR OF THE FUTURE

The first obvious thread to emerge in the tapestry of the future is a very positive one of continuing need for a professionally trained person such as the health visitor to provide the kind of service outlined by the *Report of the Committee on Nursing* and it appears that most current opinion recognizes this need for a worker with the kind of skills the present-day health visitor has.

One area which may not always receive the recognition it deserves is the health visitor's particular skill in helping to establish stable family relationships and so lay the foundations of physical and emotional health and happiness in the early years of life. It is increasingly evident, as we have seen, that a large proportion of her time is devoted to families with young children, and she possesses a unique set of skills, which could be more widely recognized in this setting, but are in danger of being eroded by other commitments which could perhaps be performed by others—*not* necessarily professionally trained workers.

Another point often unrecognized is that the health visitor is and appears likely to continue to be the one professionally trained worker with access to all homes where there are young children, who is there before crisis and breakdown situations occur and who is also able to offer anticipatory guidance.

A second thread which emerges in the future tapestry is that with the possibility of drastic changes likely in future policy concerning priorities, brought about by economic crises, resources are limited and recognition is at last being given more frequently to the value of preventive services. The health visitor of today is at a very strategic point to take up this challenge. She must, however, be open to change and be flexible according to human need. This may require the development of new skills involving a new approach to the education and training of health visitors.

It is important, however, to note that while much current thought recognizes the need for a total approach to patient care and integration of hospital and home care, this does *not*, as some would suppose, mean that one professional worker must possess and deliver all kinds of nursing and health teaching skills. The service may need to offer professionals with different kinds of expertise at different times, and there is a very specific and developing role in the future pattern of things for a person with a background of nursing experience, and specially developed skills in the application of human and social sciences and educational expertise, as Bartholomew has outlined (Reinhardt & Quinn 1973).

Educating the Health Visitor of the Future
It is not easy to predict changes in the preparation for health visiting until such time as the proposals for changes in basic nursing education and obstetric experience have been clarified. There are, however, a few straws in the wind.

With the recognition of the need for a specific post-basic preparation for health visiting, it is evident that the new statutory bodies beginning to formulate plans will, under the coordination of the Central Council, be setting up the new structure for planning and coordinating training. Health visiting courses are likely to remain firmly based in the further and higher education sector. This position may well have been enhanced by the growing popularity of all nursing-related courses in higher education, and by the establishment of courses implementing the new district nursing training in many colleges. There are now quite a substantial number of departments with a strong nursing- or health-based interest.

Since the first edition of this book was published, the working party established by the Council to investigate the principles of health visiting (CETHV 1977, 1982) has produced two reports, and continues to meet. Further issues are being examined, including the concept of a 'health visiting process'. The findings will doubtless influence future practice and education.

The Report of the Working Party on Curriculum Planning has also been circulated for comment. These reports, together with prospective structural changes in the roles of the statutory bodies, will all be reflected in future practice and education.

Naturally, an important feature in shaping future health visitor preparation will be the philosophy of the basic nursing training. It remains to be seen how the student nurse will be orientated to the community aspects of nursing care, and there are many difficulties to be negotiated, not least that of placing students in the community. Much confused thinking exists as yet about the value of the community options as they were planned in basic training. Separate 'modules' of community experience are not perhaps the best way of introducing the concept of community care, and are certainly heavy on resources.

It is hoped that a new approach can be found to introduce students more effectively to community care, and perhaps to plan a new integrated form of training, orientating students to a 'health care' model of nursing, rather than a 'sickness'-based approach. This would mean that ward sisters and tutors may need to broaden their horizons somewhat. It could, however, have significant implications for the future of health visitor education. At the time of writing, the shape of things to come is still ill-defined and speculation is difficult.

Some of the existing degree courses and the six original integrated courses described in Chapter 1 (p. 20) have experimented with an approach (Owen 1976), introducing the student to community care early in nursing experience, or following a patient's care from home to hospital and/or return to home (Chapman 1974). The original concept of an integrated course which included a health visitor's certificate was open to considerable criticism. However, research has shown that health visitors prepared in these courses had a very clearly defined awareness of their own identity and their specific role as a clinical nurse, community nurse or health visitor (Owen 1976). They also demonstrated appreciation of the roles of other workers and ability to work well in a primary health care team. They also emerged with a unique perspective on total patient care in hospital, home and community. Some of the initial criticisms that they lacked confidence were shown to be unimportant, as they very quickly 'catch up' with other students and demonstrate their ability in the clinical and particularly the teaching situation. These experiments, it would appear, had something to offer in consideration of changes in basic nursing education as a preparation for health visiting practice, or for nursing in an integrated health service.

Whatever form of preparation for health visiting does emerge, therefore, will depend greatly on the programme for basic nursing education, attitudes acquired towards community care, and the nature of the obstetric course experience.

A RESEARCH-BASED PROFESSION?

June Clark

It would not be fitting to leave speculation about future developments without some more positive comment on the need for research in health visiting. This textbook has been written along lines which, it is hoped, will stimulate students and others to develop an enquiring approach to health visiting, and a readiness to refer to research studies in any area relevant to the needs of their particular area of work.

When the first edition of this book was published in 1977, the research studies on which health visitors could draw were in general limited to the literature of allied fields such as sociology, psychology, and medicine; there was very little research literature concerned specifically with health visiting, and even less based on work undertaken by health visitors themselves. Since that time the situation has improved considerably. The preoccupation of the 1960s and the early 1970s with the superficial quantification of the health visitor's work (Clark 1981) has given way to more thoughtful analysis of health visiting skills and methods of practice. Attempts are being made to evaluate the contribution of health visiting to the care of certain vulnerable groups such as the elderly (Luker 1980) and babies at risk of 'cot death' (Battye & Deakin 1979). The development of tools which health visitors can use to evaluate their own practice is a difficult task, but progress is being made (Luker 1978; Fitton 1981). Most important of all, perhaps, is the increasing number of reports of small-scale studies undertaken by practising health visitors into subjects such as infant-feeding, child-rearing practices, and the management of problems such as sleep disturbance, milk allergy and postnatal depression; work of this kind represents the beginning of the body of knowledge on which health visiting practice needs to be based, and without which health visiting cannot claim to be a profession.

A number of health visitors are currently undertaking research in universities and polytechnics at master's or doctoral level, and the DHSS has recently funded several projects in the field of health visiting. In 1981, the CETHV appointed its first research officer.

Although progress is being made, much more research is needed. Methods of investigating and analysing health visiting practice are still rudimentary, and we have as yet neither suitable criteria nor adequate measurement tools for evaluating the effectiveness of health visiting interventions. The methods used by health visitors in their daily practice have not yet been systematically tested, and the knowledge base of health visiting still draws more heavily on 'experience' than on science. The responsibility for this work must be with health visitors themselves, although other disciplines will necessarily be involved. Equally, health visitors have a great deal to contribute to multidisciplinary research in allied fields.

The Development of Theories and Models

One of the purposes of research is the development and refinement of theory and, as the CETHV (1977) has pointed out, 'The profession has reached a stage where in order to develop further it must spell out its implicit principles which ultimately predict and guide its practice'. Nursing has only recently begun to develop its own body of theory and to make explicit the use which it makes of the theories of other disciplines for the 'unique mix' which constitutes nursing; health visiting is even less well developed in this respect than other fields of nursing. Yet, as Leonardo da Vinci is reputed to have said, 'practice without theory is like a man who goes to sea without a map in a ship without a rudder'. Of course, health visitors do use theories of many kinds in their day-to-day practice—for example the theories of child development developed by, among others, Erikson, Piaget and Bowlby. Health visitors use, indeed sometimes take for granted, such concepts as mothering, need, support, counselling, health education, and many others. What is lacking is the rigorous and systematic analysis of these concepts and the testing of these theories in the context of health visiting practice. In 1977 the CETHV made a courageous start on this task by publishing a discussion document entitled *An Investigation into the Principles of Health Visiting*, whose intention was 'to express the principles more scientifically so that they can be subjected to rigorous evaluation'.

Theories are developed by both inductive and deductive means. Inductive development involves observing, naming, and classifying health visiting experience; developing and analysing concepts used in health visiting practice; and first postulating and then testing relationships between them. By deductive means, one applies concepts and theories from other disciplines—for example the theories of child development mentioned above (McFarlane 1977). Clark (1980) has attempted to describe health visiting practice within the framework of general systems theory, and has developed a simple model (Clark 1982a) which can be used by health visitors to analyse and organize their own practice with particular clients.

The Nursing Process in Health Visiting
The systematic approach to nursing care, which has become known as the 'nursing process', offers a further framework within which health visiting can be examined and analysed. The four main stages of the nursing process—the assessment of an individual's nursing needs, the development of a plan of care based on the needs and problems identified, the implementation of the plan, and the review of the care given to see how far it matches its specified intentions— are the same steps which health visitors and others have always used as part of a more generalized problem-solving approach to the care of patients and clients. The difference is that the conscious and systematic use of such a framework requires that each step in the decision-making process is made explicit and is precisely documented; this is important to ensure consistency and continuity over the sometimes long intervals between the health visitor's contacts with a particular family. In addition, the goals must be validated with the patient or client, who thus becomes a more active participant in care, and the care given must be consciously reviewed for its effectiveness so that the plan can be modified as necessary. There is now an extensive literature describing the use of the nursing process in general nursing, district nursing, psychiatry, and mental handicap, but as yet little has been written about its use in health visiting. Luker (1979) and Clark (1982b) are among the first.

Professional Accountability
The use of the nursing process in this way makes explicit the accountability of each health visitor for her own standards of practice (Royal College of Nursing 1981), and this also is an indication of the development of health visiting as a profession, which was discussed at the beginning of this book.

THE NEW TOMORROW
Grace Owen

It is pleasing to reflect that this last section in this chapter could not have been written in 1977—there were in fact just four lines in the first edition pointing in that direction, and now research is gaining momentum. If, in the future, health visiting must continue to change, as it always has done in the past in response to changing needs, it is essential that those needs should be defined clearly and recognized in terms of priorities. Also the skills required to respond to change and maintain good practice must be defined and identified. The fact that movement is now apparent in this direction opens up hopeful new horizons for the future.

By the time the next edition of this book is due, it is likely that it will need to be rewritten completely in the context of the new administrative framework and proposals for re-designing the curriculum. Whatever shape the future takes, one thing is sure, and that is that a challenging and exciting future lies ahead for health visitors of tomorrow if they respond to change creatively and positively. It will be for the present generation of students, for whom this book is written, to interpret these ideals, and see some of the dreams realized, as they most certainly weave the tapestry of tomorrow.

REFERENCES

Battye, J. & Deakin, M. (1979) Surveillance reduces baby deaths. *Nursing Mirror*, *148*, 19, 38–40.

CETHV (1977) *An Investigation into the Principles of Health Visiting*. London.

CETHV (1982) *Health Visiting Principles in Practice*. London.

Chapman, C.M. (1974) Nurse education. *Nursing Times*, *70*, 18 (2 May).

Clark, J. (1980) A framework for health visiting. 1. The application of system theory to health visiting. 2. The nature of health visiting activity. 3. The environment and the time dimension. *Health Visitor*, *53*, 10, 418–20; *53*, 11, 487–8; *53*, 12, 533–5 and correction *54*, 1, 6.

Clark, J. (1981) *What do Health Visitors Do? A Review of the Research 1960—1980*. London: Royal College of Nursing.

Clark, J. (1982a) Theories and models on the concept of nursing. *Journal of Advanced Nursing* (in press).

Clark, J. (1982b) Using the nursing process in health visiting. *Nursing Times Community Outlook* (in press).

DHSS (1976) *Prevention and Health: Everybody's Business. A Consultative Document*. London: HMSO.

Fitton, J.M. (1981) How am I doing as a health teacher? One way of measuring the effectiveness of health visiting is by monitoring clients' responses. *Nursing Times*, 77, 85–6.

HMSO (1972) *The Report of the Committee on Nursing*. Cmnd. 5115. London.

HMSO (1976a) *Priorities of Health and Personal Social Services in England*. London.

HMSO (1976b) *'Fit for the Future'. Report of the Committee on Child Health Services*, Vol. 1. London.

HMSO (1977) *The Way Forward—Priorities in the Health and Social Services*. London.

Luker, K. (1978) Goal attainment: a possible model for assessing the role of the health visitor. *Nursing Times*, 74, 30, 1257–9.

Luker, K. (1979) The nursing process. In: *The Nursing Process*, ed. C. Kratz. London: Baillière Tindall.

Luker, K. (1980) *Health Visiting and the Elderly: An Experimental Study to Evaluate the Effects of Focused Health Visitors' Intervention on Elderly Women Living at Home*. Edinburgh University Thesis (PR D).

McFarlane, J.K. (1976) A charter for caring. *Journal of Advanced Nursing*, 1, 3 (May).

McFarlane, J.K. (1977) Developing a theory of nursing: the relation of theory to practice, education and research. *Journal of Advanced Nursing*, 2, 261–70.

Ministry of Health, Department of Health for Scotland and Ministry of Education (1956) *An Inquiry into Health Visiting. Report of a Working Party on the Field of Work, Training and Recruitment of Health Visitors*. London.

Mussallem, H.K. (1970) 2020: nursing fifty years hence. In: *Nursing Education in a Changing Society*, ed. M.Q. Innis, pp. 209–224. Toronto: University of Toronto Press.

Nuttal, P. (1976) Nursing in the year AD 2000. *Journal of Advanced Nursing*, 1, 2 (March).

Owen, G.M. (1976) *A Study of Six Courses Integrating Basic Nursing Education with Health Visiting*. Unpublished Thesis: London University Library.

Parker, K.M. (1970) Nursing circa 2020. In: *Nursing Education in a Changing Society*, ed. M.Q. Innis, pp. 225–240. Toronto: Toronto University Press.

Reinhardt, A. & Quinn, M. (eds.) (1973) *Family Centered Community Nursing*. St. Louis: Mosby. (Article by Claire Bartholomew from the Proceedings of the First Annual Conference of the Western Council on Higher Education for Nursing, March 1958, San Francisco.)

Royal College of Nursing (1981) *Towards Standards*. London.

Toffler, A. (1970) *Future Shock*. London: Pan.

FURTHER READING

CETHV (1980) *The Investigation Debate*. London.

Robinson, J. (1982) *An Evaluation of Health Visiting Practice*. London: CETHV.

Index